CASE STUDIES IN CRITICAL CARE MEDICINE

ROY D. CANE, M.B.B.Ch., F.F.A.(S.A.)

Associate Professor of Clinical Anesthesia
Northwestern University Medical School
Chicago, Illinois

BARRY A. SHAPIRO, M.D.

Professor of Clinical Anesthesia
Northwestern University Medical School
Chicago, Illinois

YEAR BOOK MEDICAL PUBLISHERS, INC.
CHICAGO

0 9 8 7 6 5 4 3 2 1

Library of Congress Cataloging in Publication Data
Main entry under title:

Case studies in critical care medicine.

  Bibliography: p.
  Includes index.
  1. Critical care medicine—Case studies,   I. Cane,
Roy D.   II. Shapiro, Barry A., 1937–   [DNLM:
1. Critical Care.   WX 218 C337]
RC86.7.C38   1984   616'.028   84–7517
ISBN 0–8151–1421–4

Sponsoring Editor: Susan M. Harter
Editing Supervisor: Frances M. Perveiler
Production Project Manager: Jack Grady
Proofroom Supervisor: Shirley E. Taylor

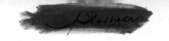

Case Studies in Critical Care Medicine

To Joe, Leslie and David

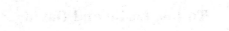

CONTRIBUTORS

Roy D. Cane, M.B.B.Ch., F.F.A.(S.A.)

Associate Professor of Clinical
  Anesthesia
Northwestern University Medical
  School
Chicago, Illinois

Richard Davison, M.D.

Associate Professor of Medicine
Northwestern University Medical
  School
Chicago, Illinois

Jeffrey Glassroth, M.D.

Assistant Professor of Medicine
Northwestern University Medical
  School
Chicago, Illinois

David Green, M.D.

Professor of Medicine
Northwestern University Medical
  School
Chicago, Illinois

Scott Greene, M.D.

Associate in Anesthesia
Northwestern University Medical
  School
Chicago, Illinois

Kerry Kaplan, M.D.

Assistant Professor of Medicine
Northwestern University Medical
  School
Chicago, Illinois

Antoun Koht, M.D.

Assistant Professor of Clinical
  Anesthesia
Northwestern University Medical
  School
Chicago, Illinois

Frank A. Krumlovsky, M.D.

Associate Professor of Medicine
Northwestern University Medical
  School
Chicago, Illinois

Paul S. Mesnick, M.D.

Assistant Professor of Clinical
  Anesthesia
Northwestern University Medical
  School
Chicago, Illinois

John P. Phair, M.D.

Professor of Medicine
Northwestern University Medical
  School
Chicago, Illinois

Nauman Qureshi, M.D.
Formerly Associate in Medicine
Northwestern University Medical
    School
Now Medical Director
Dialysis Center
Athens, Alabama

**Donald M. Sinclair, B.Sc.,
    M.B.B.Ch., F.F.A.(S.A.)**
Formerly Director Cardiac
    Anesthesia
University of Utrecht
Now Assistant Professor
    of Anesthesia
Rush Medical School
Chicago, Illinois

Tod Sloan, M.D., Ph.D.
Assistant Professor of Anesthesia
Northwestern University Medical
    School
Chicago, Illinois

Barry A. Shapiro, M.D.
Professor of Clinical Anesthesia
Northwestern University Medical
    School
Chicago, Illinois

Jeffrey Vender, M.D.
Assistant Professor of Clinical
    Anesthesia
Northwestern University Medical
    School
Chicago, Illinois

PREFACE

CRITICALLY ILL PATIENTS differ from other patients, not because of specific pathologies or therapies, but because of their unstable clinical condition which mandates the frequent reevaluation of the patient's physiologic homeostasis and adjustment of therapy. Critical care practitioners are continually required to integrate a plethora of physiologic data and make frequent therapeutic decisions. In our opinion, conventional texts do not readily convey to the reader this process of decision analysis. The case study format of this book represents an attempt to reflect the process of decision making and hopefully better instruct the reader in the application of this process in the management of critically ill patients.

We have chosen topics that describe the major problems encountered in adult intensive care units. Case histories were selected to present a mix of surgical and medical patients though obviously the principles of therapy and monitoring apply equally well to all critically ill patients. This text makes no pretense of addressing the entire body of knowledge of critical care medicine. Rather, we have focused on clinically relevant material and its application in decision analysis and management of critically ill patients.

The topics cover problems that occur with greatest frequency in critically ill patients and in which there is a reasonable body of clinically relevant information. The earlier chapters deal with therapeutic modalities that have an application to various pathologies and with simpler clinical problems involving single organ systems. The later chapters are devoted to more complex specific therapies and the clinical problem of multi-organ system disease.

Pediatric critical care has been excluded due to limitations of space and the existence of other pediatric case study texts. We chose not to address to multiple trauma or burns as specific subjects because outside of the elements of cardiopulmonary support and fluid therapy, the management of these patients is a surgical, not critical care problem. These elements of therapy and support have been discussed in this text, although not necessarily in the context of patients with traumatic disease.

We wish to thank the contributing authors for their chapters. Thanks are due to our colleagues, in particular Drs. Edward Brunner, James Eckenhoff, and Chris Chomka for their unfailing support of our endeavors. We thank Judith Stutz for her invaluable assistance in the development and preparation of the manuscript and Kelly Quinn and Mary Rivera for secretarial assistance.

ROY D. CANE

BARRY A. SHAPIRO

CONTENTS

1 / Monitoring Cardiovascular Dynamics

BARRY A. SHAPIRO, M.D.

THE MAINTENANCE OF INTERNAL respiration (oxygen and carbon dioxide exchange between blood and tissue) depends upon adequate blood flow through systemic capillaries—perfusion. Despite impressive technical advances in cardiovascular monitoring, the clinical assessment of acceptable tissue perfusion still depends on subjective criteria such as the level of consciousness and sensorium, appreciation of the amplitude of a palpated peripheral pulse, the status of capillary filling, status of skin temperature and color, and serial monitoring of urine output.

Tissue perfusion requires adequate circulation that is dependent upon generation of adequate ventricular pressure, which in turn is dependent upon appropriate venous conductance. Although reasonably reliable quantification of cardiac output is clinically available, we continue to rely upon pressure measurements to guide therapy. Vascular resistance and ventricular pressure generation are important factors to be considered in maintaining adequate flow and minimal myocardial work. Bedside assessment of cardiovascular function depends upon the thorough understanding of physiologic factors affecting flow. This is best approached by a functional analysis of factors affecting blood volume, vascular space, and myocardial function.

DISTRIBUTION OF TOTAL BODY WEIGHT

Total body water is generally expressed as a percent of body weight. Several studies have shown that approximately 70% of lean body mass consists of water.[1] Fat tissue has a much lower water content per gram than other tissue, resulting in a lower than predicted total body water content in people with excessive fat tissue.[2] Representative mean values of total body water are 60% for lean men and 50% for lean women.[3]

As illustrated in Figure 1–1, total body water expressed in liters constitutes approximately 60% of total body weight in kilograms. In the adult the

1

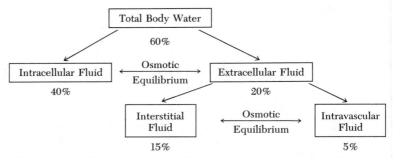

Fig 1–1.—Body fluid compartments with water percentages expressed as a percentage of ideal body weight.

intracellular fluid compartment constitutes approximately 40% of the ideal body weight, whereas the extracellular fluid compartment accounts for 20%. The extracellular fluid is distributed between the intravascular space (plasma volume) and the interstitial fluid space. The balance between intravascular and interstitial volume is determined largely by the presence of albumin and globulins, which exert a colloid osmotic pressure (oncotic pressure). Approximately 5% of ideal body weight is due to intravascular water excluding the red blood cell mass, and 15% is due to the interstitial fluid. An example of the distribution of fluid volumes within the various compartments is given in Table 1–1.

Primary Blood Volume Deficiency

Inadequate blood volume frequently results from acute blood loss. An acute blood loss of up to 10% (the amount of blood given by a blood donor) can readily be tolerated by most patients without adverse cardiovascular effects. A blood loss between 10% and 20% is usually not associated with

TABLE 1–1.—Representative Fluid Volumes

MEASURED PARAMETERS	MALE Abs. Value (% Body Weight)	FEMALE Abs. Value (% Body Weight)
Weight (kg)	80	55
Total body water (L)	48.0 (60)	2.75 (50)
Intracellular fluid (L)	32.0 (40)	18.7 (34)
Extracellular fluid (L)	16.0 (20)	8.8 (16)
Interstitial (L)	12.0 (15)	6.3 (11.5)
Intravascular (blood volume ml)	6,000 (7.5)	3,575 (6.5)
Plasma volume (ml)	4,000 (5.0)	2,475 (4.5)
RBC mass volume (ml)	2,000 (2.5)	1,100 (2.0)

significant signs of cardiovascular distress when the patient is supine. However, orthostatic changes, physical exertion, or the administration of vasodilating drugs often cause tachycardia and hypotension. An acute blood loss between 20% and 40% is usually associated with signs of cardiovascular distress including hypotension, tachycardia, marginal peripheral circulation, and inadequate tissue perfusion.[4] Once acute blood loss exceeds 40%, inadequate tissue perfusion is likely to persist despite appropriate volume replacement ("irreversible shock").

Other common causes of primarily decreased intravascular volume are dehydration and third space sequestration in the lumen of the intestinal tract or abdominal cavity. Endothelial cell dysfunction may lead to increased permeability and loss of protein from the intravascular compartment. The consequent inability to maintain adequate oncotic pressure gradients results in a primary decrease in blood volume.

Secondary Blood Volume Deficiency

Inadequate perfusion is often related to an absolute increase in the intravascular space. This phenomenon is frequently referred to as a secondary or *relative hypovolemia.*

The major arteries contain 5% to 10% of the blood volume. Arterioles are responsible for regional adjustments in the distribution of perfusion because of their ability to significantly vary resistance. The microcirculatory bed (capillaries) contain 25% to 30% of the blood volume. The distribution to individual capillary beds is greatly determined by the pre- and postcapillary sphincters which are subject to changes in smooth muscle tone secondary to the autonomic nervous system, endogenous circulatory hormones, and tissue metabolites.[5]

VENOUS CAPACITANCE

Approximately two-thirds of the total blood volume normally resides in the venous system. The high "capacitance" of these vessels refers to their ability to significantly alter their blood volume with minimal pressure changes by autonomic nervous system-mediated changes in smooth muscle tone.

A decrease in venous tone leads to a significant increase in the vascular space. If this occurs in conjunction with a "normal blood volume," a state of *relative hypovolemia* exists. This is frequently observed in patients with sepsis, acute spinal cord injury, and regional anesthetic blockade. Relative hypovolemia may also exist in patients who are aggressively treated with vasodilator drugs. The recognition of the relationship between vascular volume and vascular space is of vital importance.

VASCULAR VOLUME/VASCULAR SPACE RELATIONSHIP

Blood flow from the peripheral veins to the atrium is dependent upon a pressure gradient primarily developed by the contraction of venous smooth muscle (venous tone). Whenever the venous system contains a blood volume within its range of storage capacity, a state of *relative normovolemia* exists; when the blood volume exceeds storage capacity a *relative hypervolemia* exists; when blood volume is below the range of storage capacity a *relative hypovolemia* exists.

Figure 1–2 illustrates the relationship between changes in atrial pressure and flow as venous blood volume changes. Any time the blood volume in the venous system is below its maximum capacitance or above its minimum capacitance, reasonable blood volume changes are well tolerated. Volume additions made when maximum capacitance is exceeded result in large

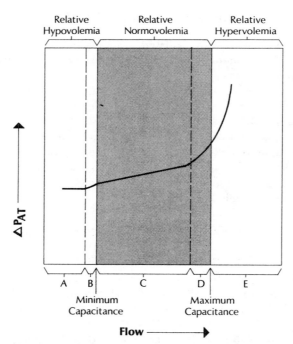

Fig 1–2.—*Model depicting the theoretic relationship between venous flow and the change in atrial pressure resulting from a specific fluid load (ΔP_{AT}). Changes in Δ_{AT} are routinely measured by a CVP catheter for the right atrium and PCWP for the left atrium. (From Shapiro B.A., Harrison R.A., Trout C.A.:* Clinical Applications of Respiratory Care, *ed. 2. Chicago, Year Book Medical Publishers, 1979. Used by permission.)*

pressure changes with very little increase in venous return. Volume removal when minimum capacitance exists results in a marked decrease in venous return.

Venous return can be improved by at least two mechanisms: (1) an increased driving pressure accomplished by an increase in venous tone while volume remains unchanged; and (2) an improved venous conductance associated with a reduction in venous tone after the addition of volume. The first mechanism is the most common initial response of the critically ill patient in an attempt to improve or maintain venous return; the second mechanism is the therapeutic approach most often used by the clinician in attempting to improve venous return.

MYOCARDIAL FUNCTION

Heart Rate

Tachycardia (>100/min) is most frequently associated with sympathetic stimulation. In the critically ill patient, insults such as hypoxemia, acidemia, hypercarbia, hyperthermia, and acute decreases in blood volume are common causes of tachycardia. Atropine-like and β-adrenergic drugs can produce pronounced tachycardia. In the elderly or critically ill patient with preexisting heart disease, an increase in heart rate to >140/min often limits ventricular filling time to the extent that cardiac output declines. Increased heart rate is associated with increases in myocardial oxygen consumption.

Bradycardia (<50/min) usually decreases cardiac output because further increases in stroke volume (SV) are limited. Myocardial hypoxia is a potentially lethal cause of bradycardia. Common causes of bradycardia in the critically ill patient are conductance disturbances, hypothermia, β-blockers (Propranolol), and anticholinesterase agents (Neostigmine or Tensilon).

Contractility

Contractility can be defined as the shortening capacity and force-generating potential of the myocardial muscle fibers making up the ventricular wall. Contractility remains an extremely difficult entity to evaluate quantitatively.[6] Diminished contractility (negative inotropism) is associated with hypoxia, acidosis, hypercarbia, poor myocardial perfusion, β-blocking agents, calcium channel blockers, and some anesthetic agents. Improved contractility (positive inotropism) is clinically correlated with enhanced states of tissue oxygenation, acid-base environment, and improved myocardial perfusion. Drugs such as the β-adrenergic catecholamines, digitalis, and calcium chloride are associated with an increase in contractility. Increased myocardial contractility is always associated with increased myocardial oxygen demands.

The majority of experimental work quantitating myocardial contractility are in vitro studies relating contractility to the velocity of muscle shortening (dl/dt), rate of pressure development (dP/dt), and maximum velocity of muscle shortening (V_{max}).[7] A decreased ejection fraction (SV:end diastolic volume) has been correlated with a decrease in contractility.[8] Gated cardiac-blood-pool studies may eventually provide a dependable bedside assessment of contractility.[9]

Preload

Preload is defined as the loading force or the end diastolic volume distending the relaxed ventricular wall. Assuming a constant myocardial compliance, as end diastolic volume is increased, end diastolic pressure must increase. Figure 1–3 clearly demonstrates that as the end diastolic pressure (preload) is increased, SV is correspondingly increased until a point is reached where further increases in preload result in a decrease in SV. There are an infinite number of pressure:volume curves, each one related to a different state of myocardial contractility.[10]

Afterload

Afterload can be defined as the force or tension developed in the ventricular wall to overcome impedance to flow in the ventricular outflow

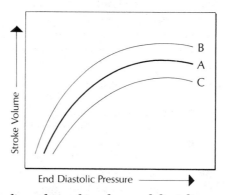

Fig 1–3.—*Frank-Starling relationship where end-diastolic pressure is directly proportional to end-diastolic volume. Curve A represents normal contractility; B, increased contractility; and C, decreased contractility. (From Shapiro, B.A., Harrison R.A., Trout C.A.:* Clinical Application of Respiratory Care, *ed. 2. Chicago, Year Book Medical Publishers, 1979. Used by permission.)*

tract. Factors causing impedance include valvular/vascular wall distensibility, major artery wall compliance, and the arteriolar resistance.

Acute afterload increases are associated with increased myocardial oxygen consumption. The most common cause of acute afterload increase is an increased vascular resistance. Two common factors are valvular disease and increased blood viscosity.[11]

BEDSIDE ASSESSMENT OF CARDIOVASCULAR FUNCTION

Tissue perfusion depends upon adequate circulation, which is dependent upon adequate ventricular contractility, preload, and afterload. Proper utilization of arterial, central venous pressure (CVP) and balloon-tipped pulmonary artery (PA) catheters allows the preload and afterload function of both ventricles to be monitored.

Contractility Assessment

History and physical examination will usually determine the patient with high probability of primary myocardial dysfunction—myocardial ischemia, ventricular failure, and valvular disease. Negative inotropic factors such as acidemia, alkalemia, hypercarbia, hypoxemia, and sepsis must be evaluated. Once primary and obvious secondary factors leading to negative inotropism have been reasonably ruled out, further evaluation of the circulation and myocardial function depend upon appropriate assessment and support of venous return.

Afterload Assessment

Under most circumstances an arterial catheter properly placed in a brachial or radial artery will measure pressures that are quantitatively close to aortic root pressure. In the critically ill patient with severely compromised myocardial function, significant errors between radial artery pressure and aortic root pressure may be present. In such circumstances it would be advisable to place a longer catheter into an artery closer to the aorta. Pulmonary artery catheters provide access for measurement of pulmonary artery pressures and hence right ventricular afterload.

Preload Assessment

The clinical assessment of venous return cannot be ascertained from a single pressure reading obtained from a CVP or PA catheter. Since neither the state of venous tone nor the degree of peripheral to central venous pressure gradient can be measured, the only alternative approach is to make serial measurements of pressure after manipulation of the volume status. This concept is embodied in the *fluid challenge principle.*

A fluid challenge consists of the administration of a finite volume over a short interval followed by correlation of serial pressure changes in either CVP or pulmonary artery occluded pressure (PAOP) readings with clinical and physiologic assessment of changes in the systemic circulation and tissue perfusion status. The following guidelines are a useful systematic approach for the application of the fluid challenge principle.

Step 1. Obtain general clinical, hemodynamic, and laboratory baseline values, especially PAOP or CVP measurement.

Step 2. Give from 50 to 200 ml of appropriate volume (crystalloid, colloid, or blood) within ten min. The amount and type of volume are dependent upon the appraisal of the patient's clinical status.

Step 3. Observe for improvement in blood pressure (BP), pulse, and peripheral tissue perfusion. Examination of the chest for evidence of pulmonary edema is essential.

Step 4. Evaluate the change in PAOP or CVP measurement and continue as outlined under conditions listed in Table 1–2.

Once the assessment of vascular volume to vascular space is completed, then the assessment of primary myocardial function is more meaningful. If necessary, more direct pharmacologic support of the myocardium can be instituted.

Cardiac Output Measurement

In the late nineteenth century, Adolph Fick described a procedure whereby the concentration of a dissolved substance in the blood (in the initial description the substance was oxygen) could be used as an indicator for determining the amount of blood flow.[12] This concept has subsequently

TABLE 1–2.—GUIDELINES FOR VOLUME ADMINISTRATION WHEN USING A FLUID CHALLENGE PRINCIPLE

CONDITIONS	↑ ΔPAOP	↑ ΔCVP
Add additional volume	≤ 3 mm Hg	≤ 2 cm H_2O
Do not add additional volume	≥ 7 mm Hg	≥ 5 cm H_2O
Wait 10 min, add smaller volumes and repeat evaluation	Between 3 and 7 mm Hg	Between 2 and 5 cm H_2O

become known as the Fick principle and, with oxygen as the dissolved substance, is described by the Fick equation. This approach has remained the standard against which newer techniques are compared. The capability of directly measuring circulation (cardiac output) has provided the clinician with an important direct link to the assessment of cardiovascular function.

THERMAL DILUTION TECHNIQUE

This is accomplished by using a PA flotation catheter with an injection port approximately 30 cm from the distal end and a thermister located at the distal end. The thermister, a device capable of sensing changes in temperature, is normally in one of the branches of the PA. The proximal port normally resides within the right atrium and is used for injection of an iced solution of which the temperature is known.

The "cold injected" can be measured by knowing the volume of injectate, the specific heat of the solution, and the temperature difference between the solution and the patient's blood. The thermister measures the changes in blood temperature from the baseline value as the cold solution ejected by the right ventricle passes the catheter tip. Therefore, because the amount of "cold injected" and the time duration and magnitude of temperature changes have all been measured, a cardiac output can be calculated.[13]

Two distinct advantages of thermodilution are availability of repeated measurements without the need for repeated blood sampling and less artifact due to the phenomenon of recirculation because of the close proximity of the sampling site to the injection site. Some of the disadvantages in the technique are related to potential incomplete mixing of the cold solution in the right ventricle, variations in the rate of injection, inaccurate sampling by the thermister in the catheter tip because of malposition, and varying losses of the "injected cold" into adjacent cardiac, vascular, and pulmonary tissues.

Derived Indices of Cardiovascular Hemodynamics

Additional information relating to cardiovascular function can be obtained by combining two or more of the measured parameters, thus deriving a new index of function.[14] Often the combination of several independent physiologic measurements will provide insight into specific aspects of myocardial function or cardiovascular relationships that are not as readily apparent by looking at a series of isolated measurements.

CARDIAC INDEX

The cardiac index (CI) is a calculation used to relate cardiac output to body size.

$$CI = \frac{\text{Cardiac output (L/min)}}{\text{Body surface area (m}^2)}$$

Normal range for CI is 2.7–4.3 L/m^2/min with a mean of 3.5 L/m^2/min.

STROKE VOLUME, STROKE WORK, AND STROKE WORK INDEX

Stroke Volume

The SV is calculated by dividing the measured cardiac output by the heart rate.

Stroke Work (SW)

Estimation of myocardial work is important since increases are associated with increased myocardial oxygen demands.[15] Even under resting conditions myocardial oxygen extraction is very large; therefore, significant increases in myocardial work present the possibility of myocardial ischemia unless myocardial blood flow can be augmented. The myocardial work per contraction can be estimated by multiplying the SV by the average pressure during systole minus the left ventricular end diastolic pressure. In practice the measurements of mean arterial pressure (MAP) minus PAOP is multiplied by the stroke volume.

$$\text{STROKE WORK} = (\text{MAP} - \text{PAOP})(\text{SV})$$

Stroke Work Index

The stroke work index (SWI) is obtained by dividing the stroke work (SW) by the body surface area (BSA).

$$SWI = \frac{SW}{BSA}$$

Rate-Pressure Product

The term "rate-pressure product" (RPP) represents a simplified approach extrapolated from the experimentally determined tension index relating ventricular wall tension and systolic intervals to myocardial oxygen consumption. In brief, it uses the well established relationship that increased heart rate and increased systolic pressure (increased afterload) cause increases in myocardial oxygen consumption. The only advantage to this index is that it does not require sophisticated monitoring equipment.

$$RPP = \text{(heart rate) (systolic BP)}$$

Values >12,000 are interpreted as indicative of significantly increased myocardial work and increased myocardial oxygen demands.

SYSTEMIC AND PULMONARY VASCULAR RESISTANCE

The resistance to flow in arteries can be expressed in the following manner:

$$\text{Resistance} = \frac{\text{Arterial pressure} - \text{Atrial pressure}}{\text{Cardiac output}}$$

Because the two ventricular pumps exist in a series arrangement with two markedly different pressures but the same average flow (cardiac output), the resistances of the two vascular beds are normally quite different.

Resistance calculations require deriving the driving pressure (pressure drop) across the circuit. For systemic vascular resistance (SVR) this is equal to the aortic root pressure (MAP) minus the right atrial pressure (CVP); for pulmonary vascular resistance (PVR) this is equal to the pulmonary artery root pressure (mean PA pressure) minus the left atrial pressure (PAOP). The units of vascular resistance are expressed in dynes/sec/cm^{-5}. In clinical practice, pressure is measured in mm Hg and cardiac output in liters per minute. Using these values and taking into account the various conversion factors, the proper units can be arrived at by introducing the number 80 into the basic equation.

$$SVR = \frac{\text{MAP (mm Hg)} - \text{CVP (mm Hg)}}{\text{Cardiac output (L/min)}} \times 80$$

$$PVR = \frac{\text{PA (mm Hg)} - \text{PAOP (mm Hg)}}{\text{Cardiac output (L/min)}} \times 80$$

Representative mean values and the normal range of values are given in Table 1–3.

TABLE 1–3.—NORMAL VALUES FOR
SYSTEMIC VASCULAR RESISTANCE (SVR) AND
PULMONARY VASCULAR RESISTANCE (PVR)

	MEAN (DYNES/SEC/CM^{-5})	RANGE (DYNES/SEC/CM^{-5})
SVR	1,200	1,000–1,600
PVR	60	50–160

CASE STUDY

A 27-year-old male passenger pulled from the right front seat of a high-speed, head-on collision arrived in the emergency room via paramedic vehicle. He had been found conscious with his seat belt fastened. An 18-gauge IV line was secured in the right forearm with normal saline running at a rapid rate. An oxygen mask was in place and the man was speaking incoherently. Skin was clammy and sweaty but not mottled. The hands and feet were cold to the touch.

His BP was 90/? mm Hg, pulse rate 130/min and regular, and respiratory rate (RR) 35/min. The patient was moving all four extremities and his head without difficulty. No apparent head, neck, or chest trauma was observed. Lung sounds were equal bilaterally and shallow and no flailing or paradoxical movements were noted. Auscultation of the heart revealed normal S_1 and S_2; no S_3, S_4, or murmurs noted. The abdomen was tense and tender and no bowel sounds were heard.

Peritoneal lavage documented the presence of intra-abdominal bleeding. Blood specimens for type and cross match, CBC, and SMA-6 were obtained. A CVP catheter was positioned via the right subclavian route and then a third IV line (14-gauge) placed in the left antecubital fossa. A urinary catheter was placed and 800 ml of blood-tinged urine evacuated. A radial arterial puncture was accomplished and a specimen for blood gas analysis obtained.

Over the next 10 min the systolic BP dropped to 60 mm Hg palpable and the CVP dropped from 5 to 1 cm H_2O. The patient became unresponsive with irregular respirations. The trachea was orally intubated with a #9 OD endotracheal tube, and positive pressure ventilation (PPV) commenced via a self-inflating hand ventilator with reservoir hose and >15 L/min oxygen flow. The BP was now 40 mm Hg palpable and the ECG monitor showed a sinus tachycardia.

Discussion

It must be assumed that the inadequate perfusion status is due to a primary blood volume deficiency, i.e., intra-abdominal bleeding. Volume resuscitation is essential. The importance of having placed the two additional IVs prior to vascular collapse is obvious. There is no indication for vasopressors at this time.

It should be noted that the perfusion status significantly deteriorated when PPV was instituted. This is undoubtedly secondary to decreased venous return and is another reason for rapid volume replacement.

All three IVs should be used to reestablish an adequate blood volume. Of course, whole blood should be administered as soon as it is available. In the interim, combinations of colloid and crystalloid solutions are appropriate depending upon availability.

Case Study Continued

Normal saline was administered through the CVP and 18-gauge line while a hetastarch solution was administered through the 14-gauge line. Fifteen minutes later after 2.5 L of saline and 1.5 L of colloid had been administered, the patient's BP was 90/40 mm Hg, pulse rate 125/min (sinus tachycardia), RR 10/min by hand ventilator (tidal volumes (V_T) approximately 1.2 L and FI_{O_2} 60%–70%), CVP 5 cm H_2O, and urine output 8 cc in the past 10 min. Extremities were still cold with thready peripheral pulses. The abdomen was very tense. The patient began to move his extremities violently and tried to extubate himself. It required three people to keep him still.

Discussion

Following successful resuscitation of acute hypovolemic shock, the patient often becomes uncooperative and confused due to reestablished cerebral perfusion. This raises the circulating catecholamine level, which increases venous tone, vascular resistance, and myocardial contractility. This sympathetic response is contributing to the maintenance of perfusion and BP. Any sedation would be expected to diminish the level of sympathetic tone and therefore increase the vascular space, creating a relative hypovolemia.

Sedation is essential to allow stabilization and transport to the operating room. Several assumptions are reasonable: (1) this patient's myocardium is strong, (2) tamponade within the abdomen has probably occurred and further hemorrhage will be slight until the abdomen is surgically opened, and (3) further volume administration to compensate for venodilation is not a problem.

Tranquilizing agents, such as diazepam, have unreliable relationships between dose and CNS and respiratory depression. Furthermore, these drugs are not reversible and have unpredictable cardiovascular side effects. By contrast, morphine sulfate has a well documented and consistent relationship between dose and CNS and respiratory depression, has no direct myocardial depressant properties, is known to be a venodilator, and is completely reversible. These pharmacologic factors make morphine the drug of choice in this circumstance.

Case Study Continued

Morphine sulfate was administered in IV aliquots of 2 mg to a total of 12 mg in 10 min. Intravenous fluid was administered to maintain a CVP >5 cm H_2O and a BP >80 systolic. A total of 1.5 L of normal saline was administered in 10 min during morphinization. The patient was quiet and unconscious if not stimulated. Ventilation was easily controllable and the vital signs were now a BP of 85/50 mm Hg, a pulse rate of 122/min (sinus tachycardia), an RR of 10/min (FI_{O_2} approximately 70%), a CVP of 6 cm H_2O, and a urine output of 6 cc in 10 min. Extremities were still cold. Arterial blood gas analysis revealed a pH of 7.32, a PCO_2 of 45 mm Hg, and a PO_2 of 277 mm Hg.

Whole blood was now available and 2 units were started through blood warmers. In the next 20 min, 4 units of whole blood and 1 L of crystalloid were administered, which resulted in a BP of 110/60 mm Hg, a pulse rate of 105/min (sinus tachycardia), a RR of 10/min, a CVP of 12 cm H_2O, and a urine output of 30 cc in 20 min. Extremities were warmer with good pulses. The abdomen was still very tense. The patient was transported to the operating room for a laparotomy.

Approximately 3 L of blood were suctioned from the abdomen. A liver laceration was oversewn and a lacerated spleen removed. No other abnormalities were found in the abdomen.

Upon arrival in the surgical intensive care unit following surgery the patient had received the following IV fluids:

Blood, whole	2,000 ml (4 units)
Blood, packed cells	2,500 ml (10 units)
Hetastarch	3,000 ml
Crystalloid, saline	5,500 ml
Crystalloid, 0.2% saline	1,500 ml
Total	14.5 L

Fluid losses for the same time period were:

Estimated blood loss	5,000 ml
Urine output	1,700 ml
Total	6.7 L

Blood pressure was 125/70 mm Hg (arterial line), pulse rate 100/min (no dysrhythmia), and RR 10/min on the mechanical ventilator (vt 1,200 ml, FI_{O_2} 35%, positive end expiratory pressure (PEEP) 5 cm H_2O) with no spontaneous ventilatory efforts. A narcotic anesthetic had been used and non-depolarizing muscle relaxant had not been reversed. Temperature was 36°C, CVP 9 cm H_2O, extremities were warm and dry, hemoglobin was 11 gm/dl, pH 7.41, PCO_2 36 mm Hg, and PO_2 77 mm Hg.

Over the next 5 hours the patient spontaneously diuresed, breathed spontaneously, and maintained acceptable perfusion and gas exchange. He was removed from ventilatory support and extubated 12 hours postoperatively. The subclavian catheter was removed 36 hours postoperatively.

On the third postoperative day, there were no bowel sounds heard and he became hypotensive and tachycardic. Assessment of intake and output revealed reasonable balance; however, his weight was 2 kg less than his presumed weight prior to the accident. He required 3 L of saline to maintain adequate BP throughout the day, and urine output remained >50 ml/hour. Electrolytes were within normal limits; however, total serum proteins were decreased. An abdominal x-ray revealed a dilated fluid-filled small bowel without air fluid levels.

Because the CVP catheter had been removed, it was elected to place a pulmonary artery catheter for further fluid and cardiovascular management. His BP was 110/80 mm Hg, MAP 90 mm Hg, pulse 120/min and regular, RR 22 and regular, core temperature 37.2°C, right atrial pressure (RA) 4 mm Hg, right ventricular pressure (RV) 18/0 mm Hg, PA 16/9 mm Hg, PAOP 7 mm Hg, CI 2.2 L/min, cardiac output 4.6 L/min, and SVR 1,520 dynes/sec/cm^{-5}.

Discussion

Third spacing fluid in the small bowel is the most likely explanation for the hypotension, i.e., a relative hypovolemia (normal or contracted vascular space with diminished vascular volume). Although total body water may be normal at this juncture, much of it is sequestered in the small bowel creating an extracellular (and intracellular) fluid deficit.

The key concept to supportive therapy is to administer adequate fluid to sustain perfusion (assure adequate preload) while assuring adequate myocardial contractility. Once the small bowel fluid begins to mobilize, adequate diuresis must be assured to prevent relative hypervolemia..

Pulmonary artery hemodynamic monitoring is essential if the myocardial status is doubtful or sepsis is suspected. Because neither is true in this case, CVP monitoring would be acceptable. However, because a new central access was necessary, the placement of a PA catheter is acceptable and justifiable.

The inadequate cardiac output is most likely due to an inadequate preload. The increased SVR and tachycardia reflect increased sympathetic tone. Appropriate fluid loading should increase venous conductance and improve cardiac output.

At least 50% of administered solution should be colloid because the bowel preferentially sequesters protein.

Case Study Continued

Two hundred milliliters of hetastarch solution was administered over 3 min without change in vital signs or PAOP. This was repeated twice without measurable changes in hemodynamics. After a total of 800 ml fluid challenge, the heart rate decreased to 105/min and the cardiac output increased to 5.8 L/min. No change in MAP or PAOP was noted and SVR was reduced to 1,120 dynes/sec/cm^{-5}.

Another 200 ml of colloid was administered and rapidly resulted in a heart rate of 95/min, the PAOP increasing to 11 mm Hg and the cardiac output to 7.2 L/min (CI 3.5 L/min). Mean arterial pressure was 95 mm Hg and SVR 1,100 dynes/sec/cm^{-5}. Further fluid administration was titrated to maintain the PAOP at approximately 11 mm Hg.

A positive balance of 6 L over the next 48 hours ensued while perfusion and hemodynamics were maintained. Thereafter, the patient began to diurese (urine output >200 ml/hour) and IV fluids were decreased to a minimum. Eleven liters negative balance ensued over 72 hours with excellent perfusion and maintained hemodynamics. The patient made an uneventful recovery.

REFERENCES

1. Widdowson E., McCance R.A., Spray C.L.M.: The chemical composition of the human body. *Clin. Sci.* 10:113–125, 1951.
2. Keys A., Brazek J.: Body fat in adult man. *Physiol. Rev.* 33:245–325, 1953.
3. Schloerb P.R., Friis-Hanson, B.J., Edelman I.S., et al.: The measurement of total body water in the human subject by deuterium oxide dilution with considerations of dynamics on deuterium distribution. *J. Clin. Invest.* 29:1296–1310, 1950.
4. Walcott W.W.: Blood volume in experimental hemorrhagic shock. *Am. J. Physiol.* 143:247–261, 1945.
5. Fulton G.P., Lutz B.R., Callahan A.B.: Innervation as a factor in control of microcirculation. *Physiol. Rev.* 40(Suppl. 4):57, 1960.
6. Weissler A., Harris W.S., Schoenfeld C.D.: Bedside techniques for the evaluation of ventricular function in man. *Am. J. Cardiol.* 23:577–583, 1969.
7. Ross J., Jr., Covell J.C., Sonnenblick E.H., et al.: Contractile state of the heart characterized by force-velocity relations in variably afterloaded and isovolemic beats. *Circ. Res.* 18:149–163, 1966.
8. Dodge H.T., Baxley W.A.: Left ventricular volume and mass and their significance in heart disease. *Am. J. Cardiol.* 23:528–537, 1969.
9. Schelbert H.R., Verba J.W., Johnson A.D., et al.: Nontraumatic determination of left ventricular ejection fraction by radionuclide angiocardiography. *Circulation* 51:902–909, 1975.
10. Sarnoff S.J.: Symposium on regulation of performance of heart; myocardial contractility as described by ventricular function curves; observations on Starling's law of heart. *Physiol. Rev.* 35:107–122, 1955.
11. Haynes R.H., Burton A.C.: Role of the non-Newtonian behavior of blood in hemodynamics. *Am. J. Physiol.* 197:943–950, 1959.
12. Fick A.: Ulber die messung des blutquantuns in dem herzventribeln. *Sitzungsb. du physmed Ges. zu Wurzburg*, 1870, p. 16.
13. Weisel R.D., Berger R.L., Hechtman H.B.: Measurement of cardiac output by thermodilution. *N. Engl. J. Med.* 292:682–684, 1975.
14. Sonnenblick E.H., Strobeck J.E.: Current concepts in cardiology: Derived indexes of ventricular and myocardial function. *N. Engl. J. Med.* 296:978–982, 1977.
15. Sonnenblick E.H., Shelton C.L.: Myocardial energetics: Basic principles and clinical implications. *N. Engl. J. Med.* 285:668–675, 1971.

2 / Principles of Mechanical Support of Ventilation

BARRY A. SHAPIRO, M.D.

PRINCIPLES OF MECHANICAL SUPPORT OF VENTILATION

Inability of the pulmonary system to adequately excrete metabolically produced CO_2 results in acute hypercarbia, a circumstance referred to as acute respiratory acidosis or acute ventilatory failure (AVF). AVF can be attributed to either a primary failure of the "ventilatory pump" due to chest cage abnormality, muscle weakness, or nervous system disorders; or inability to increase the work of breathing sufficiently when severe lung disease is present.[1]

Manipulation of airway pressures is an effective means of improving pulmonary gas exchange in acute respiratory failure. Mechanical support of ventilation has proved to be the foundation for supporting the work of breathing and reversing AVF. Such therapy must be based on a clinical discipline that allows for multiple factors to be evaluated while treatment modalities are titrated and monitored.

LUNG COMPLIANCE AND THE WORK OF BREATHING

Gas movement in and out of the pulmonary system occurs in response to pressure differences between the alveoli and the upper airway—transairway pressure gradients. Elastic forces of the lung, chest, and diaphragm are mainly responsible for *expiratory* transairway pressure gradients. Although resistance is the major factor determining expiratory flow, compliance factors may be significant.

Inspiratory transairway pressure gradients are generated by the work of the respiratory muscles creating a transpulmonary pressure gradient—the difference between upper airway and intrapleural pressure. The relationship between transairway and transpulmonary pressure gradients during inspiration is greatly determined by lung compliance. For any given transairway pressure gradient, the main factor affecting gas flow is airway resistance. Since decreased lung compliance will demand a greater transpulmonary gradient to create any given transairway pressure gradient, the work of breathing must be increased when lung compliance is diminished.

ACUTE RESTRICTIVE PULMONARY PATHOLOGY

Functional Residual Capacity

Functional residual capacity (FRC) is the combination of residual volume (RV) and expiratory reserve volume (ERV) (Fig 2–1). It represents the end-expiratory lung volume, i.e., the lung volume at which inspiration begins. Measurement of FRC is reasonably reliable in acutely ill patients because the patient's active cooperation is not required. The measurement of FRC in intensive care is presently a research tool; however, new technology may make this a clinical tool in the near future.

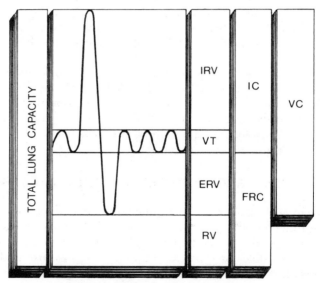

Fig 2–1.—*The divisions of total lung capacity. Total lung capacity (TLC) is the maximum amount of air the lungs can hold. The total lung capacity is divided into four primary volumes: inspiratory reserve volume (IRV); tidal volume (VT); expiratory reserve volume (ERV); and residual volume (RV). Capacities are combinations of two or more lung volumes. They are inspiratory capacity (IC), functional residual capacity (FRC), and vital capacity (VC). (From Shapiro B.A., Harrison R.A., Walton J.R.:* Clinical Application of Blood Gases, *ed. 2. Chicago, Year Book Medical Publishers, 1977. Used by permission.)*

Functional Residual Capacity and Acute Ventilatory Failure

An acute decrease in FRC leads to (1) decreased compliance of the lung-thorax complex and therefore an increased work of breathing, (2) vital capacity (VC) reduction resulting in decreased ventilatory reserves,[2] and (3) varying degrees of deadspace and shunting abnormalities. In other words, an acute restrictive disease will lead to some increased work of breathing, some diminishment of ventilatory reserve, and some inefficiency of pulmonary gas exchange (V/Q imbalance). It is the combination of these factors that often leads to AVF.

Differentiation of Acute Restrictive Pathology

Acute restrictive pathology can be divided into three theoretic types: (1) *Equal Diminishment of Lung Volumes (Type A, Fig 2–2).*—The most common lung pathologies resulting in this category are acute segmental/

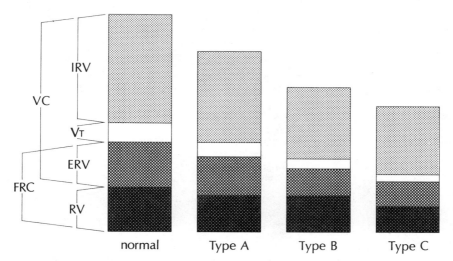

Fig 2–2.—Bar graphs of the three types of acute restrictive pathology commonly confronted in critical care medicine. RV = *residual volume;* ERV = *expiratory reserve volume;* VT = *tidal volume;* IRV = *inspiratory reserve volume;* FRC = *functional residual capacity;* VC = *vital capacity.* Type A = *equal diminishment of all lung volumes commonly seen with acute atelectasis, CNS depression, and neuromuscular disease;* Type B = *major diminishment in vital capacity commonly seen in the postoperative patient;* Type C = *major diminishment in FRC commonly referred to as the adult respiratory distress syndrome (ARDS). From Shapiro B.A., Harrison R.A., Trout C.A.:* Clinical Application of Respiratory Care, *ed. 2. Chicago, Year Book Medical Publishers, 1979. Used by permission.)*

lobar atelectasis and consolidated pneumonitis because reasonably uniform infringement of lung volumes occurs prior to eventual hyperinflation of adjacent lung. The hypoxemia that results from this zero V/Q area indirectly demands increased ventilatory work. In addition to the diminished lung compliance, pulmonary blood flow is acutely diminished to the affected lung.[3]

The most common non-pulmonary pathologies in this category are CNS depression and neuromuscular diseases (Table 2–1) that result in one or a combination of the following: (1) diminished response to afferent ventilatory stimuli, (2) ablation of normal periodic "sighs," and (3) diminished stimulation to (or response of) the diaphragm and other ventilatory muscles. Such factors alter the chest wall and diaphragm muscle tone and usually reduce all lung volumes.

(2) *Primary Diminishment of Vital Capacity (Type B, Fig 2–2).*—An injury or insult that limits expansion of the normal lung results in significant VC and FRC reduction with minimal reduction in residual volume. This is most commonly seen in postoperative abdominal and thoracic surgical patients[3] and with mild noncardiogenic pulmonary edema.[4] The decreased VC leads to an increased work of breathing.[5]

(3) *Major Diminishment of Residual Volume (Type C, Fig 2–2).*—Severe lung parenchymal disease may result in dysfunction of surfactant mechanisms that tends to increase the incidence of small alveoli emptying into larger alveoli. This results in a severe diminishment in RV and a severe

TABLE 2–1.—Neuromuscular
Disease Commonly Requiring
Respiratory Intensive Care

I. Spinal cord disease
  A. Trauma
    1. Quadriplegia
    2. Paraplegia
  B. Poliomyelitis
II. Motor nerve disease
  A. Acute idiopathic polyneuritis
    1. Guillain-Barre syndrome
    2. Landry's ascending paralysis
  B. Tick bite paralysis
  C. Porphyria
III. Myoneural junctional disease
  A. Myasthenia gravis
  B. Myasthenic syndrome
IV. Muscle-wasting disease
  A. Muscular dystrophy
  B. Congenital myotonia
V. Tetanus

decrease in lung compliance. Such pathology is commonly referred to as the adult respiratory distress syndrome (ARDS). Although the primary gas exchange alteration is severe hypoxemia, the decreased lung compliance requires significantly increased energy expenditure for ventilation.

Positive Pressure Ventilation

Consistently successful techniques for PPV were developed in the 1920s in conjunction with general anesthesia and endotracheal intubation.[6] Negative pressure methods of providing ventilatory support developed outside the operating room primarily because of the unavailability of endotracheal intubation and the desire to avoid tracheostomy.[2] Because access to the patient's body was less important on the wards than in the operating room, the negative pressure ventilator (iron lung) gained enormous popularity for supporting polio victims.[8]

The deficiencies of the negative pressure ventilator for acutely ill patients was recognized during World War II and documented during the Scandinavian polio epidemics of the early 1950s.[9] To this day, it remains true that positive pressure ventilators provide the best support for acutely ill patients as they allow necessary monitoring and nursing care. It has never been true that positive pressure ventilators are physiologically advantageous—to the contrary, the physiologic disadvantages are numerous.

PHYSIOLOGIC DETRIMENTS OF POSITIVE PRESSURE VENTILATION

Potential Diminishment of Venous Return

In comparison to spontaneous ventilation, PPV must result in increased airway pressures. Although transmission of these pressures to the intrathoracic space varies with pulmonary disease, the qualitative effect of PPV must be to increase intrathoracic pressure.[10] Thus, PPV represents a *potential* embarrassment of venous return to the heart.

Increased Deadspace Ventilation

Increasing alveolar pressure favors distribution of pulmonary blood flow to gravity-dependent portions of lung. The result is a greater portion of lung being poorly perfused but well ventilated. This phenomenon usually occurs despite the maintenance of adequate cardiac output.[11]

Increased Venous Admixture

PPV in the supine position results in decreased ventilation of the posterior lung fields.[12] This maldistribution of ventilation leads to relative underventilation of the gravity-dependent lung.[13]

CAPABILITIES OF POSITIVE PRESSURE VENTILATION

Power for Ventilation

A ventilator can provide all or part of the energy necessary to move gas into the lungs. When the patient is unable to provide this energy (or its provision is detrimental to cardiopulmonary homeostasis), PPV may maintain or reestablish adequate respiratory gas exchange. However, simply providing PPV does *not always* improve gas exchange, especially in the presence of a relative hypovolemia or left ventricular failure.

Alter Flow Pattern (Inflation Hold)

Despite much debate, there is little evidence to suggest that differing flow generators (e.g., sine wave vs. square wave) make clinically significant differences.[14] However, variations in flow pattern may significantly affect gas distribution, especially in the presence of specific pathology.[15] Specifically, the longer the interval between inspiratory volume delivery and end-inspiration, the greater will be the peripheral distribution of gas and the better the distribution to areas of low V/Q secondary to regional variation in airway resistance.[16] Thus, an end-inspiratory pause or *inflation hold* has its greatest potential in patients with significant airway resistance.[15]

MANIPULATE VENTILATORY PATTERN

Inspiratory to expiratory time relationships (I:E ratios), ventilatory rate, and tidal volume significantly affect respiratory gas exchange.[11, 17] Positive pressure ventilation can completely control or partially modify these factors.

Adjuncts to Positive Pressure Ventilators

Delivery of finite oxygen concentrations and expiratory pressure maneuvers are conveniently and reliably delivered via PPV. However, these entities can be delivered independent of the ventilator and therefore must not be considered as intrinsic capabilities of the machine.

Clinical Indications for Positive Pressure Ventilation

An attempt to categorize indications for PPV by disease entity would result in long and virtually useless lists because each disease would have to be evaluated in relation to that patient's cardiopulmonary reserves. In other words, it is not the disease per se that necessitates the ventilator, but rather the degree to which the disease's physiologic stress impinges upon the cardiopulmonary reserves. In terms of cardiopulmonary pathophysiology, commitment to PPV is indicated in three clinical circumstances: (1) apnea, (2) AVF, and (3) impending AVF.

Apnea

CNS malfunction or depression is the most common cause of apnea in the potentially salvageable patient. CNS depression may be due to primary causes such as drugs, cerebrovascular accidents, and increased intracranial pressure, or it may be secondary to cerebral hypoxia caused by cardiopulmonary deficits. In the absence of complications such as pulmonary aspiration or myocardial insult, PPV restores adequate gas exchange without excessive airway pressures or excessive inspired oxygen concentrations.

Acute Ventilatory Failure (Acute Respiratory Acidosis)

Acute ventilatory failure (AVF) may be arbitrarily defined as an arterial P_{CO_2} above 50 mm Hg coincidental with an arterial pH below 7.30. This diagnosis reflects the fact that the pulmonary system is failing to meet the organism's ventilatory metabolic demands. Although this blood gas diagnosis does not automatically or always lead to PPV, the clinical considerations and evaluation for instituting PPV are mandatory.

The availability of this blood gas measurement has undoubtedly been the single most significant advancement in ventilator management. Since metabolism produces carbon dioxide that must be excreted by alveolar ventilation (not deadspace ventilation), the arterial P_{CO_2} is almost always a reflection of the adequacy of physiologically appropriate pulmonary gas exchange in relation to the metabolic rate. Therefore, inadequate alveolar ventilation is reflected as an increased arterial P_{CO_2} (respiratory acidosis). An *acute* increase in blood P_{CO_2} must be accompanied by a corresponding decrease in pH. This mandatory chemical relationship allows arterial blood gas measurements to be reliably used as major clinical factors in ventilator commitment and management.

Impending Acute Ventilatory Failure

In the absence of AVF, the clinical assessment of (1) the work of breathing, (2) the pathogenesis of the disease process, and (3) the patient's cardiopulmonary reserves can result in the clinical judgment that AVF is inevitable or highly probable. This is often encountered when the work of breathing becomes detrimental to the maintenance of cardiopulmonary homeostasis. This is often referred to as the patient "tiring" or "fatiguing." Not infrequently this clinical impression may be documented by sequential blood gas measurements revealing increasing PCO_2 values and decreasing pH values. However, it is not unusual for patients to manifest increasing cardiopulmonary work while maintaining acceptable blood gas measurements. This increase in cardiopulmonary work is evidenced by increasing respiratory and heart rates, systolic hypertension, diaphoresis, and disorientation.

OXYGENATION AND POSITIVE PRESSURE VENTILATION

Ventilatory inadequacies are usually accompanied by an arterial oxygenation deficit while breathing room air due to the elevated alveolar PCO_2. This oxygenation deficit must be considered a "secondary" factor because restoration of adequate physiologic ventilation reverses the oxygenation deficit. Some patients with impending acute ventilatory failure may show dramatic improvements in oxygenation when PPV is instituted because the decreased energy requirements for breathing have either significantly diminished total oxygen consumption[18] or have improved cardiac function.[10]

Most "primary" arterial oxygenation deficits (hypoxemia coincident with adequate alveolar ventilation) are not significantly improved by the institution of PPV. They are best supported by means of oxygen therapy, cardiovascular therapy, bronchial hygiene therapy, PEEP therapy, or combinations of these techniques. While any or all of these therapies may be administered in *conjunction* with the ventilator, none of them *require* the use of a ventilator.

Venous Return and Positive Pressure Ventilation

Hypotension and arrhythmia following initiation of PPV are often falsely attributed to the stress or pharmacologic agents associated with the process of endotracheal intubation. Such assumptions may lead to inappropriate therapy such as vasopressors.

Hypercarbia, acidemia, and hypoxemia produce high levels of circulating catecholamines resulting in myocardial stimulation and vascular constriction. Initiation of PPV usually reverses hypercarbia and acidemia, relieves the work of breathing, and improves oxygenation—all of which results in decreased sympathetic stimulation. Most critically ill patients are unable to adequately mobilize extravascular fluid into the suddenly expanded vascular (primarily venous) space. The combination of the "relative hypovolemia" and the increased intrathoracic pressure results in diminished venous return and diminished cardiac output. In such circumstances the appropriate primary therapy is adequate fluid administration.

Positive Pressure Inspiration

Positive pressure VT from 10–20 ml/kg delivered within 0.5 to 1.5 sec demonstrates no significant differences in mean inspiratory airway pressures.[19] Thus, positive pressure ventilators can deliver approximately four times the predicted VT without significant increases in the mean inspiratory airway pressure. Such large VT: (1) are advantageous in compensating for the increased deadspace ventilation that accompanies PPV,[11] (2) appear to decrease the incidence of atelectasis when compared with smaller VT,[20] and (3) are usually better tolerated by the conscious patient. A VT of 12–15 ml/kg (approximately 3 times predicted) delivered in one second has become the standard in patients without *chronic* restrictive pathology. Variations depend upon clinical judgment, physiologic monitoring, and personal preference.

FULL VENTILATORY SUPPORT

Control Mode Ventilation

Spontaneous ventilation is defined as the *patient* providing all inspiratory power while determining both frequency and depth of VT. Control mode ventilation (CMV) may be defined as a *positive pressure ventilator* providing all inspiratory power and determining both frequency and depth of VT. The patient takes no physiologically significant role in either the ventilatory cycle or the maintenance of ventilatory homeostasis.

Keeping inspiratory dynamics constant, the slower the ventilator rate the lower the mean airway pressure. Relatively slow rates (<12/min) should have minimal effects on venous return, while relatively large VT (12–15 ml/

kg) minimize deadspace and optimize alveolar ventilation. The relationship of inspiration to expiration (I : E ratio), vt, and the frequency of ventilatory cycles make up the "ventilatory pattern." With the exception of providing all the energy required for ventilation, the success and adequacy of control mode ventilation is primarily due to the total manipulation of the ventilatory pattern.[2, 14, 17, 21]

It is obvious that CMV provides full ventilatory support. However, it may be stated that any circumstance in which the ventilator is providing all the energy required for maintaining CO_2 homeostasis may be considered full ventilatory support.[22]

Eucapneic Ventilation

Acid-base stability should be sought from the moment the patient is placed on the ventilator. *Eucapneic ventilation* encompasses the principle of artificially supporting the arterial PCO_2 in the range normally maintained by the patient so that optimal acid-base and electrolyte balance can be achieved. Since normal kidneys will take 24–36 hours to compensate for a respiratory alkalosis,[23] hyperventilation on the ventilator means that the cardiovascular, hepatorenal, and central nervous systems must function in an alkalemic milieu and its associated electrolyte environment.[24] Among other factors, the respiratory alkalemia is associated with cardiac electrophysiologic instability and altered autonomic receptor response to exogenous drugs. If one persists in hyperventilating patients on PPV, it must be remembered that cerebral vasoconstriction is predictable.[25, 26] Although desirable for limited periods of time in acute head trauma, the resulting decrease in cerebral blood flow is potentially detrimental in critically ill patients without cerebral edema.

"Fighting the Ventilator"

The patient's active attempt to diminish flow while the ventilator is in the inspiratory cycle is referred to as "fighting the ventilator" or being "out of phase." At minimum, this maneuver increases intrathoracic pressure and diminishes effective ventilation. The most common reasons for fighting the ventilator are (1) inadequate ventilation (hypercarbia), (2) acidemia, (3) inadequate oxygenation, (4) CNS malfunction, and (5) pain and anxiety.

Patients will often make ventilatory efforts during the expiratory cycle of the ventilator. This phenomenon has little, if any, detrimental effects in most patients and may actually be physiologically beneficial in some circumstances. In general, the patient who is out of phase during the *inspi-*

ratory cycle must be manipulated to come into phase; whereas, the patient who is out of phase during the *expiratory* cycle most often may be left alone if an IMV circuit is provided.

TECHNIQUES OF FULL VENTILATORY SUPPORT

Control mode ventilation is a technology for providing full support but often requires heavy sedation and paralyzation to keep the patient in phase. Since a positive pressure minute ventilation two to three times greater than predicted values should provide adequate alveolar ventilation in most patients, it is reasonable to assume that ventilator rates greater than 8/min in conjunction with a vt of 12–15 ml/kg should provide full ventilatory support in most instances. Two technologies (assist/control and IMV) are presently available to allow full ventilatory support without the inflexibility of the control mode. (See Fig 2–1.)

Assist/Control Mode

This technology has been available for over 30 years. The ventilator initiates inspiration when the patient creates a sub-baseline pressure in the circuitry. It was observed many years ago that many patients unable to tolerate CMV could readily receive full ventilatory support if allowed to initiate inspiration. A backup control rate of at least 8/min should be set to assure full support if spontaneous ventilation abates.

Intermittent Mandatory Ventilation

Intermittent Mandatory Ventilation (IMV) is the result of technology that allows the patient to breathe spontaneously through the ventilator circuit without increased resistance. At predetermined intervals, a positive pressure vt is provided by the ventilator completely independent of the patient's spontaneous breathing pattern. Most patients requiring full ventilatory support will tolerate the required positive pressure breaths while being allowed to make whatever spontaneous ventilatory efforts they desire.

There is little difference between these technologies when full ventilatory support is being appropriately provided. Thus, most of the "assist/control vs. IMV controversy" is meaningless because they are comparable methods of providing full support, while only the IMV technology allows partial support.[22]

PARTIAL VENTILATORY SUPPORT

Partial ventilatory support occurs when both the patient and the ventilator contribute physiologically significant roles toward maintaining CO_2 homeostasis.[22] With a VT of 12–15 ml/kg, the ventilator rate must be less than 8/min and the patient must be spontaneously breathing.

Theoretic advantages of partial ventilatory support center around the concept that spontaneous ventilation is a physiologic advantage (improved cardiac output and V/Q) compared to PPV. If the patient is capable of providing energy for a significant portion of the required ventilation, it should be advantageous to provide only the remaining portion by artificial means. Additionally, there is ample evidence to support the statement that PEEP is best provided in conjunction with as much spontaneous ventilation as the patient can reasonably provide.[27-29]

There is no direct evidence that spontaneous breathing efforts in conjunction with PPV are detrimental, although some suggest this may be so in the *severe* COPD patient.[30] Present data and the preponderant clinical experience support the thesis that spontaneous ventilation in conjunction with PPV is desirable in most patients. Future alterations to that statement must await future investigation.

IMV

The only technology presently available to accomplish partial ventilatory support is IMV. Intermittent mandatory ventilation has the advantage of providing the same temperature, humidity, and oxygen concentration for all inspired gases while being technically feasible and nearly universally adaptable.

IMV was initially presented in 1973 as a "weaning technique."[31] Although a convenient and workable weaning technique, it has not been demonstrated that IMV significantly reduces weaning time. When IMV is considered as a mode for partial ventilatory support, it appears to provide a marked improvement in supporting respiratory gas exchange.[32-34] The simplicity, flexibility, and reliability of IMV have become a cornerstone of modern respiratory care. It is to date the most dependable means of providing partial ventilatory support.

Synchronized IMV

Synchronized intermittent mandatory ventilation (SIMV) is a technology in which the patient is allowed to breathe on his own (usually through a demand valve ventilator circuit), and at predetermined intervals the next spontaneous breath is assisted by the machine. Various techniques (and varying terminology) have been developed to provide SIMV, for example, intermittent demand ventilation (IDV)[35] and intermittent assisted ventilation (IAV).[36] At present, SIMV has not been documented to be of significant advantage over IMV[37, 38]; in fact, SIMV may have significant technical disadvantages and at best should be considered a sophistication of IMV.

VENTILATOR DISCONTINUANCE

Ventilator discontinuance should commence once the following determinations have been appropriately assessed: (1) the underlying disease process is significantly reversed, (2) mechanical measurements of the cardiopulmonary reserves are adequate to maintain spontaneous ventilation, and (3) general clinical examination and laboratory measurements present no contraindications to maintaining both adequate spontaneous ventilation and cardiopulmonary homeostasis.

Assessment of Cardiopulmonary Reserve

Assessment of cardiopulmonary reserve in a previously normal individual may be accomplished by evaluating some or all of the following: (1) a VC >15 ml/kg is desirable, but >12 ml/kg is acceptable; (2) VT >4 ml/kg are desirable but difficult to evaluate prior to breathing spontaneously for a period (Immediate VT >2 ml/kg are encouraging.); (3) spontaneous ventilatory rates of less than 25/min are encouraging, and faster rates require reevaluation; (4) significant tachycardia on the ventilator is discouraging because the work of breathing will place an additional stress on the heart; (5) hypotension on the ventilator is discouraging, while hypertension must be evaluated carefully; (6) cardiac arrhythmias must be evaluated; (7) hemoglobin content should be at least 10 gm%; (8) arterial blood gas measurements must be acceptable on the ventilator; (9) no evidence of significant acute deadspace ventilation should be present; and (10) intrapulmonary shunt calculations should be <30% and preferably <20%.

Methodology of Discontinuance

Most patients can be given one breath every 30 sec with a hand ventilator (with adequate $F_{I_{O_2}}$). After 10 min they will be spontaneously breathing with stable vital signs and adequate blood gases. Others may require rapid step-down in IMV rates so that spontaneous ventilation is accomplished over several hours. There is nothing magic about the way a ventilator can be manipulated to accomplish discontinuance. Better than 75% of patients can be removed from the ventilator within several hours once the primary indications for PPV have been reversed.

Do not equate ventilator discontinuance with extubation. After the patient has demonstrated the ability to spontaneously ventilate, the airway should be independently evaluated for extubation.

Weaning from the Ventilator

Failure of the patient to maintain an adequate cardiopulmonary status with spontaneous breathing must be carefully evaluated. The mechanical device through which the patient is breathing must be examined, and it must be ascertained that narcotics, sedatives, and muscle relaxants have been completely reversed. When these factors have been ruled out and the physiologic parameters of cardiopulmonary reserve still indicate that the patient should be able to breathe on his own, either the patient is unable to come off the ventilator because the disease is not adequately reversed for his general body reserves or psychologic dependence exists.

Most "weaning problems" are due to either (1) attempting to discontinue ventilation too early in the disease course, (2) improper ventilation maintenance, or (3) preexisting chronic disease that severely limits reserves. In the absence of these, the next most common problem is psychologic dependence.

CASE STUDY 1

A 47-year-old female entered the intensive care unit after evacuation of a right subdural hematoma suffered in a motor vehicle accident. There were no other apparent injuries. An oral endotracheal tube was in place and no spontaneous breathing efforts were present.

The patient was placed on a volume-cycled PPV with an IMV/SIMV capability. A V_T of 1,000 ml (13 ml/kg) was set to be delivered at a rate of 10/min with an F_{IO_2} of 40. The patient had a BP of 140/100 mm Hg, a pulse of 100/min, and an EKG showed sinus tachycardia. Arterial blood gas (ABG) analysis revealed a pH of 7.44, a P_{CO_2} of 32 mm Hg, and a P_{O_2} of 110 mm Hg.

The neurosurgeons requested the P_{CO_2} be maintained at 30–34 mm Hg

because they were concerned about cerebral edema and wanted to be notified of any change in neurologic status.

Two hours later the patient began to make spontaneous breathing efforts at a rate of 30 to 40/min and to "fight" the positive pressure breaths. This resulted in a BP of 190/140 mm Hg and a tachycardia to 130/min. Manually assisted ventilation with a self-inflating ventilator and F_{IO_2} approximately equal to 70% did not alter the spontaneous pattern and resulted in a pH of 7.54, a P_{CO_2} of 26 mm Hg, and a P_{O_2} of 340 mm Hg. Spontaneous V_T varied from 100 to 200 ml with poor breath sounds. After 90 sec of spontaneous breathing, it was clinically obvious she would not maintain adequate ventilation spontaneously.

Discussion

CNS dysfunction is resulting in a ventilatory pattern that is incompatible with spontaneous ventilation. Hyperventilation with hand assist does not alter the breathing pattern which is typical of "central hyperventilation." It can be anticipated that whether assist/control or IMV modes are used, the patient will fight the positive pressure breaths because the respiratory center is not responsive to afferent stimuli. Because the spontaneous respiratory efforts are incompatible with adequate maintenance of pulmonary gas exchange, either paralysis or CNS depression is warranted. It is doubtful whether sedatives or narcotics will alter the respiratory pattern short of levels of general anesthesia, a situation that will render neurologic evaluation impossible.

The best solution to this dilemma is to use a non-depolarizing muscle relaxant (e.g., Pavulon [Pancuronium]) and temporarily reverse the neuromuscular blockade with Tensilon (edrophonium bromide) when neurologic evaluation is required. Ten to twenty milligrams of Tensilon will sufficiently reverse the neuromuscular blockade for 3–5 min during which a neurologic examination may be conducted under acceptable, albeit less than ideal, conditions. Muscurinic (vagal) stimulation is uncommon with Tensilon but may be blocked with atropine sulfate which should be readily available.

This is a situation where full ventilatory support is required but neither assist/control nor IMV are adequate, i.e., CMV is required.

Case Study Continued

Five milligrams of Pavulon were administered and within 3 min the hemodynamics and ventilatory status had stabilized. The patient was appropriately maintained at a ventilator rate of 8/min. Over the next 24 hours the patient required 2 mg of Pavulon on three occasions to maintain CMV.

On two occasions the patient was given 10 mg of Tensilon to allow neurologic assessment by the neurosurgeon. Manually assisted ventilation was administered during these periods and the patient tolerated the transient reversal of muscular blockade without serious sequelae. At the second examination the neurologic status was markedly improved and the spontaneous respiratory pattern was noted to be around 20/min. No further Pavulon was administered and the spontaneous efforts were allowed to return over the next several hours.

Four hours after the last Pavulon dose, the ventilator rate was decreased to 4/min with an IMV circuit. The patient's spontaneous breathing rate was 20–22/min with a VT of 2 ml/kg. The ABGs on 30% oxygen were a pH of 7.49, a PCO_2 of 31 mm Hg, and a PO_2 of 120 mm Hg. The ventilator rate was decreased to 2/min and after one hour the patient was placed on a T-piece after evaluation. Spontaneous ventilation remained adequate. The endotracheal tube remained in place for airway protection and suctioning because the patient was still comatose.

CASE STUDY 2

Following a severe myocardial infarction, a previously healthy 53-year-old man was severely hypotensive and required placement on an aortic counterpulsating balloon pump to restore a borderline acceptable cardiac output (CI = 2.2 L/min). He complained of dyspnea and was found to have a RR of 35/min and a VT of 400 ml (MV = 14 L). ABGs on .50 $F_{I_{O_2}}$ showed a pH of 7.32, a P_{CO_2} of 45 mm Hg, and a P_{O_2} of 52 mm Hg.

After explaining the procedure for nasotracheal intubation to the patient and accomplishing adequate topical anesthesia, an 8 mm nasotracheal tube was placed without incident. Assisted ventilation by manual self-inflating ventilator ($F_{I_{O_2}}$ approximately 0.70) resulted in abatement of the patient's spontaneous breathing efforts.

Discussion

The significant increase in deadspace ventilation (MV = 14 L with an arterial P_{CO_2} of 45 mm Hg) must be attributed primarily to diminished pulmonary perfusion secondary to the low cardiac output.[39] The increased deadspace resulted in an increased ventilatory effort that increased total oxygen consumption. This increased work of breathing was causing the patient considerable discomfort and anxiety. The decision was made to relieve the work of breathing, thus decreasing oxygen consumption and hopefully improving myocardial function.

The awake nasal intubation allowed airway placement without stress or sedation. If the patient were to become uncooperative during the procedure, small increments of IV morphine or valium may prove beneficial. However, at the first sign of stress, the nasal intubation should be abandoned and an oral endotracheal tube established following appropriate sedation and paralysis.

The fact that the patient stopped breathing when PPV was initiated is a good indication that the work of breathing was significant. Full ventilatory support can now be administered by either IMV or assist/control techniques. Any decrease in cardiac output may be due to decreased venous return and should be treated with an appropriate fluid challenge.

Case Study Continued

The patient was placed on assist/control mode of ventilation (8/min), a VT of 14 ml/kg, and an $F_{I_{O_2}}$ of .40 with resultant blood gases of pH 7.38, a P_{CO_2} of 39 mm Hg, and a P_{O_2} of 61 mm Hg.

Cardiac output remained unchanged while the ventricular rate significantly decreased. Urine output remained at 45 ml/hour.

Twelve hours later the patient began

to make spontaneous breathing efforts at a rate of 12/min. ABGs at this point were a pH of 7.42, a P_{CO_2} of 35 mm Hg, and a P_{O_2} of 63 mm Hg. Over the next 6 hours the patient was tapered

off the balloon pump with good cardiovascular dynamics and essentially unchanged blood gases. It was now decided to see if the ventilator could be discontinued.

Discussion

There are at least two reasons why a short transition period of partial ventilatory support would be more desirable than abrupt discontinuance in this patient: (1) reassumption of the work of breathing may significantly increase myocardial demands, and (2) removal of PPV may result in a significant increase in venous return and precipitate ventricular failure. Although assist/control has adequately provided full ventilatory support, the same could have been provided by IMV. The desirability of partial ventilatory support now requires changing from assist/control to IMV. Although this change is seldom troublesome, it is always time-consuming and requires a period of evaluation once the change is made. This is the main reason why IMV techniques are preferable—not because they are better than assist modes for full support, but because they can provide *both* full and partial support.

Case Study Continued

The patient was placed on SIMV at 8/min and hemodynamic studies obtained after 30 min which revealed a MAP of 80 mm Hg, a pulse of 95/min, a spontaneous RR of 16/min (V_T 75 ml), a PPV of 8/min (V_T 900 ml), a cardiac output of 3.7 L/min (CI 2.4 L/min), a PAOP of 17 mm Hg, a pH of 7.42, a P_{CO_2} of 37 mm Hg, and a P_{O_2} of 64 mm Hg ($F_{I_{O_2}}$ 40%).

After explaining the procedure to the patient, the SIMV rate was decreased to 6/min without distress to the patient. Fifteen minutes later the patient had a MAP of 80 mm Hg, a pulse of 95/min, a spontaneous RR of 12/min (V_T 200 ml),

PPV of 6/min (V_T 900 ml), a cardiac output of 3.7 L/min (CI 2.4 L/min), a PAOP of 17 mm Hg, a pH of 7.43, a P_{CO_2} of 36 mm Hg, and a P_{O_2} of 61 mm Hg ($F_{I_{O_2}}$ 40%).

When the SIMV rate was decreased to 4/min, the patient indicated he was aware of the need to breathe on his own and was reassured. Cardiopulmonary assessment revealed a MAP of 90 mm Hg, a pulse of 102/min, a spontaneous RR of 12/min (V_T 400 ml), a PPV of 4/min (V_T 900 ml), a cardiac output of 4.4 L/min (CI 2.6 L/min), a PAOP of 14 mm Hg, a pH of 7.39, a P_{CO_2} of 39 mm Hg, and a P_{O_2} of 56 mm Hg ($F_{I_{O_2}}$ 40%).

Discussion

Reassumption of a portion of the work of breathing results in increased myocardial work. The drop in PAOP may be due solely to a diminished mean intrathoracic pressure. However, it is prudent to remain on partial ventilatory support for a period.

Case Study Continued

The patient continued to improve and 12 hours later was removed from partial ventilatory support. He was subsequently extubated after remaining in stable condition breathing spontaneously via the endotracheal tube for another 3 hours.

REFERENCES

1. Roussos C., Macklem P.T.: Respiratory Muscles: The vital pump. *N. Engl. J. Med.* 78:753–758, 1980.
2. Emerson H.: Artificial respiration in the treatment of edema of the lungs: A suggestion based on animal experimentation. *Arch. Intern. Med.* 3:368–371, 1909.
3. Johansen S.H., Osgood P.: Ventilatory reserve in the dog during partial curarization. *Anesthesiology* 33:322–327, 1970.
4. Wilson R.H., Ebert R.V., Borden C.W., et al.: The determinations of blood flow through non-ventilated portions of the normal and diseased lung. *Am. Rev. Tuberc.* 68:177–187, 1953.
5. Caro C., Butler J., DeBois A.B.: Some effects of restriction of chest cage expansion on pulmonary function in man: An experimental study. *J. Clin. Invest.* 39:573–578, 1960.
6. Shapiro B.A., Cane R.D.: Metabolic malfunction of lung: Noncardiogenic edema and adult respiratory distress syndrome. *Surg. Ann.* 13:271–298, 1981.
7. Waters R.M.: Simple methods for performing artificial respiration. *J.A.M.A.* 123:559–561, 1943.
8. Drinker P., Shaw L.A.: An apparatus for the prolonged administration of artificial respiration. I. A design for adults and children. *J. Clin. Invest.* 7:229–247, 1929.
9. Lassen H.C.: A preliminary report on the 1952 epidemic of poliomyelitis in Copenhagen with special reference to the treatment of acute respiratory insufficiency. *Lancet* 1:37–41, 1953.
10. Werko L.: The influence of positive-pressure breathing on the circulation in man. *Acta. Med. Scand.* (Suppl.) 193:1–125, 1947.
11. Motley H.L., Werko L., Cournand A., et al.: Observations on the clinical use of positive pressure. *J. Aviat. Med.* 18:417–435, 482, 1947.
12. Froese A.B., Bryan A.C.: Effects of anesthesia and paralysis on diaphragmatic mechanics in man. *Anesthesiology* 41:242–255, 1974.
13. Lyager S.: Ventilation/perfusion ratio during intermittent positive pressure ventilation: Importance of no-flow interval during the insufflation. *Acta Anesthesiol. Scand.* 14:211–232, 1970.
14. Jansson L., Jonson B.: A theoretical study on flow patterns of ventilators. *Scand. J. Respir. Dis.* 53:237–244, 1972.
15. Dammann J.F., McAslan T.C., Maffeo C.T.: Optimal flow pattern for mechanical ventilation of the lungs. I. The effect of a sine versus square wave flow pattern with and without an end-inspiratory pause on patients. *Crit. Care Med.* 6:293–310, 1978.
16. Dammann J.F., McAslan T.C.: Optimal flow pattern for mechanical ventilation of the lungs: Evaluation with a lung model. *Crit. Care Med.* 5:128–136, 1977.
17. Knelson J.H., Howatt W.F., DeMuth G.R.: Effect of respiratory pattern on alveolar gas exchange. *J. Appl. Physiol.* 29:328–331, 1970.
18. Henning R.J., Shubin H., Weil M.H.: The measurement of the work of breathing for the clinical assessment of ventilator dependence. *Crit. Care Med.* 5:264–268, 1977.
19. Bergman N.A.: Effects of varying respiratory waveforms on gas exchange. *Anesthesiology* 28:390–395, 1967.

20. Latimer R.G., Dickman M., Day W.C., et al.: Ventilatory patterns and pulmonary complications after upper abdominal surgery determined by preoperative and postoperative computerized spirometry and blood gas analysis. *Am. J. Surg.* 122:622–632, 1971.
21. Lyager S.: Influence of flow pattern on the distribution of respiratory air during intermittent positive pressure ventilation. *Acta Anesthesiol. Scand.* 12:191–211, 1968.
22. Shapiro B.A., Cane R.D.: AMV-IMV controversy: A plea for classification and redirection. *Crit. Care Med.* (editorial) 12:472–473, 1984.
23. Levinsky N.G.: Acidosis and alkalosis, in Thorne G.W., Adams R.D., Braunwald E., et al. (eds.): *Harrison's Principles of Internal Medicine*, ed. 8. New York, McGraw-Hill Book Co., 1977, pp. 375–382.
24. Giebisch G., Berger L., Pitts, R.F., et al.: The extrarenal response to acute acid-base disturbances of respiratory origin. *J. Clin. Invest.* 34:231–245, 1955.
25. Phelps M.E., Grubb R.L., Jr., Ter-Pogossian M.M.: Correlation between $Paco_2$ and regional cerebral blood volume by x-ray fluorescence. *J. Appl. Physiol.* 35:274–280, 1973.
26. Wollman H., Smith T.C., Stephen G.W., et al.: Effects of extremes of respiratory and metabolic alkalosis on cerebral blood flow in man. *J. Appl. Physiol.* 24:60–65, 1968.
27. Shad D.M., Newell J.C., Dutton R.E., et al.: Continuous positive airway pressure versus positive end expiratory pressure in respiratory distress syndrome. *J. Thorac. Cardiovasc. Surg.* 74:557, 1977.
28. Downs J.B., Douglas M.E., Sanfelippo P.M., et al.: Ventilatory pattern, intrapleural pressure and cardiac output. *Anesth. Analg.* 56:88, 1977.
29. Venus B., Jacobs H.K., Mathru M.: Hemodynamic responses to different modes of mechanical ventilation in dogs with normal and acid aspirated lungs. *Crit. Care Med.* 8:620, 1980.
30. Roussos C., Fitley M., Gross D., et al.: Fatigue of inspiratory muscles and their synergistic behavior. *J. Appl. Physiol.* 46:897, 1979.
31. Downs J.G., Klein E.F., Jr., Desutels D., et al.: Intermittent mandatory ventilation: A new approach to weaning patients from mechanical ventilators. *Chest* 64:331–335, 1973.
32. Downs J.B., Perkins H.M., Modell J.H.: Intermittent mandatory ventilation: An evaluation. *Arch. Surg.* 109:519–523, 1974.
33. Civetta J.M.: Intermittent mandatory ventilation and positive end-expiratory pressure in acute ventilatory insufficiency. *Int. Anesthesiol. Clin.* 18(2):123–142, 1980.
34. Fairley H.B.: Critique of intermittent mandatory ventilation. *Int. Anesthesiol. Clin.* 18(2):179–189, 1980.
35. Shapiro B.A., Harrison R.A., Walton J.R.: Intermittent demand ventilation (IDV): A new technique for supporting ventilation in critically ill patients. *Resp. Care* 21:521–525, 1976.
36. Harboe S.: Weaning from mechanical ventilation by means of intermittent assisted ventilation (IAV): Case reports. *Acta Anesthesiol. Scand.* 21:252–256, 1977.
37. Heehan T.J., Downs J.B., Douglas M.E., et al.: Intermittent mandatory ventilation: Is synchronization important? *Chest* 77:598–602, 1980.
38. Hasten R.W., Downs J.B., Heenan T.J.: A comparison of synchronized and non-synchronized intermittent mandatory ventilation. *Resp. Care* 25:554–557, 1980.
39. Shapiro B.A., Harrison R.A., Walton J.R.: *Clinical Application of Blood Gases*, ed. 3. Chicago, Year Book Medical Publishers, 1982.

3 / Arrhythmias and Cardiac Failure

RICHARD DAVISON, M.D.
KERRY KAPLAN, M.D.

ARRHYTHMIAS AND CONGESTIVE HEART FAILURE

Continuous monitoring of the heart rhythm is inseparably intertwined with the concept of critical care medicine. Any time that there is cardiac pathology, arrhythmias will occur and will need to be identified and dealt with. Furthermore, cardiac arrhythmias are to be anticipated whenever any of the following circumstances are present: (1) dysfunction of the central and/or autonomic nervous system, (2) organ failure resulting in significant alteration of the metabolic and/or electrolytic internal milieu, (3) use of a variety of vaso-active or membrane-active drugs, and (4) placement of indwelling, intracardiac devices. Of course, the majority of seriously ill patients will exhibit several of the above conditions and therefore be prone to arrhythmias.

But the detection of a disturbance in cardiac rhythm should not reflexly lead to an attempt at its correction. There are three aspects of the management of arrhythmias in an intensive care unit setting to be considered. First, when should attempts be made to terminate an ongoing arrhythmia? With the obvious exceptions of ventricular asystole or fibrillation, the treatment—or nontreatment—of an arrhythmia will be dictated primarily by the impact that the rhythm disturbance has on the patient's physiology. More harm may be done by the pharmacologic interventions than by the arrhythmia they are directed at.[1]

A second issue that is frequently neglected in the haste to initiate antiarrhythmic therapy is the possibility that the arrhythmia may not be an expression of primary cardiac pathology but rather secondary to "extra cardiac" factors. Some of the more commonly encountered circumstances are hypokalemia producing ventricular ectopy; sinus bradycardia as an expression of severe hypoxemia; congestive heart failure (CHF) presenting as atrial tachyarrhythmias; and the wide spectrum of drug-induced arrhythmias.

The third question is not as easily settled. When is an arrhythmia a harbinger of more serious events and therefore an indication for the initiation of suppressive therapy? Unfortunately there are no hard and fast rules. In general the propensity for a rhythm disturbance to develop into a life-threatening arrhythmia is directly proportional to the magnitude of the underlying cardiac pathology. It is very difficult to induce ventricular fibrillation in a normal heart.[2] Another important consideration is the trend displayed by the arrhythmia. Corrective measures should be more promptly initiated to treat a rapidly worsening disturbance than for what may be a more alarming but stable rhythm. For example, ventricular premature beats that progress from rare and isolated to frequent and in couplets may require earlier and more aggressive treatment than ventricular triplets that have not changed in frequency over several days.

Once therapy is started, what should its aim be? Total suppression, or is "better" good enough? If total eradication of the rhythm disturbance can be accomplished without inordinate side effects, then that should be the goal. It is often wiser to settle for partial improvement. There is good evidence that the administration of antiarrhythmic drugs in doses that only *reduce* ectopic activity still lessen the chance of a lethal tachyarrhythmia.[3]

Congestive heart failure is the consequence of a persistent impairment in left ventricular function, with or without associated right ventricular involvement. In order to be clinically evident, it must be of sufficient severity to activate compensatory mechanisms that in turn are responsible for the majority of symptoms. It is a condition that, because of its chronic, slowly progressive course and the predictability of manifestations, should rarely be the primary reason for admission to an intensive care unit. Yet, because of the high incidence of hypertensive and ischemic heart disease, CHF very commonly complicates the care of the critically ill patient. Furthermore, the previously stable clinical status of a patient with CHF may take a sudden and dramatic turn for the worse with the development of complications such as arrhythmias, pulmonary embolism, and transient myocardial ischemia. These are basically reversible events that usually respond well to advanced supportive measures.

The same rationale should not be applied to patients with end-stage CHF where the introduction of intensive care techniques results in an ephemeral improvement that only lasts for as long as the measures are continued. As with other chronic organ failures, the final phase of CHF is due to an irreversible loss of function, a problem that is not appropriately dealt with in an intensive care unit setting.

CASE STUDY

A 58-year-old white male is brought to the emergency room with a 3-hour history of rapidly progressive shortness of breath. Prior to the onset of the respiratory distress, he had noted a "fast heartbeat" for several hours. The patient gave a history of "heart failure" for the past 10 years for which he was receiving a "digitalis" pill and a diuretic. On admission to the emergency room, the patient was sitting up in marked respiratory distress. The skin was cool, pale, and sweaty. His respiratory rate was 40/min, respirations were labored with prominent wheezing and "gurgling" noises; pulse rate was 160/min and regular, and BP by cuff measured 120/90 mm Hg. Neck veins were distended to the angle of the jaw and had prominent pulsations. Fine and coarse moist rales and wheezes were heard throughout both lungs. A sustained apical impulse was visible and palpable over the fifth and sixth intercostal spaces, 13 cm lateral to the midsternal line. On auscultation, heart tones were distant and difficult to identify but a gallop rhythm was clearly present. Examination of the abdomen revealed an enlarged liver (spanning 13 cm) that was tender to palpation. Peripheral pulses were thready but symmetrical. There was 2+ pitting edema of both ankles.

Arterial blood gases (room air) showed a P_{O_2} of 42 mm Hg, a P_{CO_2} of 45 mm Hg, and a pH of 7.12. Routine chemistries were normal except for mildly elevated BUN, SGOT, and LDH. The chest x-ray revealed bilateral alveolar infiltrates and pulmonary venous redistribution and congestion, compatible with pulmonary edema. There was marked cardiomegaly. The ECG is shown in Figure 3–1.

Oxygen was given by ventimask at an $F_{I_{O_2}}$ of 0.4, and the patient received 40 mg of furosemide and 4 mg of morphine sulphate intravenously. His respiratory distress lessened and repeat blood gases were improved. The ECG was read as showing ventricular tachycardia. A bolus of 100 mg of IV lidocaine was given but the bedside monitor showed persistence of the abnormal cardiac rhythm. Because of the lack of response to lidocaine, the original interpretation was questioned and a supraventricular tachycardia with aberrant intraventricular conduction postulated. Five milligrams of IV verapamil were given. The arrhythmia persisted but the BP declined to 90/65 mm Hg. The patient was transferred to the intensive care unit.

Discussion

The patient presents to the emergency room with what appears to be an acute decompensation of chronic CHF precipitated by a tachyarrhythmia. Although the patient is in florid pulmonary edema, arterial BP and cerebral perfusion are adequate. Had either of them been seriously impaired, proper management would have required immediate electrical cardioversion. Therapy is initiated, including the administration of morphine sulphate, which is *not* contraindicated when CO_2 retention and respiratory acidosis are directly attributable to cardiac pulmonary edema.[4]

The ECG poses a dilemma that one faces often in acute cardiac crisis: the differential diagnosis of "wide-QRS" tachycardia. Wellens, Bar, and Lie[5] have identified those findings that suggest a ventricular origin for

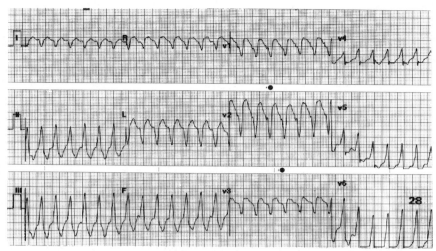

Fig 3–1.—"Wide-QRS" tachycardia: ventricular versus supraventricular with aberrancy.

these tachyarrhythmias. They are summarized in Table 3–1. The ECG reproduced in Figure 3–1 does not fit several of the criteria listed, yet a ventricular origin for the tachycardia—later confirmed by electrophysiological testing—is strongly suggested by the very wide and bizarre QRS.

Lidocaine (Xylocaine) has few deleterious effects on the cardiovascular system and, therefore, is a wise choice as the initial agent for a therapeutic trial in a suspected ventricular arrhythmia. Unfortunately, in the case under discussion effective blood levels were probably never achieved because of an inadequate loading dose. A total of 3–4 mg/kg of lidocaine, given in divided doses over 10 min, will usually result in therapeutic blood levels and is associated with a very low incidence of toxicity. After the loading dose, a maintenance infusion must be initiated at a dose as outlined in Table 3–2. Even with a continuous infusion of lidocaine, blood levels will initially decline due to redistribution of the drug. When this occurs, it is

TABLE 3–1.—FINDINGS SUGGESTIVE
OF VENTRICULAR TACHYCARDIA

Heart rate 130–170
Atrioventricular dissociation
QRS width >0.14 seconds
Left axis deviation
If RBBB: Mono- or biphasic complexes in V_1
If LBBB: qR or QS complexes in V_6

TABLE 3–2.—INTRAVENOUS ANTIARRHYTHMICS

DRUG	LOADING DOSE	MAINTENANCE DOSE	MAIN TOXICITY
Lidocaine	3–4 mg/kg	Normal: up to 55 µg/kg/min CHF:† up to 25 µg/kg/min Shock: up to 10 µg/kg/min	Dizziness Dysarthria Obtundation and/or Agitation
Procainamide	Up to 15 mg/kg (100 mg q. 5 min)	30–60 µg/kg/min	Hypotension, IVCD*
Bretylium tosylate	5–30 mg/kg	1–2 mg/min	Postural hypotension, emesi

*IVCD: intraventricular conduction disturbances
†CHF: congestive heart failure

common to see a recrudescence of the original arrhythmia, and one or more small boluses (12.5–25.0 mg) will be required to restore suppressive levels.[6]

In the event that lidocaine fails to control the ventricular arrhythmia, the next parenteral drug of choice is procainamide (Pronestyl). Intravenous loading with this agent is achieved by giving a 100 mg bolus (injected over 2 min) every 5 min until either the arrhythmia is suppressed, a total of up to 15 mg/kg is given or a side effect supervenes.[7] Close attention must be given to the development of hypotension and/or widening of the QRS. An increase in the duration of the QRS of more than one third over control values should be construed as a warning that toxic blood levels are being reached. Maintenance infusion rates will vary between 30 and 60 µg/kg/min and may initially require supplementation with small 50 mg boluses.

Bretylium tosylate (Bretylol), originally marketed for the treatment of ventricular fibrillation, is now considered a second-line drug for the treatment of other ventricular arrhythmias. The initial dose is 5 mg/kg given as an IV bolus that may be injected rapidly if the patient is unresponsive. In the alert patient, unless it is given slowly, vomiting will promptly follow. Up to 30 mg/kg can be administered as a loading dose and followed with a maintenance infusion of 1–2 mg/min. The only common side effect is postural hypotension. It is important to know that the antiarrhythmic effect of bretylium may be delayed for 30–120 min.[8]

Following an apparent lidocaine failure, the alternate diagnosis of supraventricular tachycardia with aberrant intraventricular conduction was entertained and a therapeutic trial attempted with verapamil.[9] This substance, a calcium antagonist, has depressant effects on the atrioventricular and sinoatrial nodes, is a powerful arterial vasodilator, and exerts a considerable anti-inotropic effect. In a dose of 0.15 mg/kg, divided into 2 IV boluses as needed, it is currently the agent of choice for the abolition of paroxysmal supraventricular tachycardia. Verapamil is also very effective when a prompt reduction of the ventricular response to atrial fibrillation or flutter is desired, although it will not commonly terminate these rhythms. On the other hand, our example illustrates a use of verapamil that is *not recommended*. In the setting of a patient that is hemodynamically impaired by an ill-defined tachyarrhythmia, the administration of verapamil—which has little effect on ventricular arrhythmias—may result in further cardiovascular deterioration. In comparison to other available antiarrhythmics, verapamil has myocardial and vascular depressant actions that are much too potent to allow its use as a safe "diagnostic" tool.

Case Study Continued

On arrival in the intensive care unit, the patient received another 150 mg of IV lidocaine in divided doses and reverted to a sinus tachycardia at a rate of 130. On auscultation moist rales were present over most of both lung fields, and a loud holosystolic murmur was heard at the apex with radiation to the axilla. The foley catheter had yielded 30 cc of urine over the last hour. Repeat blood gases demonstrated a Po_2 of 58 mm Hg, a Pco_2 of 38 mm Hg, and a pH of 7.30 on a Fi_{O_2} of 0.4. A repeat ECG showed non-specific repolarization abnormalities suggestive of digitalis effect and was compatible with left ventricular hypertrophy and left atrial disease. There were no changes suggestive of acute myocardial ischemia.

Eighty milligrams of furosemide were given IV. Shortly thereafter the monitor indicated the development of atrial fibrillation with a ventricular response of 145 beats/min and frequent "aberrantly conducted" beats (Fig 3–2). With this there was little change in the clinical status. Blood pressure was 110/85 mm Hg. Two doses of 0.125 mg of IV digoxin were given over the next 3 hours and the ventricular response slowed to 110–120/min. During this time, the urine output that had briefly risen to 120 cc/hour in response to the diuretic had again declined to 20–30 cc/hour. Furosemide was again administered, 120 mg by IV push. Within the next 15 min the pulse rate was noted to again rise to 140/min, the RR increased, and the patient was observed to become more agitated and diaphoretic. Blood pressure was recorded at 90 mm Hg systolic by palpation, and preparations for the insertion of a pulmonary artery catheter were begun.

Discussion

The onset of atrial fibrillation poses several questions. First, could it be a manifestation of digitalis toxicity? Atrial fibrillation develops as a consequence of excess digitalis only exceptionally, and when it does the ventricular response is *always slow* because of the associated atrioventricular block. In this instance, the atrial fibrillation is more likely related to dilatation of the atria secondary to the high filling pressures required by the failing ventricles.

The second question is, should synchronized electrical cardioversion be used to terminate the atrial fibrillation? Although electrical cardioversion

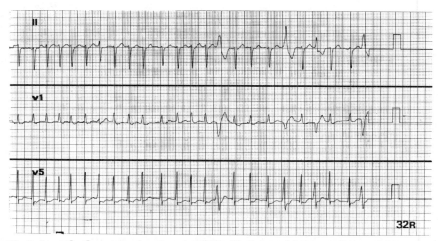

Fig 3–2.—*Rhythm strip showing atrial fibrillation and frequent beats with a bizarre configuration. Intraventricular aberrant conduction (Aschman's) rather than ventricular premature beats is suggested by (1) the degree of aberrancy that is cycle dependent (i.e., it is greater with a long-short RR pattern); (2) lack of fixed coupling intervals; and (3) variable morphology.*

can be performed safely in patients with no clinical evidence of digitalis toxicity,[10] the risk of inducing malignant ventricular arrhythmias may be heightened by concurrent hypoxemia and acidemia. But even more important, it serves no useful purpose to abolish a tachyarrhythmia unless the underlying precipitating factor(s) are also eliminated or at least modified. In the case under discussion, had cardioversion succeeded in restoring a sinus mechanism, it is highly probable that atrial fibrillation would have recurred promptly.

The final query is, how to reduce the ventricular response to atrial fibrillation in a patient that is already "digitalized." Atrial fibrillation provides us with a unique end point to assess the degree of "digitalization": the ventricular response. Digitalis should be "pushed" gently in order to minimize the risk of toxicity. This is done by giving several small doses frequently since the effect of IV digoxin peaks at 2–4 hours. If the higher levels of digitalis are not well tolerated, the addition of small doses of a β-blocker (i.e., propranolol, 5 mg p.o. 3 or 4 times a day) or of verapamil[11] may result in adequate slowing. Obviously these drugs are best avoided in patients with severe cardiovascular impairment, such as the case in discussion.

One of the harder decisions that frequently comes up in acute cardiac care is whether wide and bizarre QRS complexes detected during atrial fibrillation are ventricular premature beats or aberrantly conducted impulses, the so-called Aschman phenomenon. This dilemma is compounded by the fact that extra digitalis doses are usually being considered in an effort to slow the heart rate. Our first recommendation is that a 12 lead ECG be obtained before rendering an opinion. Monitor strips are good to document arrhythmias but not to diagnose them. Table 3–3 lists the criteria most commonly used in this differential diagnosis.

TABLE 3–3.—DIFFERENTIAL BETWEEN VPB AND ABERRANCY

CRITERION	VPB	ABERRANCY
Initial QRS deflection	Opposite to normal beat	Same as normal beat
Configuration in V_1	Atypical RBBB (R or RS), or LBBB	Typical RBBB (RSR')
Fixed coupling	Diagnostic if present	Never present
"Long-short" pattern*	Not present	Present
Fusion beats	Diagnostic if present	Never present

*Long-short pattern refers to the tendency for the QRS that closes a short R-R interval after a long R-R interval to be aberrantly conducted. Figure 3–2 is a good example of this phenomenon.

Case Study Continued

A Swan-Ganz catheter was placed and the initial hemodynamic information obtained is listed in Table 3–4 (column titled "Baseline"). The twice normal A/V O_2 difference reflects a marked desaturation of the central venous blood and confirms the accuracy of the measurement of a very low CI. Because the patient had received agents that dilate the veins (morphine and furosemide) as well as the arteries (verapamil), it was reasonable to assume that relative hypovolemia may have occurred. The filling pressures were indeed considerably lower than expected for an individual with long-standing CHF. Therefore, volume expansion with normal saline was initiated and 1,200 cc given over the next hour. This was attended by an improvement in the clinical status with slowing of the heart rate and decreased agitation and respiratory distress. A re-peat set of hemodynamic parameters (Table 3–4, "After Volume Loading") demonstrated improvement but the urine output remained depressed. Sodium nitroprusside was started at an initial dose of 0.25 μg/kg/min. After 30 min, there was no significant change in the vital signs and the dose was doubled. In the next hour, the urine output increased to 100 cc and the final set of hemodynamic data were obtained (Table 3–4, "On Nitroprusside"). The patient's clinical status continued to improve over the next 24 hours. Oral hydralazine was started and the sodium nitroprusside gradually tapered and stopped. The lidocaine was discontinued after several doses of oral procainamide and good control of the ectopic activity was maintained. The patient was ambulated under monitored surveillance and sent home in good condition.

TABLE 3–4.—HEMODYNAMIC DATA*

	BASELINE	AFTER VOLUME LOADING	ON NITROPRUSSIDE
Mean right atrial pressure	10	13	8
Pulmonary artery pressures	50/16	65/22	45/14
Mean pulmonary artery pressure	27	36	24
Mean pulmonary artery occluded pressure	15	22	13
Mean arterial pressure	80	92	86
A/V O$_2$ diff. (vol %)	10.5	8.0	5.8
Cardiac output (1/min)	2.2	3.2	5.8
Cardiac index (1/min/m^2)	1.3	1.9	2.8

*All pressures are expressed in mm Hg.
A/V O$_2$ diff = arteriovenous oxygen content difference.

Discussion

If in the course of treating CHF the administration of IV furosemide is followed shortly by signs of deteriorating tissue perfusion, then it is very likely that the venodilating action of this drug has caused a critical reduction in the venous return to the heart.[12] The ensuing fall in preload adversely affects SV and leads to reflex peripheral arterial constriction. As in the case under discussion, if measurements of the pulmonary artery occluded pressure are taken at this time, they are often found to be within the normal range. This finding in a chronically failing ventricle is evidence of relative hypovolemia. One is then placed in the apparently paradoxical situation of ordering volume expansion in a patient that up to that point was being vigorously treated for pulmonary edema and who, in fact, may still demonstrate moist rales on auscultation. This scenario results from a return of the ventricular function to baseline after the insult that precipitated pulmonary edema is overcome. A hypertrophied and dilated ventricle may then find that the same measures used to moderate the filling pressures at a time when they were acutely elevated are now responsible for suboptimal diastolic volumes.

The coexistence of physical findings compatible with pulmonary venous hypertension with measurements that are within the normal range is simply due to the normal delay in the clearing of excessive interstitial fluid by the lymphatics of the lungs. Exemplified here is a circumstance where the clinical assessment of the patient's cardiovascular status has been obscured by therapeutic interventions, making the placement of a pulmonary artery catheter virtually mandatory.

As expected, improvement was brought on by the higher filling pressures achieved with fluid administration. However, further volume expansion was precluded by the risk of making pulmonary congestion worse. At this point, additional circulatory support could be achieved in one of three ways: intra-aortic balloon counterpulsation, IV catecholamines, or afterload reduction (AR). The primary indication for intra-aortic counterpulsation is an acute cardiovascular decompensation that is potentially amenable to surgical correction or amelioration. This is certainly not true in the case at hand. Catecholamines are a valid option, but a word of caution is timely. Short of a rare instance of response to oral ephedrine sulfate,[13] there is currently no evidence that a positive inotropic effect with catecholamines can be provided *other than parenterally.* A patient who responds well to an IV agent may not always be successfully "weaned" from it, which may result in one being caught in the quandary of chronic support of the circulation with an IV preparation. For these reasons and others, we favor an initial trial with AR. The purpose of this intervention is to reduce the peripheral arterial resistance with a vasodilator, enhance left ventricular emptying, and increase cardiac output. For many years it was feared that hypotension would be a limiting factor. However, when AR is successful, the drop in resistance is associated with a compensatory increase in flow and BP changes little.[14] In short, AR attempts to transform a high-resistance, low-flow system into a low-resistance, high-flow system. The patient under discussion had evidence of a condition that makes AR an especially attractive alternative: mitral incompetence.[16] Reduction of the resistance in the outflow tract of the left ventricle will "redirect" flow and reduce the fraction of cardiac output that is regurgitated into the left atrium through the incompetent valve. For similar reasons, AR is also of special benefit in aortic valvular insufficiency and acute ventricular septal defects.

Therefore, AR should be entertained whenever low cardiac output is associated with any of the following: (1) cardiomegaly; (2) mitral regurgitation, (3) aortic insufficiency; (4) acute ventricular septal defects. As a general rule, the higher the calculated systemic vascular resistance, the better the results.* However, because there is considerable overlap between responders and non-responders, only a therapeutic trial provides the answer in an individual case.

Sodium nitroprusside (SN) is the drug most often used for AR.[16] It offers the following advantages: (1) it has a very brief duration of action which permits flexible titration; (2) it dilates both arteries and veins (a "balanced" vasodilator) thus reducing both afterload and preload; and (3) it has no effects other than those resulting from the vasodilation. Because it influences preload, the adequacy of filling pressures must be ascertained before it is administered for AR. The same limitation does not exist when SN is used

---

*Systemic vascular resistance = (mean arterial pressure − mean right atrial pressure/ cardiac output) × 80. Normal values 1,200 +/− 180 dynes/sec/cm^{-5}.

in the management of hypertensive emergencies where BP is the main parameter monitored. Toxicity from SN is only observed in two circumstances: (1) when very large doses are given over a short period of time (such as with controlled hypotension techniques), the ability of the liver to detoxify cyanide into thiocyanate may be exceeded and poisoning of the cellular respiratory enzymes occur; and (2) prolonged infusion in patients with severely limited renal function may lead to thiocyanate accumulation. The manifestations of thiocyanate intoxication are nausea, vomiting, psychosis, and convulsions; they are usually seen with serum levels of 10 μg percent or more.

Nitroprusside is a very powerful drug that requires careful titration. The recommended starting dose for AR (0.25 μg/kg/min) is lower than that used in the treatment of hypertension. It should be escalated cautiously by increments of 50% until a change is noted in the circulatory parameters. These changes include a lowering of the pulmonary artery occluded or mean arterial pressures, a mild increase in the heart rate, or signs of clinical improvement such as an increase in the urine output. At that point, measurements of cardiac output and arterial and venous oxygen content should be done to document the beneficial effects. A successful application of AR should lead to (1) clinical improvement, (2) an increase in cardiac output, (3) only minor changes in mean arterial pressure and heart rate, and (4) a lowering of the pulmonary artery occluded pressure. Occasionally a disproportionate fall in pulmonary artery occluded pressure prevents infusion rates from becoming effective enough to reduce afterload. In this setting, volume expansion will restore the filling pressures and permit further increases in the SN infusion.[17] In patients with pulmonary pathology and significant ventilation/perfusion imbalance, SN may cause a worsening of intrapulmonary shunting. It does so by dilating pulmonary vessels and increasing perfusion to poorly ventilated areas.

As a safety measure it is wise to infuse the SN through a separate IV line that is not used for the administration of other intravenous medication. A bolus injection of another drug, given through tubing that is filled with an SN solution, can deliver enough of this agent to produce catastrophic hypotension.

Intravenous nitroglycerin is now available as an alternative to SN, although its main action is exerted on the venous side of the circulation. Finally, there are several agents that permit an easy transition from parenteral to oral AR. Hydralazine is the most recommended agent, but prazosin and more recently captopril have also proved effective.[18, 19]

REFERENCES

1. Smith W.M., Gallagher J.J.: "Les Torsades de Pointes": An unusual ventricular arrhythmia. Ann. Intern. Med. 93:578–584, 1980.

2. Josephson M.E., Seides S.F.: *Clinical Cardiac Electrophysiology.* Philadelphia, Lea & Febiger, 1979, p. 56.
3. Winkle R.A., Alderman E.L., Fitzgerald J.W., et al.: Treatment of recurrent symptomatic ventricular tachycardia. *Ann. Intern. Med.* 85:1–7, 1976.
4. Aberman A., Fulop M.: The metabolic and respiratory acidosis of acute pulmonary edema. *Ann. Intern. Med.* 76:173–184, 1972.
5. Wellens H.J.J., Bar F.W.H.M., Lie K.I.: The value of the electrocardiogram in the differential diagnosis of a tachycardia with a widened QRS complex. *Am. J. Med.* 64:27–33, 1978.
6. Collinsworth K.A., Kalman S., Harrison D.C.: The clinical pharmacology of lidocaine as an antiarrhythmic drug. *Circulation* 50:1217–1230, 1974.
7. Giardina E.G.V., Heissenbuttel R.H., Bigger J.T., Jr.: Intermittent intravenous procaine amide to treat ventricular arrhythmias. Correlation of plasma concentration with effect on arrhythmia, electrocardiogram and blood pressure. *Ann. Intern. Med.* 78:183–193, 1973.
8. Heissenbuttel R.H., Bigger J.T., Jr.: Bretylium tosylate: A newly available antiarrhythmic drug for ventricular arrhythmias. *Ann. Intern. Med.* 91:229–238, 1979.
9. Stone P.H., Antman E.M., Muller J.E., et al.: Calcium channel blocking agents in the treatment of cardiovascular disorders. Part II. Hemodynamic effects and clinical applications. *Ann. Intern. Med.* 93:886–904, 1980.
10. Ditchey R.V., Karliner J.S.: Safety of electrical cardioversion in patients without digitalis toxicity. *Ann. Intern. Med.* 95:676–679, 1981.
11. Klein H.O., Kaplinsky E.: Verapamil and digoxin: Their respective effects on atrial fibrillation and their interaction. *Am. J. Cardiol.* 50:894–902, 1982.
12. Kiely J., Kelly D.T., Taylor D.R., et al.: The role of furosemide in the treatment of left ventricular dysfunction associated with acute myocardial infarction. *Circulation* 58:581–587, 1973.
13. Franciosa J.A., Cohn J.N.: Hemodynamic effects of oral ephedrine given alone or combined with nitroprusside infusion in patients with severe left ventricular failure. *Am. J. Cardiol.* 43:79–85, 1979.
14. Miller R.R., Vismara L.A., Williams D.O., et al.: Pharmacological mechanisms for left ventricular unloading in clinical congestive heart failure. Differential effects of nitroprusside, phentolamine, and nitroglycerin on cardiac function and peripheral circulation. *Circ. Res.* 39:127–133, 1976.
15. Goodman D.J., Rossen R.M., Holloway E.L., et al.: Effect of nitroprusside on left ventricular dynamics in mitral regurgitation. *Circulation* 50:1025–1032, 1974.
16. Palmer R.F., Lasseter K.C.: Sodium nitroprusside. *N. Engl. J. Med.* 292:294–296, 1975.
17. Miller R.R., Vismara L.A., Zelis R., et al.: Clinical use of sodium nitroprusside in chronic ischemic heart disease. Effects on peripheral vascular resistance and venous tone and on ventricular volume, pump and mechanical performance. *Circulation* 51:328–336, 1975.
18. Chatterjee K., Ports T.A., Brundage B.H., et al.: Oral hydralazine in chronic heart failure: Sustained beneficial hemodynamic effects. *Ann. Intern. Med.* 92:600–604, 1980.
19. Levine T.B., Franciosa J.A., Cohn J.N.: Acute and long-term response to an oral converting-enzyme inhibitor, captopril, in congestive heart failure. *Circulation* 62:35–41, 1980.

4 / Nutrition

Roy D. Cane, M.D.
Scott Greene, M.D.

NUTRITION

Malnutrition in the critically ill patient is extraordinarily common. It is caused by several factors that include (1) inadequate intake of nutrients due both to anorexia and dysfunction of the gastrointestinal tract; (2) increased demand for nutrients secondary to hypermetabolic catabolic states; and (3) preexisting depleted nutritional status commonly associated with chronic disease. The impact of an inadequate nutritional status on the critically ill patient's ability to recover from acute disease is variable and, in particular, involves host immune defenses and wound healing.

Metabolic Responses to Starvation and Stress

The critically ill have metabolic adjustments in substrate utilization due to starvation and the stress of an acute illness which involve the central nervous and endocrine systems. In simple starvation a progressive decrease in energy requirements and nitrogen loss occurs.[1] Initially carbohydrate stores are used to provide glucose substrates to those organs dependent on obligatory carbohydrate metabolism. The major alternate energy substrate is provided by mobilization of fat stores to produce ketone bodies. Glycerol is used to synthesize glucose; however, the majority of the patient's glucose requirements are met by gluconeogenesis of amino acids derived from somatic protein components.[2] The shift from glucose as a predominant energy substrate to fat is associated with a decrease in the resting metabolic rate. In the early stages of starvation, 2.8 gm of fat are metabolized to provide energy for each gram of protein metabolized. Once starvation adaptation has occurred 7.5 gm[3] of fat will be catabolized per gram of protein metabolized in starvation. The body decreases activity in those organs requiring a high rate of protein synthesis. Demand for amino acids decreases and by decreasing metabolic synthetic activities, energy requirements diminish.[4] Further amino acid conservation is achieved by increasing degra-

48

dation of spent protein and shuttling amino acids from one site to an alternate site for protein synthesis.[5] These adaptations have high energy requirements. Survival of the organism in starvation is guaranteed by conservation of lean body mass at the expense of fat stores.

Acute illness produces metabolic changes thought to be due to the control exerted by the endocrine system on intermediary metabolism.[6] Alterations in the neuro-endocrine milieu following acute stress (summarized in Figure 4–1) result in a functional hypoinsulinemia. The metabolic response to acute stress differs from starvation and initially manifests a rapid depletion of carbohydrate stores following which protein degradation increases

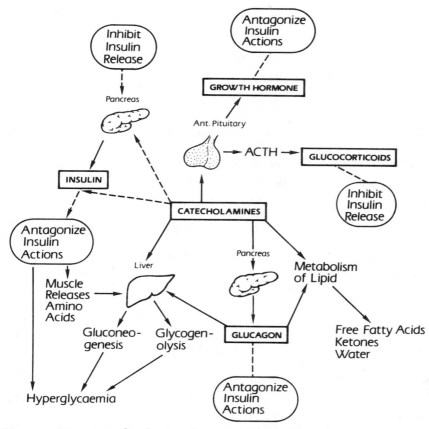

Fig 4–1.—The principal endocrine changes and their effects on energy substrate utilization following trauma. **Straight line** *represents stimulation;* dotted line *represents inhibition. (From Beal J.M.:* **Critical Care for Surgical Patients,** *MacMillan Publishing Co., 1982. Used by permission.)*

to provide intermediates for hepatic gluconeogenesis, thereby maintaining a carbohydrate energy supply. When deaminated, most amino acids become glucogenic or yield carbohydrate intermediates.[5] Fatty acids can provide substrate for general tissue energy requirements but are unable to provide sufficient glucose precursors to meet the high metabolic demand of the critically ill patient. Reparative tissue processes and metabolic processes of brain and red cells are obligatory carbohydrate metabolic processes with respect to energy source. The metabolic adjustments to stress result in a greater loss of nitrogen and lean body mass. Catabolism of more than 30% of lean body mass will have an impact on the survival of the individual.[6] Starved catabolic patients with an adequate premorbid nutritional state can develop a state of protein calorie malnutrition within five to seven days.

NUTRITIONAL SUPPORT

The nutritional management of the critically ill patient is based on two major principles: removal of those factors inducing or prolonging the catabolic neuro-endocrine response of the patient and provision of adequate amounts of appropriate metabolic substrates in a suitable form to maintain and restore the composition of the body. Therefore the basic principles of patient care such as treatment of pain, hemorrhage, tissue necrosis, and sepsis, must be undertaken either before or concomitantly with the initiation of nutritional support.

Assessment of the Patient

Nutritional assessment can be performed at the bedside in conjunction with laboratory investigations. It must be appreciated, however, that this assessment is at best gross and subject to error due to the specific changes commonly encountered in cardiopulmonary function, microcirculatory endothelial cell function, and water metabolism in the critically ill patient.

The somatic and visceral protein and fat components of the body are assessed by anthropometric and laboratory measurements.

Somatic Protein Compartment and Fat Stores

Skeletal muscle mass is assessed by (1) the ratio of the arm size and fat content and (2) the creatinine-height index.

(1) The mid-upper-arm circumference is measured and compared to the normal range to determine the degree of deficit which is usually expressed as the percent of standard. Fat stores are assessed by the triceps skin fold test (TSF). The triceps skin fold of the non-dominant arm is measured with

calipers. Skeletal muscle mass can then be calculated from the following formula:

Arm muscle circumference

$$= \text{Arm circumference} - (0.314 \times \text{TSF in mm})$$

(2) Creatinine-Height Index (CHI). A linear relationship exists between the quantity of creatinine excreted and skeletal muscle mass under conditions of steady state renal function.[7] A 24-hour urine creatinine measurement is made and compared to the values expected for nutritionally normal persons of the same height at ideal body weight and reported as percent of the expected standard.

$$\text{CHI} = \frac{\text{Actual mgm urinary creatinine}}{\text{Ideal creatinine from table}} \times 100\%$$

The reliability of this measurement in the critically ill patient is questionable as catabolism increases creatinine production and loss.[5]

Visceral Protein Compartment

Various visceral protein concentrations can be measured and correlated with the degree of nutritional deficit. Serum transferrin, total iron binding capacity, serum albumin, and lymphocyte count have been shown to be reliable indicators of the visceral protein compartment. The following values correlate with the degree of depletion: (1) Moderate depletion: serum transferrin <200 mgm%, total iron binding capacity <250 mgm%, serum albumin <3.5 gm% and lymphocyte count <1,500/mm^{-3} when total WBC is corrected to 10,000/mm^{-3}. (2) Severe depletion: serum transferrin <170 mgm%, serum albumin <3.0 gm%, lymphocyte count <900/mm^{-3} when total WBC is corrected to 10,000/mm^{-3}. Changes in water balance and endothelial cell function or the administration of colloid occur commonly in critically ill patients and may limit the usefulness of these measurements. Retinol-binding protein and thyroxine-binding prealbumin are rapidly effected by changes in nutritional state and are not directly altered by catabolism and, therefore, may be more reliable indicators of the visceral protein compartment status.[8]

Cell-Mediated Immunity

Depression of the delayed hypersensitivity reaction to specific antigens may indicate severe depletion of the somatic and visceral protein compartment. The competence of cell-mediated immunity (CMI) is assessed by application of four recall antigens injected intradermally. Streptokinase/streptodornase (SK/SD), ppd, mumps, and candida are commonly used. A normal skin test will produce a 15 mm induration at 24–48 hours; 5 mm or less indicates immune incompetence (anergy). A negative response to all four of the recall antigens is associated with an anergic state. If the anergic state is due to malnutrition only, it may be reversed with adequate nutritional support. The existence of an anergic state secondary to malnutrition requires immediate, aggressive nutritional support to minimize a high rate of sepsis-related morbidity and mortality.[9, 10] Remember, however, that anergy can be produced by pathology other than malnutrition.

Nitrogen Balance

Measurement of the daily nitrogen balance is useful in the assessment of malnutrition. Ninety percent of the nitrogenous products of protein catabolism are excreted in the urine as urea. A nitrogen balance is determined by measurement of all nitrogen losses in a 24-hour period and correlated with the total nitrogen intake for the same time period. A positive nitrogen balance (i.e., more nitrogen absorbed than lost) implies an anabolic state. To achieve an anabolic state, the patient's total energy requirements must be met by provision of adequate non-protein calories (CHO, fat) concomitantly with sufficient amino acids for tissue synthesis.

MONITORING OF NUTRITIONAL SUPPORT

Measurement of nitrogen balance, visceral protein concentrations, and CMI provide reliable indices of the efficacy of the nutritional support the patient is receiving. (1) Nitrogen balance should be assessed daily until a positive balance is achieved. Positive balances of 4–6 gm of nitrogen/day are required for lean tissue synthesis. Once positive balance is achieved, this assessment can be made every 3–4 days. If the patient develops any major changes in the disease process or therapy is changed, a new nitrogen balance should be obtained. (2) Visceral protein concentrations should be measured weekly. (3) Changes in the CMI or anthropometric measurements may be expected after 2–3 weeks. Anergy due to malnutrition may be expected to reverse after 10–14 days of adequate intensive nutritional support.

A full nutritional assessment including skin tests performed weekly provides an objective means to evaluate the efficacy of nutritional therapy.

NUTRITIONAL REQUIREMENTS

Calorie Supply

Nitrogen retention is a function not only of the rate of supply of amino acids but also a function of caloric supply. Sufficient calories must be supplied as non-protein calories in order to optimize anabolic utilization of amino acids supplied to the patient. The optimal calorie:nitrogen ratio is 150–200 calories/gm of nitrogen. There are no clear data concerning the relative ratio of lipid or carbohydrate sources for these nonprotein calories.

The desired ratio of carbohydrates and fat sources for nonprotein calories will vary with respect to several factors such as the ventilatory reserve of the patient, the fluid volume the patient will tolerate, and the available routes of access for delivery of these nutrients. The metabolism of carbohydrate energy sources has a respiratory quotient (RQ) of 1 and is associated with an increase in carbon dioxide production and demand on the ventilatory system.[11] In patients with chronic pulmonary disease or those requiring ventilatory support, provision of the bulk of the patient's caloric requirements via a carbohydrate source may adversely affect ventilatory function and the ability to wean patients off mechanical ventilatory support. Metabolism of fat has an RQ of 0.7, and addition of fat to a diet allows maintenance of a calorie supply with lower CO_2 production and hence less demand on the ventilatory system.

Fat emulsions can provide more calories in smaller isotonic volumes than carbohydrate solutions and can be administered via peripheral veins. A certain minimal amount of fat is required to prevent the development of essential fatty acid deficiencies especially linoleic acid. Twenty grams of linoleic acid should be provided per day to prevent development of a deficiency state.[12] The carbohydrate:fat calorie ratio derived from dietary intake in relatively normal people ranges from between 60:30 and 30:55.[13] Whether these ranges are applicable to the IV support of nutrition in the critically ill patient is unclear. It is reasonable to state that a minimum of 10% and a maximum of 55% of total caloric intake may be provided as fat.[13]

Protein Requirements

As one of the prime reasons for parenteral nutrition is the prevention of depletion of body protein stores, it is essential that adequate protein be supplied to the patient. Provision of adequate protein substrate will ensure maintenance of nitrogen balance and promote protein synthesis for tissue repair, wound healing, and the synthesis of hormones and enzymes necessary for the control of biochemical and physiologic activities and the regulation of metabolic processes.

The recommended dietary allowances for young adults is 50 gm of protein/day (approximately 0.8 gm/kg body weight/day) to maintain nitrogen balance.[14] Expressed as grams of nitrogen, this is approximately 8.0 gm/day. Older people may require increases in protein intake, although the data are inconclusive.[15, 16] The total nitrogen need of adult patients requiring parenteral nutrition is 8–16 gm/day irrespective of their age. Twelve to thirteen gm/day have been found adequate to maintain positive nitrogen equilibrium in most critically ill patients except those with severe trauma, such as patients with major burns and sepsis.[17]

Patients with liver disease or chronic renal failure require lesser amounts of protein. Patients with chronic renal failure receiving 1.5–4 gm nitrogen/day in the form of essential amino acids with adequate caloric supply have achieved equilibrium and weight gain.[13]

An essential amino acid is one whose carbon skeleton cannot be synthesized by the organism in amounts adequate to provide for optimal growth and maintenance. Absence of any one of the essential amino acids will result in failure of growth, weight loss, and death. The amino acids thought to be essential for healthy adults are listed in Table 4–1. The classification of amino acids as essential or non-essential is not absolute as certain disease states are known to require specific amino acids normally considered nonessential. In patients with uremia and chronic renal failure, histidine increases nitrogen retention following intravenous hyperalimentation. Premature infants require cysteine. Therefore histidine and cysteine may be considered to be essential amino acids in these conditions.[5]

A particular protein will be synthesized only if all of the amino acids required for its synthesis are provided in sufficient amounts. Deficiency of

TABLE 4–1.—ESSENTIAL AND
NONESSENTIAL AMINO ACIDS

AMINO ACID	ABBR.	ESSENTIAL
Alanine	Ala	No
Arginine	Arg	No
Asparagine	Asn	No
Aspartic acid	Asp	No
Cysteine	Cys	No
Glycine	Gly	No
Glutamic acid	Glu	No
Glutamine	Gln	No
Histidine	His	Semi
Isoleucine	Ile	Yes
Leucine	Leu	Yes
Lysine	Lys	Yes
Methionine	Met	Yes
Phenylalanine	Phe	Yes
Proline	Pro	No
Serine	Ser	No
Threonine	Thr	Yes
Tryptophan	Trp	Yes
Tyrosine	Tyr	No
Valine	Val	Yes

any component amino acid may limit the synthesis of a particular protein. The amino acid composition of tissues varies, and synthesis of a large amount of a particular protein may selectively increase demands for particular amino acids. The amino acid composition of commercially available amino acid solutions differs. Hence, the adequate supply of particular amino acids may depend on the choice of amino acid preparation. An additional factor that may limit protein synthesis is the supply of sufficient nonprotein calories to meet the energy requirements of protein synthesis.

The weight of the essential amino acids divided by the total nitrogen content of any amino acid mixture has been termed the E/T ratio. It has been shown in man that the best nitrogen balance is associated with an E/T ratio of 2.22:1, i.e. approximately 30% of the amino acids administered are essential amino acids.[18] The amino acid solution used should be sufficient to provide each of the amino acids necessary to meet requirements. Solutions containing <10% essential amino acids would probably not provide sufficient quantities of these amino acids. Diets containing >50% essential amino acids may produce adverse effects on diet and growth rate, causing amino acid imbalance, antagonism, or toxicity.[12]

Vitamin Requirements

Some disease processes increase the critically ill patient's requirements for vitamins. Gastrointestinal hemorrhage, jaundice, and cirrhosis may be accompanied by Vitamin K deficiency. Biliary tract obstruction decreases concentration of bile salts in the gut which leads to decreased absorption of the fat-soluble vitamins.

Thiamin, riboflavin, and pyridoxine deficiencies are associated with alcoholism due to inadequate dietary intake and interference with absorption.[19] Therefore, cirrhotic patients will probably have increased requirements. Thiamin requirements are proportional to caloric intake and increase with the increased energy demands of the critically ill patient. Folate deficiency[22] in critically ill patients may produce platelet dysfunction.

The production of normal collagen for tissue repair requires ascorbic acid. Burns or extensive trauma increase requirements for this vitamin enormously.[20] Vitamin C deficiency may be associated with deficient wound healing leading to dehiscence or nonhealing of cutaneous ulcers.

Administration of 10,000 to 40,000 IU of Vitamin A has been reported to reduce the incidence of stress ulcers from 63% to 18% in patients with large surface area burns,[21] an effect possibly mediated by the role of Vitamin A in maintaining epithelial integrity.

Overwhelming sepsis may result in marked increase of all vitamin requirements. The metabolic rate and nutrient requirements of the patient are increased, and the bacteria compete with the infected host for the same vitamins to maintain their own metabolic functions.

METHODS OF NUTRITIONAL SUPPORT

For specific details regarding proprietary alimentation solutions currently available, the reader is referred to other general nutrition texts.[5, 23, 24] Two routes of access for nutritional support are available—enteral or parenteral.

Enteral Route

Ideally if the patient has a functional gastrointestinal (GI) tract, it should be used to provide nutritional support as enteral feeding avoids the septic and technical complications of parenteral feeding. Ileus, GI bleeding, and gastric retention are not uncommon in the critically ill and may limit the use of the enteral route. As intolerance of the GI route for nutritional support may produce emesis and diarrhea with the concomitant risk of pulmonary aspiration, it is important to initiate enteral feeding slowly and sequentially increase administration of nutrients as GI tolerance develops.

Small caliber Silastic and polyurethane nasogastric and nasoduodenal feeding tubes are easy to place and are well tolerated. Duodenal feeding is preferable to gastric feeding as feeding past the pylorus is less likely to result in pulmonary aspiration. Continuous feeding is preferable to bolus feeding as the gut appears to empty and adjust to the osmolarity of the feeding, resulting in better patient tolerance and less morbidity. If patient status permits, the head of the bed should be elevated to enhance gastric emptying.

Surgical access by gastrostomy or jejunostomy are alternate means of providing enteral feedings and are probably best reserved for those critically ill patients who are undergoing abdominal exploration for problems other than malnutrition. Gastrostomy feedings are not well tolerated by the critically ill patient.[5] However, jejunal feeding is well tolerated, particularly if proximal decompression of the stomach by gastrostomy or nasogastric sump suction is provided. The technique of needle-catheter-feeding jejunostomy has an acceptably low complication rate and can be rapidly performed. Continuous infusion of low-viscosity tube feedings can be given by this needle-catheter jejunostomy even in the immediate postoperative period.[25]

As many patients will have some GI function, an approach using both enteral and parenteral routes may be adopted. With this approach the patient can be rapidly placed on parenteral feeding, and with time enteral feedings are initiated and increased depending on the patient's tolerance. Once the enteral feedings have been increased to a level sufficient to support the patient, the parenteral feedings can be gradually weaned and discontinued.[5]

Parenteral Route

Intravenous hyperalimentation (IVH) by the central venous route has developed to a degree of safety and efficacy such that reports of technical and septic complication rates below 3% are common.[26, 27]

Catheterization of the subclavian vein by sub- or supraclavicular percutaneous puncture is the preferred route for intravenous alimentation.[28] Alternate routes include subclavian catheterization via the median basilic vein, internal and external jugular veins. It is imperative that IV feeding catheters are placed under conditions of strict asepsis. The line should be dedicated solely to alimentation. Meticulous aseptic technique should be followed for all catheter care after insertion. Silicone catheters are less thrombogenic than PVC or teflon. Use of a clear, water-permeable, bacteria-impermeable, polyurethane dressing allows for direct inspection of the catheter site and is associated with less than 1% of catheter-induced sepsis.[29]

Available solutions for IV alimentation include carbohydrate mixtures (40%–70% dextrose), fat emulsions, and amino acid solutions. Several different commercial preparations are available. The specific mix of these solutions and additives should be determined for each patient and prepared under aseptic conditions.

COMPLICATIONS OF NUTRITIONAL SUPPORT

Experience with nutritional support has led to a significant reduction in the incidence of complications. Metabolic complications occur with either parenteral or enteral feeding and are largely caused by excessive or inadequate administration of specific components of the diet. Parenteral feedings are specifically associated with technical and septic complications related to the intravenous catheter. Enteral feedings are associated with technical problems secondary to delivery of large volumes of hyperosmolar solutions into the GI tract and also a significant risk of pulmonary aspiration.

Metabolic Complications

Frequent evaluation of the metabolic, fluid and electrolyte, and acid-base status of the patient is of fundamental importance.

Volume replacement and cardiovascular resuscitation should be accomplished prior to initiating nutritional support. Correction of fluid and electrolyte as well as acid-base abnormalities may take place concomitantly with hyperalimentation.

Electrolyte and Acid-Base Problems

Critically ill patients with normal renal function commonly show depletion of potassium, chloride, and magnesium stores secondary to the widespread use of diuretics and increased gastrointestinal drainage. Cellular depletion because of decreased nutrient intake and increased catabolism also contribute to these losses and may be associated with depletion of phosphate stores.

The electrolyte status of the patient receiving nutritional support should be monitored by serial determinations of serum electrolytes, BUN, glucose, magnesium, phosphate, and calcium. Alimentation solutions should be modified as indicated. Trace element deficiencies such as zinc and copper should be corrected with addition of trace element solutions.

Bicarbonate cannot be added to IV solutions because an alkaline pH is likely to result in precipitation of calcium salts. The acetate salts of sodium and potassium may be used to provide the patient with substrate that can be metabolized to bicarbonate. Metabolic alkalosis due to loss of fixed acid from the gut or urinary tract contraindicates the use of acetate salts.

A hypokalemic metabolic alkalosis may be corrected by administration of large amounts of potassium chloride and alkalinization of the urine with sodium acetazolamide.

Glucose Intolerance

The critically ill patient frequently manifests glucose intolerance. Persistent glycosuria produces an osmotic diuresis and often leads to nonketotic hyperosmolar dehydration and coma in nondiabetic patients[30, 31] and a ketoacidotic state in the diabetic patient. The addition of small amounts of regular insulin to IVH solutions enables control of blood sugar despite a significant loss of insulin due to adherence to the glass and plastic of the infusion apparatus.[32, 33] If prompt control of hyperglycemia is not obtained, it may be necessary to change the major calorie source from carbohydrate to fat.

Chromium deficiency has been reported as an uncommon cause of glucose intolerance.[34] Chromium trichloride may be added to the IV solutions in a dose of 10 μg day to maintain normal serum chromium levels.

Other Metabolic Complications

A discussion of all fluid and electrolyte abnormalities is beyond the scope of this chapter and the reader is referred to other texts.[23, 24, 35]

Technical Complications

The primary technical complications of IVH relate to catheter insertion and include inadvertent carotid or subclavian artery catheterization, pneumothorax, pneumomediastinum, and venous thrombosis.

Volume overload can be a problem, particularly in patients with cardiac disease and those requiring mechanical ventilatory support. Positive pressure ventilation results in changes in ADH secretion, renal perfusion, and water balance so that the patient tends to retain water.[36]

Septic Complications

Because critically ill patients are prone to develop sepsis, the differential diagnosis of sepsis after the introduction of a central venous catheter and initiation of IV hyperalimentation is important. The search for a septic focus requires cultures of blood, urine, sputum, and any removed catheters for bacteria and fungi. The incidence of catheter-induced sepsis is 3% to 7%.[37]

The mainstay of preventing the development of catheter-related sepsis is meticulous attention to aseptic technique in the placement of parenteral catheters, catheter dressings, and IV fluid preparation. The catheter used for IVH should never be used for any other purpose.

CASE STUDY

A 64-year-old male with an 8-year history of chronic obstructive pulmonary disease presented to the emergency room with a complaint of increasing shortness of breath and coughing for 2 days' duration. The patient has had two previous admissions in the last 18 months for pneumonia. He normally produces small quantities of whitish sputum but has been producing approximately half a cup per day of thick yellow sputum over the last two days. Further questioning revealed loss of appetite and a weight loss of 30 lb over the last 6 months associated with severe depression following the death of his wife.

On examination he was noted to be markedly cachectic and weighed 55 kg. His heart rate was 115/min with occasional ventricular ectopic beats, and his BP was 160/90 mm Hg. Extremities were cyanotic and the fingernails were clubbed. There was no evidence of jugular venous distension or peripheral edema. Auscultation of the heart revealed a marked P2 component to the second heart sound, and no murmurs were heard. His RR was 35/min with VT of 300 ml and the patient was using accessory ventilatory muscles. The anteroposterior diameter of his chest was enlarged and the chest was hyperresonant to percussion. Diaphragmatic excursion was minimal and rhonchi and fremitus were noted in the right middle and lower lobe regions. The rest of the physical examination was unremarkable.

Initial laboratory investigations revealed a serum sodium of 143 mEq/L, a potassium of 4.8 mEq/L, a chloride of 90 mEq/L, a bicarbonate of 36 mEq/L, a serum glucose of 270 mg%, and a BUN of 28 mg%. The patient's hemoglobin concentration was 17 gm% and WBC was 18,000 mm^{-3} with a leftward shift. Arterial blood gases on room air revealed a pH of 7.51, a P_{CO_2} of 45 mm Hg, and a P_{O_2} of 40 mm Hg. Gram staining of the sputum showed the presence of many WBC and gram-positive diplococci. A sputum sample was sent for a culture and sensitivity. Urinalysis was within normal limits. The ECG showed sinus tachycardia with occasional ventricular premature beats. Chest x-ray revealed infiltrates in the right, middle, and lower lobe, flattened diaphragms, and hyperinflation. A preliminary diagnosis of acute bacterial pneumonia superimposed on chronic obstructive pulmonary disease was made, and the patient's poor nutritional status noted.

The patient was started on penicillin for his presumed pneumococcal pneumonia and given 24% oxygen via an air entrainment mask, which resulted in arterial blood gases with a pH of 7.50, a P_{CO_2} of 45 mm Hg, and a P_{O_2} of 44 mm Hg. The $F_{I_{O_2}}$ was increased to 0.28 with resultant improvement in the arterial oxygenation, decrease in heart rate, BP, and a change in respiratory pattern to a rate of 28/min with VT of 350 ml and a VC of 1.1 L. Arterial blood gases on 28% oxygen showed a pH of 7.46, a

P_{CO_2} of 50 mm Hg, and a P_{O_2} of 52 mm Hg. Chest physical therapy was ordered to help the patient mobilize secretions, and the nutritional support service was requested to review the patient's nutritional status. Three hours later the patient was noted to have increasing RR, heart rate, and systemic blood pressure. Blood pressure and repeat arterial blood gases on 28% oxygen revealed a pH of 7.32, a P_{CO_2} of 68 mm Hg, and a P_{O_2} of 43 mm Hg. The patient was deemed to be developing AVF and was ventilated with a manual resuscitator and face mask in preparation for naso-tracheal intubation to facilitate mechanical ventilatory support. Following uneventful placement of a naso-tracheal tube, the patient was put on a mechanical ventilator at a rate of 8 breaths/min, mechanical VT of 1,000 ml, and 40% oxygen with +5 of PEEP, which resulted in an arterial pH of 7.42, a P_{CO_2} of 53 mm Hg, and a P_{O_2} of 71 mm Hg. At this time the patient was noted to have no spontaneous respiratory efforts at all and was resting quietly. Sputum cultures confirmed the diagnosis of pneumococcal pneumonia.

Assessment of the patient's nutritional status revealed the following:

Anthropometric Measurements

- Mid-upper-arm circumference (MAC) —15.2 cm (60% of standard),
- Triceps skin fold thickness (TSF)—7.5 mm (60% of standard),
- Arm muscle circumference (MAC)— (0.0314 × TSF) = 15.0 cm (60% of standard.)

Laboratory Measurements

- Serum albumin—2.9 gm%, serum total iron binding capacity—175 mg%.
- Serum transferrin—100 mg%, WBC—18,000 mm^{-3} with 6% lymphocytes.

- Correcting lymphocyte number to a total white cell of 1,000 mm^{-3} = 600 lymphocytes/mm^{-3}
- Serum magnesium—15 mg%, serum calcium—7.0 mg%.
- Serum calcium—7.0 mg%.
- Serum phosphorus—2.5 mg% and urine urea nitrogen—2 mg%.
- Cell-mediated immunity—total anergy.
- Liver and renal function—normal.

On the basis of these measurements, the patient was deemed to have severe depletion of somatic and visceral protein compartments and a mixed marasmus and kwashiorkor-like state of malnutrition.

The patient's ideal body weight was 70 kg and therefore it was determined that he required 2,450 kcal per day (35 kcal/kg) and 105 gm of protein (1.5 gm protein/kg per day). It was decided to start the patient on enteral feedings administered via a nasogastric tube as the patient had no evidence of abnormal GI function. Fifty cc of full strength isocal were administered per hour via the nasogastric tube. Gastric residual volumes, urine glucose, and acetone were checked every four hours. This diet gave the patient 1,200 calories per day with 41 gm of protein in a volume of 1.2 L/day.

The patient was tolerating mechanical ventilatory support and required 2 mg of IV morphine every 2–4 hours for sedation. The 50 cc per hour nasogastric feedings were well tolerated in the first 24 hours with no sugar or acetone noted in the urine. The following day the feedings were increased to 75 cc per hour, and four hours later gastric residual was noted to be 150 cc. Examination of the patient revealed decreased bowel sounds and slight abdominal distension. Feedings were cut back to 50 cc per hour and the patient was started on 10 mg of IV metaclopramide every 6 hours. On day 4, feedings were again increased to 75 cc per hour, which resulted in marked abdominal distension, nausea, vomiting, and a gastric residual of 200 cc after 4 hours. A flat plate x-ray of the abdomen was taken and was consistent with an ileus.

Discussion

The initial premise that the patient's GI function was adequate to enable enteral feedings was clearly incorrect. The probable causes for this ileus include the morphine sedation and the initiation of mechanical ventilatory support. Metaclopramide enhances GI motility and has an anti-emetic action. Although it helps increase tolerance for enteral feedings, metaclopramide was ineffective for this patient. Fifty cc per hour of isocal feedings are insufficient to provide the patient's caloric and protein requirements. Therefore, it is necessary to either stop the feedings until the factors producing the ileus can be corrected or switch the patient to IV alimentation. In view of the severe degree of the patient's nutritional depletion and the probability that this nutritional depletion will adversely impact on the patient's response to infection and the ability to resume spontaneous ventilation, it was decided to switch the patient to IV alimentation.

Case Study Continued

A right subclavian silicone catheter was placed under aseptic technique to enable IV hyperalimentation. A chest x-ray taken after placement of the line confirmed the position of the line and revealed no evidence of pneumothorax or hemothorax. The patient's WBC at this time had decreased to 11,000 mm^{-3} and the patient was normothermic with a normal temperature curve. Intravenous alimentation was started with a mixture of 60% dextrose and 8.5% amino acid solution with additional electrolytes, trace elements, and vitamins. The infusion was started at a rate of 50 ml/hour with the goal of increasing it over time to 100 cc/hour, which would provide the patient with 2,448 calories and 102 gm of protein per day. To prevent development of essential fatty acid deficiencies, 500 ml of a 10% lipid emulsion were administered twice a week which would provide an additional 1,100 calories per week. The patient tolerated the IV alimentation at 50 cc/hour with no acetone or glucose in the urine. After 24 hours of IV alimentation, the rate was increased to 75 cc/hour which resulted in 0.1% glucose detected in the urine by clini-test and no acetone, and a serum glucose of 180 mg%. On the third day of IV alimenta-

tion, the infusion rate was increased to 100 ml per hour which resulted in a 1% urinary glucose and a serum glucose of 325 mg%. Fifteen units of regular insulin were added to each liter of hyperalimentation solution and resulted in a lowering of serum glucose to 120 mg% with no glucose or acetone detected in the urine.

Over the next 48 hours the patient continued to tolerate IV feedings and a routine monitoring arterial blood gas on 40% oxygen revealed a pH of 7.52, a Pco$_2$ of 53 mm Hg, and a Po$_2$ of 71 mm Hg.

The chest x-ray showed no significant changes in the infiltrates at this time. The patient remained afebrile. The serum potassium was noted to have decreased to 3.6 mEq/L with a serum chloride of 90 mEq/L. Additional potassium chloride was added to the patient's IV fluids bringing it to a total of 40 mEq/L. On the eighth day of IV alimentation (12th hospital day), serum potassium was 4.3 mEq/L and arterial blood gases on full ventilatory support with an F$_{IO_2}$ of 0.4 showed a pH of 7.43, a Pco$_2$ of 54 mm Hg, and a Po$_2$ of 83 mm Hg. The urinary urea nitrogen (UUN) was 7 gm per day and a calculated nitrogen balance was +5.3 gm.

Discussion

Metabolic disturbances are common during hyperalimentation. Close attention must be paid to monitoring serum electrolytes and glucose concen-‐ trates because most of these problems are easily corrected.

The following formula is used to calculate nitrogen balances:

$$\text{Nitrogen balance} = \text{Nitrogen in} - \text{Nitrogen out}$$

$$\text{Nitrogen balance} = \frac{\text{Protein intake}}{\text{Gm usable N2}} - (\text{UUN} + 4)$$

The usable nitrogen per gram of protein is 6.25 and the factor of 4 added to the UUN represents 2 gm for non-urea urinary nitrogen, 1 gm for fecal nitrogen, and 1 gm for nitrogen lost from desquamation of skin and epithelial surfaces. A nitrogen balance of 0 to $+4$ gm/day is indicative of anabolism equal to catabolism. Nitrogen balances of $+4$ to $+6$ indicate anabolism occurring at a rate sufficient to restore nutritional status and promote growth.

This patient has now been in the hospital for 12 days and has received a full course of antibiotics and 8 days of appropriate nutritional support. He is in positive nitrogen balance, though only for a short period of time. It would be reasonable to assess the patient with the objective of attempting to wean him from mechanical ventilatory support. Before attempting to wean, it is essential to determine first that the primary reason for the development of ventilatory failure has been corrected and second that there are no other acutely correctable factors that may limit the patient's ability to ventilate spontaneously. These factors would include: electrolyte disturbances, hemodynamic imbalances, acid base imbalances, and inadequate hemoglobin concentrate. As this patient is a known CO_2 retainer, he may in part depend on a hypoxic drive to maintain spontaneous ventilation. Therefore, the inspired oxygen concentration should be decreased to return the arterial oxygenation to a level closer to that which is normal for this patient with chronic lung disease.

Case Study Continued

Assessment of the patient revealed marked improvement on the chest x-ray and clinical findings implying resolution of his pneumonia. Electrolyte status was within normal limits. The patient was afebrile and in positive nitrogen balance. The F_{IO_2} was decreased to 25% resulting in the following arterial blood gases: a pH of 7.42, a P_{CO_2} of 51 mm Hg, and a P_{O_2} of 55 mm Hg. The patient was noted to have some spontaneous ventilation at a rate of 20 breaths/min with V_T of 250 cc. His measured VC was 900 ml. The patient was placed on a free flowing CPAP system at $+5$ cm of water and an F_{IO_2} of 0.25. He had a heart rate of 115 beats/min and a BP of 130/90 mm Hg. The patient felt comfortable. Over the next four hours his heart rate increased steadily to 130 beats/min, and his BP rose to 170/100 mm Hg. The patient complained of shortness of breath, and repeat arterial blood gases revealed a pH of 7.33, P_{CO_2} of 64 mm Hg, and a P_{O_2} of 49 mm Hg on an F_{IO_2} of 0.25. Mechanical ventilatory support was reinstituted and the patient's condition stabilized on the ventilator at 8 breaths/min with V_T of 1,000 ml.

Repeat measurement of serum albumin revealed a concentration of 3 gm% and the serum phosphorus concentration was 2.2 mg%. The patient was given IV potassium phosphate and on the following day the serum phosphorus had risen to 3.8 mg%. Carbon dioxide production was measured and found to be 320 ml/min.

Discussion

Hypophosphatemia is associated with ventilatory failure, although the onset of ventilatory failure is usually only seen with levels of phosphorus below 1.8 mg%. It is not clear whether the low phosphorus measured in this patient was a significant factor in his failure to be weaned from mechanical ventilatory support. However, it was deemed wise to correct this deficiency as it may have played a part in the failure to wean.

The high carbon dioxide production measured in this patient probably reflects the high caloric intake of a carbohydrate source. Carbohydrate energy substrates are metabolized with a respiratory quotient of 1 and are associated with marked increase in CO_2 production and minute ventilatory requirements.[11] The metabolic demand on the ventilatory system can be decreased by reducing the total number of calories given to a patient or by reducing the carbohydrate source of those calories and replacing it with fat. Fats are metabolized with a lower respiratory quotient of 0.7 and a lower CO_2 production. In addition, if patients are overfed with carbohydrates, excess carbohydrate will be converted to fats. This process of lipogenesis has a respiratory quotient of 7.0 and is therefore associated with a high CO_2 production.[38]

Case Study Continued

The patient's IV alimentation was changed to a mixture of 40% dextrose and 8.5% amino acid solution with 25 cc of 20% lipid emulsion per hour added to provide the appropriate number of calories. This change gave the patient a total of 2,506 calories of which 1,200 were derived from lipids and 1,306 from carbohydrate sources with 102 gm of protein per day. The patient was maintained on mechanical ventilatory support and the new alimentation regimen for two days. Carbon dioxide production was remeasured. At this time carbon dioxide production had decreased to 210 cc/min and the nitrogen balance was found to be +4.3. Once again the patient was removed from mechanical ventilatory support and allowed to breathe spontaneously on a free flowing CPAP system with essentially the same result of a rising arterial P_{CO_2} and a falling pH. No immediately correctable reason for the patient's inability to ventilate spontaneously could be identified, and it was felt that he required further nutritional repletion. A tracheostomy was performed. The patient was maintained on mechanical ventilatory support with the intention of providing two weeks more of IV alimentation before further attempts at weaning would be undertaken.

Twenty-four hours later the patient spiked a fever to 102.2°F rectally. He had been afebrile for the preceding seven days.

Discussion

Acceptance of the need for strict aseptic technique in catheter placement and maintenance has led to a fall in catheter-related sepsis to 3% from 7%.[37] Alimentation catheters must be placed under conditions of surgical sterility and dedicated solely to infusion of alimentation solutions. When a patient receiving IV alimentation develops a fever, a full fever work-up should be performed. In addition, the alimentation catheter tip and fluids must be cultured. Inspection of the catheter site often provides useful information. If the catheter grows organisms, then another catheter must be inserted in a new site. If the catheter is found to be uninfected, then alimentation can be reinstituted via the existing site.[39]

Case Study Continued

Blood, urine, and sputum samples were collected and sent for culture and sensitivity. A WBC was measured. Blood was drawn through the alimentation catheter and sent for culture and sensitivity, and the IV alimentation solution was returned to the pharmacy for culture and sensitivity. The skin site of the subclavian catheter was inspected and looked clean. The subclavian catheter was removed after a guide wire had been inserted through it and the catheter tip sent for culture and sensitivity. A fresh catheter was introduced over the guide wire and hyperalimentation fluids discontinued while the patient received 10% dextrose and water through the new catheter. All the cultures were negative and 24 hours later the patient's fever had subsided. Intravenous alimentation was recommenced at this time. As the patient's ileus had resolved, it was decided to attempt to reinstitute enteral feedings. A Dobhoff naso-enteral tube was passed. Once the position of the Dobhoff tube had been verified by x-ray to be in the duodenum, enteral feedings of Isocal were instituted. Over a period of several days, the rate of enteral feedings was increased while the IV alimentation was decreased. During this period the relative volumes and concentrations of enteral and parenteral feedings were adjusted to maintain the same daily delivery of protein, calories, and volume that the patient had been receiving when on full parenteral alimentation. After four days the patient was tolerating 125 ml/hour of enteral feedings and the IV alimentation was discontinued. The patient was maintained on this regimen for twelve more days and remained afebrile during this period. The chest x-ray was clear and the WBC was 7,000/mm^{-3}. Electrolytes were appropriate for a patient with chronic obstructive pulmonary disease and the arterial blood gases on 30% oxygen showed a pH of 7.41, a P_{CO_2} of 52 mm Hg, and a P_{O_2} of 72 mm Hg. Remeasured carbon dioxide production was 190 ml/min and the patient had been in positive nitrogen balance for three weeks. Serum albumin was 3.8 gm%, total iron binding capacity 300 mg%, serum transferrin 250 mg%, and serum magnesium, calcium, and phosphorus were all within normal limits. Skin antigen testing revealed an appropriate response—the mid-upper-arm circumference was 27.3 cm, triceps skin fold thickness 12.5 mm, and arm muscle circumference 23.4 cm, which are all within normal limits.

Once again the F_{IO_2} was reduced to 0.24 and the patient's PaO_2 on this inspired oxygen concentration was 53 mm Hg. Ventilatory support was discontinued and the patient was maintained on a free flowing CPAP system with +5 cm of water pressure. His spontaneous ventilatory rate was 22/min with a V_T of 280 ml. Vital capacity was 1.1 L. The patient was comfortable and maintained this level of ventilation. Heart rate was 95/min with a BP of 130/90 mm Hg. The extremities remained warm and the patient continued to pass urine. After 24 hours off mechanical ventilatory support, the tracheostomy tube was replaced with a fenestrated tracheostomy tube which was subsequently corked enabling the patient to breathe through the upper airway. The patient developed no further problems and two days later the trachea was decannulated without event.

REFERENCES

1. Keys A., Brozek J., Henschel A.: *The Biology of Human Starvation*. Minneapolis, University of Minnesota Press, 1970, 2 vols.
2. Coleman J.E.: Metabolic interrelationship between carbohydrates, lipids and proteins, in Bondy P.K., Rosenberg L.E. (eds.): *Duncan's Disease of Metabolism*. Philadelphia, W.B. Saunders Co., 1969, pp. 89–198.
3. Cahill G.F., Jr.: Starvation in man. *N. Engl. J. Med.* 282:668–675, 1970.
4. Addis T., Poo L.J., Lew W.: The quantities of protein lost by various organs and tissues of the body during a fast. *J. Biol. Chem.* 115:111–116, 1936.
5. Vazquez R.M.: Nutritional support systems for care of the critically ill surgical patient, in Beal J.M., (ed.): *Critical Care for Surgical Patients*. New York, MacMillan Publishing Co., 1982, pp. 188–213.
6. Moore F.D., Brennan M.F.: Surgical injury: Body composition, protein metabolism and neuroendocrinology, in Ballinger W.F., Collins J.A., Drucker W.R., et al. (eds.): *Manual of Surgical Nutrition*. Philadelphia and London, W.B. Saunders Co., 1975, pp. 169–222.
7. Bistrian B.R., Blackburn G.L., Sherman M., et al.: Therapeutic index of nutritional depletion of hospitalized patients. *Surg. Gynecol. Obstet.* 141:512–516, 1975.
8. Shetty P.S., Jung R.T., Watrasiewicz A., et al.: Rapid-turnover transport proteins: An index of subclinical protein-energy malnutrition. *Lancet* 2(8136):230–232, 1979.
9. Mullen J.L., Gertner M.H., Busby G.P., et al.: Implications of malnutrition in the surgical patient. *Arch. Surg.* 114:121–125, 1979.
10. Pietsch J.B., Meakins J.L., MacLean L.D.: The delayed hypersensitivity response application in clinical surgery. *Surgery* 82:349–355, 1977.
11. Askanazi J., Rosenbaum S.H., Hyman A.L., et al.: Effects of parenteral nutrition on ventilatory drive. *Anesthesiology* 53:5185, 1980.
12. Jeejeebhoy K.N.: Total parenteral nutrition. *Ann. R. Coll. Phys. Surg. Can.* 9:287–300, 1976.
13. Meng H.C.: Parenteral nutrition: Principles, nutrient requirements, techniques and clinical applications, in Schneider H.A., Anderson C.E., and Coursin D.B. (eds.): *Nutritional Support of Medical Practice*. New York, Harper & Row, 1977, pp. 152–183.
14. Recommended Dietery Allowances. A Report of the Food and Nutrition Board, National Research Council, National Academy of Science, ed. 8, 1974.
15. Kountz W.B., Hofstatter L., Acerman P.G.: Nitrogen balance studies in four elderly men. *J. Gerontol.* 6:20, 1951.
16. Moore F.D.: Surgical nutrition—parenteral and oral, in Committee on Preoperative and Postoperative Care of the American College of Surgeons: Manual of Preoperative and Postoperative Care. Philadelphia, W.B. Saunders Co., 1967.
17. Van Way C.W., III, Meng H.C., Sandstead H.H.: An assessment of the role of parenteral nutrition in the management of surgical patients. *Ann. Surg.* 177:103, 1973.

18. Furst P., Josephson B., Vinnars E.: The effect on nitrogen balance of the ratio of essential/nonessential amino acids in intravenously infused solutions. *Scand. J. Clin. Lab. Invest.* 26:319–326, 1970.
19. Dreyfus P.M., Victor M.: Effects of thiamin deficiency on the central nervous system. *Am. J. Clin. Nutr.* 9:414–425, 1961.
20. Levenson S.M., Green R.W., Taylor F.H., et al.: Ascorbic acid, riboflavin, thiamin and nicotinic acid in relation to injury, hemorrhage, and infection in humans. *Ann. Surg.* 124:840–856, 1946.
21. Chernov M.S., Cook F.B., Wood M., et al.: Stress ulcer: A preventable disease. *J. Trauma* 12:831–833, 1972.
22. Mant M.J., Connolly T., Gordon P.A., et al.: Severe thrombocytopenia probably due to acute folic acid deficiency. *Crit. Care Med.* 7:297–300, 1979.
23. Schneider H.H., Anderson C.E., Coursin D.B.: *Nutritional Support of Medical Practice.* New York, Harper & Row, 1977.
24. Halpern S.L.: *Quick Reference to Clinical Nutrition.* Philadelphia, J.B. Lippincott, Co., 1979.
25. Page C.P., Ryan J.A., Haff R.C.: Continual catheter administration of an elemental diet. *Surg. Gynecol. Obstet.* 142:184–188, 1976.
26. Lumb P.O., Dalton B., Bryan-Brown C.W., et al.: Aggressive approach to intravenous feeding of the critically ill patient. *Heart Lung* 8:71–80, 1979.
27. Ryan J.A., Abel R.M., Abbott W.M., et al.: Catheter complications of total parenteral nutrition. *N. Engl. J. Med.* 290:757–761, 1974.
28. Dudrick S.J., Long J.M., Steiger E., et al.: Intravenous hyperalimentation. *Med. Clin. North Am.* 54:577–589, 1970.
29. Vazquez R.M.: Tracheostomy and subclavian catheterizations. *Surg. Gynecol. Obstet.* 152:342–343, 1980.
30. Kaminski M.V.: Hyperosmolar hyperglycemic non-ketonic dehydration: Etiology, pathophysiology and prevention during total parenteral nutrition. Proceedings of the International Symposium on Intensive Therapy. Rome, 1975, pp. 290–305.
31. Brenner W.I., Lansky Z., Engleman R.M., et al.: Hyperosmolar coma in surgical patients. *Ann. Surg.* 178:651–654, 1973.
32. Oh T.E., Dyer H., Wall B.P., et al.: Insulin loss in parenteral nutrition systems. *Anaesth. Intensive Care* 4:342–346, 1976.
33. Weber S.S., Wood W.A., Jackson E.A.: Availability of insulin from parenteral nutrient solutions. *Am. J. Hosp. Pharm.* 34:353–357, 1977.
34. Freund H., Atamian S., Fischer J.E.: Chromium deficiency during total parenteral nutrition. *J.A.M.A.* 241:496–498, 1979.
35. *Manual of Surgical Nutrition.* In Committee on Preoperative and Postoperative Care of the American College of Surgeons. Ballinger W.F., Collins J.A., Drucker W.R., et al. (eds.): Philadelphia, W.B. Saunders Co., 1975.
36. Cane R.D.: Fluid balance and parenteral intravenous support systems, in Beal J.M. (ed.): *Critical Care for Surgical Patients.* New York, MacMillan Publishing Co., 1982, pp 172–187.
37. Copeland E.M., MacFayden B.V., McGowan C., et al.: The use of hyperalimentation in patients with potential sepsis. *Surg. Gynecol. Obstet.* 138:377–380, 1974.
38. Saltarauh A., Salyano J.V.: Effect of carbohydrate metabolism upon respiratory gas exchange in normal man. *J. Appl. Physiol.* 30:228, 1971.
39. Blackburn G.L.: Hyperalimentation in the critically ill patient. *Heart Lung* 8:67–70, 1979.

5 / Drug Overdose

ROY D. CANE, M.D.

DRUG OVERDOSE

The definition of a poison is as imprecise as are the statistics on the incidence of both accidental and deliberate poisoning. Poisoning may be defined as exposure to a substance in sufficient quantity that it will produce untoward effects in the majority of individuals thus exposed. This chapter will deal with poisoning due to drug overdose with particular reference to sedatives and narcotics. The reader is referred to other texts for more general information regarding the wider range of poisons.[1, 2, 3]

EPIDEMIOLOGY OF DRUG OVERDOSE

Analysis of 121,077 reports of drug overdoses from hospital emergency rooms revealed that 177,586 drugs had been taken. Of these, benzodiazepines made up 19%, ethanol 11%, opium 11%, major tranquilizers and antidepressants 10%, barbiturates 8%, general sedatives 6%, aspirin 4%, amphetamines 2%, and acetaminophen 1%.[4] Three-quarters of overdosed patients are under the age of thirty and the incidence of overdose with suicidal intent is higher in women than in men.[5] In adolescents and adults, drug overdose occurs as a deliberate act in 65%–90% of instances.[6, 7] Eighteen percent of fatally drug-overdosed individuals reach hospitals alive, and only 8% survive the first 12 hours following hospitalization.[2] In the last decade the frequency of drug overdose has increased considerably while the in-hospital deaths from drug overdose have been dramatically reduced.[8, 9, 10] The causes of death from drug overdose are due primarily to depression of vital functions with consequent respiratory and circulatory failure. Aspiration of gastric contents is a significant cause of morbidity and may produce deaths. Aspiration pneumonia may be the most common preventable complication in acute drug overdose. (See Chapter 8.)

DIAGNOSIS OF DRUG OVERDOSE

The diagnosis of drug overdose will depend on history, physical examination, and laboratory evaluation. The signs and symptoms of overdose will vary depending on both the nature of the agent that has been ingested and also on the quantity and timing of such ingestion.

History

Valuable information can be obtained from careful questioning of the patient and the patient's family, friends, neighbors, and physician. Frequently the patient will be admitted to the hospital comatose and history can only be obtained from secondary sources. A detailed family history and psychological assessment of the patient can be invaluable as preexistent psychosocial problems are common in poisoning victims.[6, 11–13] Knowledge of medications prescribed for other family members may help identify a putative drug. Certain substances require immediate specific therapy. Therefore, direct questioning concerning possible exposure to substances such as acetaminophen, ethylene glycol, lead, lithium, methanol, or salicylates is mandatory.[2]

Physical Examination

It is imperative when dealing with the comatose patient suspected of drug overdose that immediate assessment of the adequacy of cardiopulmonary function be undertaken prior to any further examination or therapy. In addition to clinical observation of peripheral perfusion, skin temperature, color, urine output, and BP, this assessment should always include arterial blood gas analysis. Alveolar hypoventilation cannot readily be documented on clinical observation alone.

When examining a patient examine the skin and the mucosa and look for bullae at pressure points which may occur in overdose with barbiturates, opioids and other sedatives.[2] The patient may have stigmata of drug abuse that can be identified by careful physical examination of the extremities. A detailed neurologic examination is essential. It is important to check for evidence of cervical injuries before attempting to move the head. Practically any neurological finding can occur in drug overdoses[14] and, furthermore, the clinical picture can be obscured because of head injury, intracranial bleeding, and generalized or localized CNS ischemia superimposed on drug overdose.

The differential diagnosis of coma[14] is very extensive and beyond the scope of this text. However the two important conditions to rule out immediately are an intracranial lesion and meningitis. If an intracranial lesion is suspected, computerized tomography will invariably help make a diagnosis. Meningitis can be detected by an evaluation of intracranial pressure and cerebrospinal fluid analysis.

Laboratory Tests

Laboratory investigations can be of value in identifying a specific drug and may be of use in guiding therapy. The laboratory can undertake screening in suspected drug overdoses for common agents, but it is important to remember that the range of potential drugs that could have been abused is very large. The presence of drugs can be sought in gastric contents, blood, urine or feces. Laboratories commonly employ chromatographic and mass spectrometric techniques to identify substances in bodily fluids. The routine use of a laboratory for toxicology screening is difficult to justify because of the enormous cost and the relatively low yield. Furthermore, the laboratory may detect the presence of substances routinely prescribed to patients for therapeutic reasons and not present in the patient because of ingestion of excessive quantities.

Serum Electrolytes

Use of the clinical laboratory for measurement of serum electrolytes may help confirm the suspicion of a drug overdose. Estimation of serum osmolality from measured serum electrolytes when compared to a measured osmolality may identify the presence of a significant concentration of occult osmoles which would suggest the possibility of poisoning with an alcohol. This discrepancy in estimated and measured osmolality can be misleading in patients given glycerol, mannitol, or isosorbide, and in the face of a significant lipemia.[2] Assessment of the anion gap may be useful as occult anions may result from tissue hypoxia secondary to poisoning with cyanides or sulfides, the formation of acid metabolites of methanol and ethylene glycol, or from the lactic acidosis produced by substances that inhibit oxidative cellular metabolism.

Serum Drug Concentration

Laboratory measurement of specific drug serum concentrations is of limited value as serum levels will rise following ingestion of a drug and then subsequently decline with time. A particular level on the upswing is far more significant than the identical level on the downswing of that particular drug serum concentration curve. When evaluating any particular drug serum level, it is important to consider the timing at which the blood sample was taken relative to ingestion of the drug, history of prior drug exposure, interactions among detected drugs, and the influence of age and disease. Serum drug concentrations are of little prognostic value because with appropriate care and support almost all patients will survive poisoning with therapeutic drugs. Trends in serum drug concentrations can be of qualitative value in assessing and managing an acute overdose.

The laboratory was shown to be useful in identifying toxins in 58% of 235 patients with a clinical diagnosis of drug overdose.[15] The correlation between drug level and clinical state was poor. Of these 235 patients, only 21 required active therapy and in no instance was this therapy influenced by the toxicological analyses. Similar results have been reported by other workers.[16, 17]

MANAGEMENT OF DRUG OVERDOSE

The management of drug overdose involves supportive therapy and specific measures aimed at decreasing the absorbence of the ingested drug, enhancing removal of the ingested drug, or antagonizing the specific effects of an ingested drug.

Supportive therapy should be aimed at guaranteeing airway maintenance and protection, tissue perfusion, and ventilation. Consideration must be given to the correction of any significant disturbances of arterial oxygenation and acid-base balance.

Decreasing Drug Absorbence

Most drug overdoses result from oral ingestion of the substance and, therefore, most measures are aimed at removal of the drug from the GI tract. Parenteral self-administration of drugs is less common. Most ingested drugs will have left the stomach within the first four hours[18]; however, some drugs may in themselves directly decrease or inhibit gastric and intestinal motility thereby vastly prolonging the period of time in which there is potential access to the drug in the stomach. This is particularly true for glutethimide and salicylates and, in fact, may account for the fluctuating levels of consciousness observed with glutethimide. As there is no specific interval after drug ingestion that makes recovery of drug from the stomach unlikely,[19] it is wise to give serious consideration to lavage or emesis in all suspected drug overdoses.

Lavage

Lavage and emesis can be effective in removing drugs contained in the stomach; however, both are associated with significant risks of pulmonary aspiration and esophageal rupture. It is of vital importance to assess the patient's airway and their ability to protect their airway before undertaking lavage or inducing emesis. If there is any doubt as to the patient's ability to protect their airway, it is imperative that a cuffed endotracheal tube be placed prior to attempting lavage or induction of emesis. In patients with adequate airway protection reflexes, it is important to continually reassess these reflexes during the period of lavage or emesis. The patient may lose this ability to protect their airway with time if the drug concentration in the brain is still rising. Introduction of large volumes of fluid to the stomach will promote emptying of the stomach into the intestine and, therefore, should be avoided.[20] Lavage should be undertaken with small volumes or via double lumen tubes that allow continuous drainage while fluid is being introduced into the stomach. Lavaging should be continued until such time as the fluid returned is clear of any drug or food particles. Lavaging with tap water can lead to water intoxication but there is only a minimal risk of increasing gastric emptying, which occurs more readily with large volumes of isotonic fluids. If large volumes of lavage fluid are required, body-temperature saline is probably the wisest fluid to use. Gastroscopy offers an additional means of identifying and removing tablets and drug masses from the stomach.

Emesis

Many emetics have been described, although most are associated with toxicity of their own and probably should be avoided.[21] Syrup of ipecac and apomorphine are effective in emptying the stomach and are the agents of choice for the induction of emesis.[22, 23] Apomorphine may be associated with hypoventilation and sedation due to central depression. The effects of central depression can be antagonized with naloxone. A common misconception in relation to the use of emetics is that large volumes of fluid should be given to the patient to enhance emesis. Administration of fluid does not enhance vomiting[24] and may in itself promote emptying of the stomach and, therefore, should be avoided.[20] Emetics are safer to use in children than adults and are generally more effective than lavage because of the technical difficulties of lavage in small children.

Adsorbents

The administration of an adsorbent to a patient is probably safer and is at least as effective as emetics.[25, 26, 27] Charcoal is the principal adsorbent used and will effectively decrease absorption from the gut of most drugs with the exception of organic solvents and inorganic salts.[28] It may be necessary to repeat the administration of adsorbent in patients who have taken drugs excreted in bile and returned to the gut or in patients who have active metabolites excreted in bile. Cathartics such as castor oil or osmotic cathartics are less effective than adsorbents in preventing absorption of drugs from the gut and will decrease the efficacy of activated charcoal.[29, 30]

Enhancing Removal of Drugs

Specific measures aimed at hastening elimination of the drug include forced diuresis, dialysis, hemoperfusion, exchange transfusion, and the use of antibodies.

Many drugs are excreted in the urine, and forced diuresis may facilitate drug removal. It is important to remember, however, that the efficacy of diuresis is limited by renal perfusion and it may be necessary to enhance renal perfusion with a dopamine infusion. Osmotic diuretics are effective in increasing the excretion of barbiturates, salicylates, and phencyclidine, whereas the efficacy of furosemide and thiazides have not yet been established.[2] The degree of drug ionization is in some instances a function of urinary pH. Alkalinization of the urine can enhance renal clearance of some drugs, particularly barbiturates and salicylic acid. Acidification of the urine generally enhances excretion of basic substances such as phencyclidine, amphetamine, and quinidine.

Peritoneal dialysis is generally ineffective in clearing drugs because the rate of exchange of dialysis fluid is slow, and peritoneal blood flow and diffusion of drug across the peritoneum is not great. Hypertonic dialysis and alkaline dialysis can enhance peritoneal removal of some drugs but have associated risks.[31]

Hemodialysis is considerably more effective than peritoneal dialysis. Provided the patient's BP is adequate, it is the preferred method for removing drugs by dialysis. Drugs with high lipid solubility may be more effectively Dialyzed out by employing a lipid dialysate; however, the data to substantiate this claim are not strong.[31, 32, 33]

Hemoperfusion against an adsorbent is usually more effective than hemodialysis. Hemoperfusion employing oil, hydrocarbons, charcoal, and other resins has the advantage of increasing the surface area of contact between blood and the sorbent. For most drugs charcoal hemoperfusion is approximately twice as effective as aqueous hemodialysis and half as effective as XAD-4 resin hemoperfusion.[31, 34, 35] Charcoal and resin hemoperfusion cartridges will also adsorb platelets and white cells, an undesirable effect that may be controlled with administration of thromboxane and prostacyclin. Anuria constitutes an important indication for hemoperfusion as it may represent the only possible means of eliminating the drug.

Exchange transfusion may be useful in clearing drugs in small children but is of little value in adults. Specific antibodies to individual drugs administered intravenously bind the drug and the antibody-drug complex is then excreted, thereby greatly enhancing removal of a drug from the blood.[2] Unfortunately, there are very few specific drug antibodies presently available.

Techniques to enhance removal of the drug from the blood are probably most effective if implemented early during the phase of rising blood concentration secondary to absorption of drug from the gut. The more aggressive forms of management such as hemodialysis or hemoperfusion probably should be used in patients who have taken very large doses of drugs or who have high blood concentrations of drug.

Antagonizing Drug Effects

Specific antidotes can be given in cases of overdose with certain agents. These antidotes are given to (1) modify drug metabolism, (2) antagonize drug actions, e.g., opioids, cholinergic agents, or (3) bind or chelate drugs and their metabolites, e.g., cyanide, heavy metals. Some of the more commonly encountered toxic substances and their antidotes are listed in Table

TABLE 5–1.

AGENT	ANTIDOTE
Acetaminophen	Sulfates, dimercaprol, methionine, N-acetyl cysteine
Acid, corrosive	Weak alkali
Alkali, caustic	Weak alkali
Alkaloids	Potassium permanganate
Amphetamine	Phenothiazine
Anticoagulants, oral	Phytonadione
Atropine	Physostigmine, pilocarpine
Cholinesterase inhibitors	Atropine sulfate, pralidoxime
Cocaine	Propranolol
Codeine	Naloxone
Coumadin derivatives	Phytonadione
Cyanide	Sodium thiosulfate, hydroxycobalamin
Diazepam	Physostigmine
Ethylene glycol	Ethyl alcohol
Heparin	Protamine sulfate
Heroin	Naloxone
Meperidine	Naloxone
Methadone	Naloxone
Methyl alcohol	Ethyl alcohol
Morphine	Naloxone
Opium alkaloids	Naloxone
Phenothiazine tranquilizers	Diphenhydramine
Physostigmine	Potassium permanganate
Scopolamine	Physostigmine
Tricyclic antidepressants	Physostigmine

5–1. For a more comprehensive list of drug and toxin antidotes, the reader is referred to the work of Arena.[1, 3] Modifications of drug metabolism may prevent the formation of toxic metabolites, hasten the production of harmless metabolites, or bind and inactivate toxic metabolites.

PROGNOSIS

With appropriate supportive, specific therapy and good general nursing care, the prognosis in most instances of drug overdose is good. Almost all patients will survive poisoning with therapeutic drugs if they reach the hospital alive. Measurement of serum drug concentrations or EEG studies have little or no prognostic value.[36] Elderly patients or those with significant cardiorespiratory disease will not tolerate a period of coma as well as a younger, healthier individual and therefore warrant greater consideration for more aggressive therapy.

As drug overdose is frequently a result of suicidal intent, the long-term outlook for these patients is poor. Adults who have previously attempted to kill themselves have a 4–20 fold increase in their predicted death rates as a result of further suicide attempts.[2, 37] Psychiatric care will reduce the incidence of repeated suicide attempts[38] and it has been shown that such care can be as effectively delivered by general physicians as by psychiatrists.[39]

CASE STUDY 1

A 38-year-old white male was admitted to the emergency room after he had been found unresponsive and cyanotic on the floor of his apartment following a call from his estranged wife. She had not been able to contact him for 24 hours after he had threatened to take an overdose of Glutethimide. He had a past history of chronic sedative abuse and two previous episodes of deliberate sedative drug overdose. On examination he was well developed and well nourished but unresponsive to deep pain. Pulse rate was 120/min, BP 140/60 mm Hg, and the RR was 50/min and shallow. Pupils were at midpoint and sluggishly reactive to light. No nystagmus was noted. Examination of the chest revealed coarse rhonchi bilaterally, though it was more marked on the right than the left. Heart rate was regular, heart sounds normal, and no S_3 S_4, or murmurs were heard. The abdomen was scaphoid and had hypoactive bowel sounds. Peripheral perfusion was adequate.

Examination of the skin revealed multiple areas of pressure necrosis over the ankles and elbows. Evaluation of the airway demonstrated obtunded protective reflexes. The initial arterial blood gas obtained in the emergency room on room air revealed a pH of 7.40, a P_{CO_2} of 36 mm Hg, and a P_{O_2} of 41 mm Hg.

Discussion

Two immediate problems have been identified by initial evaluation: (1) lack of airway protection and (2) severe hypoxemia. Airway protection must be provided by intubation with a cuffed endotracheal tube prior to initiation of any specific therapy. The most likely explanation of the hypoxemia is pulmonary aspiration. The patient should receive oxygen therapy and further pulmonary evaluation concomitantly with specific therapy for the drug overdose.

Case Study Continued

A cuffed endotracheal tube was passed nasally, 50% oxygen given, and gastric lavage with activated charcoal initiated. Lavage returned greenish material consistent with Glutethimide tablets. A chest x-ray was obtained which showed a right basilar infiltrate. The patient was admitted to the intensive care unit and placed on 5 cm H_2O CPAP with a FI_{O_2} of 50%. Arterial blood gas analysis revealed a pH of 7.41, a PCO_2 of 36 mm Hg, and a PO_2 of 60 mm Hg. Routine laboratory tests revealed normal serum electrolytes and hemoglobin concentration and a WBC of 18,000/ mm^{-3}. Fiberoptic bronchoscopy was performed and copious yellow-green secretions were observed in the right lower and middle lobes. No particulate matter was identified. Secretions were suctioned during the bronchoscopy, and following bronchoscopy a chest physical-therapy treatment was given to the patient. Repeat arterial blood gases following these interventions revealed a pH of 7.44, a PCO_2 of 32 mm Hg, and a PO_2 of 73 mm Hg with a FI_{O_2} of 0.5.

Discussion

Aspiration is a frequently encountered cause of morbidity in patients following sedative drug overdose. Not all aspirations are associated with an infective pneumonitis (see Chapter 8); however, the nature of the secretions seen on bronchoscopy in conjunction with an elevated WBC strongly suggest a pneumonia. A sputum culture and sensitivity should be performed prior to commencing antibiotic therapy. The patient may have developed a pneumonia due to secondary bacterial infection superimposed on either the chemically induced lung injury of aspiration or because of hypostasis and retention of pulmonary secretions.

A bronchoscopy was performed to determine whether the patient had aspirated drug masses. If aspirated particles of large size are found, consideration needs to be given to repeat the bronchoscopy with a rigid bronchoscope to remove these particles. Chest physical therapy is indicated to facilitate the suctioning and removal of retained secretions.

Case Study Continued

Gram staining and a culture of the aspirated sputum revealed a *pseudomonas* organism and the patient was started on appropriate antibiotic therapy. The patient's condition stabilized. He maintained good urine output and was maintained on 5 cm H_2O CPAP with an $F_{I_{O_2}}$ of 0.5 and continued to receive antibiotic and chest physical therapy. His arterial oxygenation steadily improved and the $F_{I_{O_2}}$ was decreased to 40%. Fourteen hours later arterial blood gases revealed a pH of 7.43, a P_{CO_2} of 36 mm Hg, and a P_{O_2} of 78 mm Hg with a $F_{I_{O_2}}$ of 40%. Eight hours later the patient was still unconscious but now responded to noxious stimuli. Twelve hours later the patient regained consciousness.

Discussion

Glutethimide intoxication may be associated with the clinical phenomenon of waxing and waning levels of consciousness. This phenomenon may be due to one of several mechanisms. First, glutethimide prolongs gastric emptying time, and drug masses in the GI tract may break down releasing more drug for absorption. This can cause a consequent secondary rise in serum and subsequently in brain drug concentration. Second, the drug may be metabolized to a pharmacologically active metabolite that in itself will depress CNS function. Third, the primary drug or an active metabolite may be excreted in the bile and, hence, be returned to the GI tract and reabsorbed; a process termed enterohepatic recirculation. Finally, highly lipid-soluble drugs will accumulate in fatty tissues in large concentrations. They will be released into the serum following an acute reduction in serum concentration secondary to dialysis or hemoperfusion, resulting in a secondary rise in serum concentration. Therefore, consideration has to be given to the possibility that this patient may relapse into unconsciousness with possible loss of ability to protect his airway. If the patient is tolerating the endotracheal tube, the wisest course of action is to leave the patient intubated for a further 4 to 8 hours. In the event that the endotracheal tube is not being tolerated, the patient can be extubated, maintained on nil per mouth, and frequently reevaluated with respect to level of consciousness and ability to protect his airway.

Case Study Continued

The patient was not tolerating the endotracheal tube and was extubated. Following extubation while receiving 40% oxygen via face mask, arterial blood gas analysis revealed a pH of 7.42, a P_{CO_2} of 34 mm Hg, and a P_{O_2} of 77 mm Hg.

The patient did not lose consciousness again and his pneumonia resolved over the next two days. He was subsequently transferred from the intensive care unit to the psychiatric ward for long-term management of his drug abuse problem and suicidal tendencies.

CASE STUDY 2

A 24-year-old female was brought to the emergency room by her roommate after she had been found confused and barely rousable. An empty medication vial marked codeine was found by the patient's bedside. The patient's friend volunteered the information that the patient had recently broken off her engagement with her boyfriend. She was not aware of any previous suicide attempts on the part of her friend.

On examination the patient was noted to be a well nourished female of approximately 55 kg weight who was obtunded but could be aroused with difficulty. Her RR and vт were 8/min and 300 ml respectively. Heart rate was 60/min and regular BP was 90/60 mm Hg. An arterial blood sample was sent for blood gas analysis and the patient given 40% oxygen to breathe via an air entrainment mask. While awaiting the results of blood gas analysis, further examination showed pinpoint pupils which reacted sluggishly to light. Tendon reflexes were symmetrically depressed. The patient showed none of the stigmata of IV drug abuse. The rest of the examination revealed a sluggish gag reflex and hypoactive bowel sounds but no other demonstrable abnormalities. Arterial blood gas analysis revealed a pH of 7.28, a PCO_2 of 55 mm Hg, and a PO_2 of 65 mm Hg ($FI_{O_2} = 0.21$). An IV line was established and 0.4 mg of Naloxone administered by slow IV injection. The patient's level of consciousness improved and her RR increased to 18/min with a vт of 420 ml. Pulse rate was 85/min and regular and BP was 110/60 mm Hg. The patient was hostile and refused to answer questions. Repeat arterial blood gas analysis at this time on 40% oxygen revealed a pH of 7.38, a PCO_2 of 45 mm Hg, and a PO_2 of 170 mm Hg. The oxygen mask was bothering the patient and was replaced with a nasal cannula with an oxygen flow of 2 L/min. Routine laboratory investigations revealed a normal serum chemistry and blood count. The chest x-ray was normal. The patient was now adequately protecting her airway. A nasogastric tube was placed and the aspirate contained white material consistent with codeine tablets. Gastric lavage with saline was performed and activated charcoal administered. The patient was transferred to the intensive care unit for observation and further evaluation.

Discussion

The single most important aspect of management in acute narcotic overdose is cardiopulmonary support. Direct respiratory center depression will result in hypoventilation and acute ventilatory failure. It is imperative that blood gas analysis be performed to assess the adequacy of alveolar ventilation and that ventilatory support be provided when indicated until the respiratory depression can be reversed with a narcotic antagonist. The cardiovascular effects of narcotic overdose include bradycardia and hypotension. The hypotension is secondary to venodilatation and will respond to administration of IV fluids and usually will reverse following administration of a narcotic antagonist. In this patient the degree of hypoventilation and hypotension were such that it was appropriate to administer an antagonist as a primary step. If the degree of CNS obtundation had been greater, then mechanical ventilatory support would have to have been initiated as a primary step. The safest way to provide this is by endotracheal intubation with a cuffed endotracheal tube and ventilation with a manual resuscitation bag or a mechanical ventilator.

Naloxone is the narcotic antagonist of choice as it has little intrinsic narcotic activity. It is important to remember that the duration of action of the narcotic may exceed that of the antagonist and that repeat doses of antagonist may be required. For this reason, patients should be closely monitored for evidence of renarcotization for at least 12 hours. The other problem that may be encountered with the administration of a narcotic antagonist is acute narcotic withdrawal. This is usually seen in individuals who habitually take narcotics. This patient showed none of the stigmata associated with chronic narcotic abuse and, hence, withdrawal phenomena were not anticipated. Lavage is helpful only in removing unabsorbed drug, thereby limiting any further rise in serum and brain drug concentration.

Case Study Continued

The patient's friend who had returned to their apartment telephoned to report finding an empty container of a proprietary preparation of acetaminophen in the bathroom. She did not know how many tablets had been in the bottle. Repeat questioning of the patient confirmed that she had taken these tablets in addition to the codeine. She denied taking any other medications, substances, or alcohol. Blood was immediately sent to the toxicology laboratory for measurement of acetaminophen concentration. Two grams of methionine were immediately administered to the patient orally and orders were written to repeat this every 4 hours for a total of 4 doses. The patient's serum acetaminophen concentration was 120 mg/L. Blood was sent for measurement of serum bilirubin, enzymes, albumin, methemoglobin, and a coagulation profile. Urine was sent for measurement of hemoglobin. Serum bilirubin, enzymes, albumin, and coagulation studies were all normal. The urine contained no hemoglobin and serum methemoglobin concentration was 1.5% of total hemoglobin.

Discussion

Acetaminophen is a commonly used analgesic marketed as a safe alternative to aspirin. Unfortunately, it is anything but safe when used in larger doses. Five grams will produce liver damage and 10 gm may be lethal.[2] The toxicity of the drug is related to its metabolites. Normal metabolism of acetaminophen by mixed-function oxidase systems results in the formation of a highly reactive compound that binds to liver cell proteins, thereby disrupting hepatic function. These metabolites are normally bound to the sulfhydral group of glutathione which renders them harmless. Overdose of acetaminophen, induction of the oxidase enzymes, or depletion of glutathione may all result in the formation of larger amounts of these toxic metabolites and produce liver damage.

Other than nausea, there are no early signs or symptoms of acetaminophen intoxication. This is one circumstance where the toxicology laboratory is of paramount importance as hepatotoxicity is accurately predicted by serum concentration of acetaminophen. Concentrations >200 mg/L 4 hours after ingestion or 80 mg/L 12 hours after ingestion will be associated with hepatotoxicity.[2] The half-life of acetaminophen is approximately 2½ hours, though this can be prolonged by liver damage to 7–8 hours.

Active therapy aimed at reducing the concentration of toxic metabolites will effectively prevent liver damage if initiated promptly. Administration of sulfate will enhance conjugation of acetaminophen. The preferred and more effective approach is to increase the availability of sulfhydral groups to bind these metabolites. Methionine, N-acetylcysteine, or cysteamine are useful. Untreated acetaminophen poisoning will result in liver damage in 70% of patients, while prompt administration of methionine will reduce the incidence to 10%.[2] There may be slight toxicity due to the antidote, which includes nausea and vomiting or rashes. Administration of an antidote is the cornerstone of therapy; however, activated charcoals and lavage are indicated to reduce further absorption of drug.

Other problems that may be encountered in acetaminophen overdose include hemolysis and rarely the formation of methemoglobin. Hemolysis is more frequently encountered in chronic abuse of the drug but may occur in an acute overdose in individuals with red blood cell glucose-6-phosphate dehydrogenase deficiency.

Case Study Continued

Three hours after the initial dose of Naloxone, the patient was noted to be more somnolent and a second dose of 0.2 mg Naloxone was given IV, which resulted in a prompt improvement in level of consciousness. Serum acetaminophen concentration measured 4 hours after the initial measurement was 50 mg/L. Treatment with methionine was completed as originally ordered. No further problems developed and the patient was transferred from the intensive care unit to the psychiatric unit 24 hours later.

REFERENCES

1. Arena J.M.: The treatment of poisoning. *Clin. Symp.* Vol 3–38, 1978.
2. Thompson W.L.: Poisoning: The twentieth century black death, in Shoemaker W.C., Thompson L. (eds.): *Critical Care State of the Art.* Chapter N, Society of Critical Care Medicine, California, 1980.
3. Arena A.M.: Poisoning: Toxicology-symptoms-treatment. 4th ed. Springfield, IL, Charles C. Thomas, 1978.
4. Ungerleider J.T., Lundberg G.B., Sunshine I., et al.: The drug abuse warning network (DAWN) program: toxilogic verification of 1,008 emergency room "mentions." *Arch. Gen. Psych.* 37:106–109, 1980.
5. Robertson J.: The epidemiology of self-poisoning. *Public Health* 91:75–82, 1977.
6. McIntire M.S., Angle C.R.: The taxonomy of suicide as seen in poison control centers. *Pediatr. Clin. North Am.* 597–706, 1970.
7. McIntire M.S., Angle C.R.: "Suicide" as seen in poison control centers. *Pediatrics* 48:914–922, 1971.
8. Vale J.A.: The epidemiology of acute poisoning. *Acta Pharmacol. Toxicol.* (Suppl.) 41:443–458, 1977.
9. Graham J.D.P., Hitchens R.A.N., Marshall R.W., et al.: Self-poisoning—a decennial survey from Cardiff. *Public Health* 93:223–229, 1979.
10. Proudfoot A.T., Park J.: Changing pattern of drugs used for self-poisoning. *Br. Med. J.* 1:90–93, 1978.
11. White H.C.: Self-poisoning in adolescents. *Br. J. Psychiatry* 124:24–35, 1974.
12. McIntire M.S., Angle C.R.: Psychological "biopsy" in self-poisoning of children and adolescents. *Am. J. Dis. Child* 126:42–46, 1973.
13. Bancroft J., Skrimshire A., Casson J., et al.: People who deliberately poison or injure themselves: Their problems and their contacts with helping agencies. *Psychol. Med.* 7:289–303, 1977.
14. Plum F., Posner J.B.: *The Diagnosis of Stupor and Coma,* ed. 2. Philadelphia, F.A. Davis, Co., 1972.
15. Qirbi A.A., Poznanski W.J.: Emergency toxicology in a general hospital. *Can. Med. Assoc. J.* 116:884–888, 1977.
16. Bobik A., McLean A.J.: Drug analysis in the overdosed patient: Its application to clinical toxicology. *Med. J. Aust.* 1:367–369, 1977.
17. Wiltbank T.B., Sine H.E., Brody B.B.: Are emergency toxicology measurements really used? *Clin. Chem.* 20:116–118, 1974.
18. Nimmo W.S.: Drugs, diseases and altered gastric emptying. *Clin. Pharmacokinet.* 1:189–203, 1976.
19. Blake D.R., Bramble M.G., Evans J.G.: Is there excessive use of gastric lavage in the treatment of self-poisoning? *Ann. Intern Med.* 87:721–722, 1977.
20. Henderson M.L., Piccioni A.L., Chin L.: Evaluation of oral dilution as a first aid measure in poisoning. *J. Pharm. Sci.* 55:1311–1313, 1966.
21. Manno B.R., Manno J.E.: Toxicology of ipecac: A review. *Clin. Toxicol.* 10:221–242, 1977.
22. Corby D.G., Decker W.J., Moran M.J., et al.: Clinical comparison of pharmacologic emetics in children. *Pediatrics* 42:361–364, 1968.
23. MacLean W.C., Jr.: A comparison of ipecac syrup and apomorphine in the immediate treatment of ingestion of poisons. *J. Pediatr.* 82:121–124, 1973.
24. Friday K.L., Powell S.H., Thompson W.L., et al.: Emetics in poisoned dogs: Efficacy independent of ingested volume. *Crit. Care Med.* 8:233, 1980.
25. Lipscomb D.J., Widdop B.: Studies with activated charcoal in the treatment of drug overdosage using the pig as an animal model. *Arch. Toxicol.* 34:37–46, 1975.
26. Decker W.J.: In quest of emesis: Fact, fable and fancy. *Clin. Toxicol.* 4:383–387, 1971.
27. Chin L.: Induced emesis—a questionable procedure for the treatment of acute poisoning. *Ariz. Med.* 30:28–30, 1973.

28. Greensher J., Mofenson H.C., Piccioni A.L., et al.: Activated charcoal updated. *J.A.C.E.P.* 8:261–263, 1979.
29. Powell S.H., Van deGraaff W.B., Thompson W.L., et al.: Charcoals, emetics and cathartics in care of poisoned patients. *Crit. Care Med.* 8:233, 1980.
30. Scholtz E.C., Jaffe J.M., Colaizzi J.L.: Evaluation of five activated charcoal formulations for inhibition of aspirin absorption and palatability in man. *Am. J. Hosp. Pharm.* 35:1355–1359, 1978.
31. Winchester J.F., Gelfand M.C., Knepshield J.H., et al.: Dialysis and hemoperfusion of poisons and drugs—update. *Trans. Am. Soc. Artif. Intern. Organs* 23:762–842, 1977.
32. von Hartitzch B., Pinto M.H., Mauer S.M., et al.: Treatment of glutethimide intoxication: An *in vitro* comparison of lipid aqueous and peritoneal dialysis with albumin. *Proc. Clin. Dial. Transplant Forum* 3:102, 1973.
33. Kopelman R., Miller S., Kelly R., et al.: Camphor intoxication treated by resin hemoperfusion. *J.A.M.A.* 241:727–728, 1979.
34. Winchester J.F., Gelfand M.C., Knepshield J.H., et al.: Present and future uses of hemoperfusion with sorbents. *Artif. Organs* 2:353–358, 1978.
35. Winchester J.F., Gelfand M.C., Tilstone W.J.: Hemoperfusion in drug intoxication: Clinical and laboratory aspects. *Drug Metab. Rev.* 8:69–104, 1978.
36. Bird T.D., Plum F.: Recovery from barbiturate overdose coma with a prolonged isoelectric electroencephalogram. *Neurology* 18:456–460, 1968.
37. Lonnqvist J., Niskanen P., Achte K.A., et al.: Self-poisoning with follow-up considerations. *Suicide* 5:39–46, 1975.

6 / Smoke Inhalation

PAUL S. MESNICK, M.D.

SMOKE INHALATION

Injury to the pulmonary system by inhalation of thermal gaseous or particulate products of combustion is generically referred to as *smoke inhalation*. The United States has the highest rate of fire deaths among the industrialized nations that record fire statistics. The majority of these deaths are attributed to asphyxia and the inhaled products of combustion.[1] The synergistic lethal relationship between body surface area burn and pulmonary injury secondary to smoke inhalation is well documented. The chemical and particulate nature of a specific fire produces a potential complexity of direct and indirect effects on the pulmonary system that frequently makes it impossible to determine the specific nature of an airway or pulmonary injury.[2] Smoke inhalation may be considered in terms of immediate manifestations (carbon monoxide poisoning, airway injury, and lung burn) occurring within minutes to hours and the delayed effects occurring within days to weeks.

EARLY MANIFESTATIONS OF SMOKE INHALATION

Carbon monoxide poisoning and the onset of upper airway obstruction are the earliest and most life-threatening problems associated with smoke inhalation. The toxic, gaseous products of combustion include numerous pulmonary irritants which may produce bronchoconstriction and various degrees of non-cardiogenic pulmonary edema, which may occur hours after the initial exposure.

Carbon Monoxide Poisoning

Smoke inhalation may be considered a form of carbon monoxide poisoning complicated by the addition of gaseous and particulate materials of combustion superimposing their direct and indirect chemical effects upon the pulmonary system. Carbon monoxide gas is a product of incomplete hydrocarbon combustion that lacks a characteristic odor. It is tasteless and non-irritating. Clinical and experimental data indicate that carboxyhemoglobin levels measured shortly after injury are proportional to an inhaled dose of smoke.[3, 18, 19]

Inhaled carbon monoxide combines readily with hemoglobin to form carboxyhemoglobin (HbCO), a compound 210 times more stable than normal oxyhemoglobin. Not only does HbCO diminish the blood's oxygen carrying capacity, it also shifts the oxygen dissociation curve (Fig 6–1) to the left which means the "unloading" of oxygen at the tissue level is impaired. It is important to realize that in the presence of an arterial PO_2 above 80 mm Hg, the available hemoglobin moieties (those not saturated with carbon monoxide) will be fully saturated with oxygen. Tissue hypoxia may occur because the hemoglobin is less capable of "giving up" oxygen to the tissues.

The peripheral chemoreceptors (aortic and carotid bodies) respond chiefly to deficits in arterial oxygen tensions rather than to arterial oxygen content. A patient suffering from carbon monoxide poisoning usually has an adequate arterial PO_2 and therefore may not have a cardiopulmonary response to tissue hypoxia until lactic acidemia occurs.[4, 5]

In addition to the well documented effects of carbon monoxide on oxygen transport and delivery, a number of studies suggest that carbon monoxide may have a disrupting effect on cellular oxidative metabolism by interfering with the function of intracellular cytochrome oxidase systems.[6, 7] This may account for occasional discrepancies between the severity of the patient's clinical status and the measured level of blood carboxyhemoglobin.

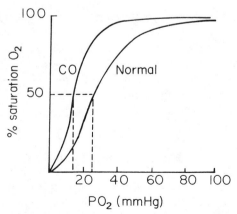

Fig 6–1.—Hemoglobin:oxygen dissociation curve showing leftward shift of curve for HbCO. CO = carbon monoxide.

DIAGNOSIS OF CO POISONING

The clinical diagnosis of carbon monoxide poisoning is usually based on a history of exposure to smoke or exhaust fumes. The classical textbook description of "cherry red" facial coloration is rarely seen in clinical practice. The milder symptoms of carbon monoxide poisoning, e.g., headache, nausea, fatigue and occasional breathlessness (Table 6–1) are rarely seen below carboxyhemoglobin levels of 15%. Symptoms of confusion, disorientation, and dizziness are seen in patients who remain in contaminated atmospheres after initial symptoms develop.

Carbon monoxide manifests its effects primarily on the CNS by producing a stupor that leads to an eventual loss of consciousness and death. Various phases of disorientation, athetosis, and paresis have all been reported.[8, 9, 10] Of course, tissue hypoxia secondary to carbon monoxide poisoning may cause irreversible damage and further aggravate preexisting cardiovascular or cerebrovascular disease.

The definitive diagnosis of carbon monoxide poisoning is accomplished by measurement of the percent of total hemoglobin that is saturated with carbon monoxide, i.e., carboxyhemoglobin (HbCO). These levels are readily determined by a multiple band spectrophotometer such as the IL 232 Co-Oximeter, an instrument that should be available in any appropriately equipped laboratory providing blood gas measurements. An HbCO >20% is usually considered carbon monoxide poisoning. Because most smoke inhalation victims are receiving oxygen therapy prior to their arrival at the

TABLE 6–1.—CO POISONING SIGNS,
SYMPTOMS WITH % HbCO

HbCO %	SIGNS and SYMPTOMS
0–10	None
10–20	Tightness across forehead; slight headache; dilatation of cutaneous blood vessels
20–30	Throbbing headache
40–50	As above with possibility of syncope; increased respiratory and pulse rates
50–60	Syncope; increased respiratory and pulse rates; coma with intermittent convulsions; Cheyne-Stokes respiration
60–70	Coma with intermittent convulsions; depressed cardiovascular and respiratory function; possible death
70–80	Weak pulse, slow respiratory rates; respiratory failure and death

hospital, an HbCO level >40% assumes the patient has had a severe exposure. It is at these levels >40% HbCO that the more severe neurologic sequelae of ataxia, cortical blindness, and behavioral disturbances manifest themselves. Levels in excess of 50% HbCO may produce irreversible CNS damage.

The use of a pH-PO_2 nomogram to calculate an assumed oxyhemoglobin (HbO_2) saturation will be totally misleading in the presence of significant HbCO because the nomogram assumes all hemoglobin is either reduced or saturated with oxygen. When the HbO_2 is measured, the diagnosis of carbon monoxide poisoning may be suggested by the presence of a significantly lower oxyhemoglobin saturation than would be predicted from the arterial PO_2 level. In other words, a discrepancy between expected HbO_2 and measured HbO_2 may be due to the presence of HbCO.

Arterial PCO_2 may be normal, decreased, or elevated in carbon monoxide poisoning depending on the patient's CNS, pulmonary, and acid base status. Severely poisoned patients frequently exhibit a lactic acidemia secondary to tissue hypoxia. The resulting metabolic acidemia frequently stimulates minute ventilation and a lower than normal $PaCO_2$ is then produced.

TREATMENT OF CO POISONING

The definitive treatment of carbon monoxide poisoning is to facilitate elimination of the gas via the lungs. Because the hemoglobin affinity for carbon monoxide is so great, less than 2 mm Hg PCO will result in greater than 50% HbCO. This means that even after the victim is removed from the carbon monoxide source and the alveolar PCO approaches zero, there is an extremely small carbon monoxide tension gradient from blood to alveolar gas. The elimination of carbon monoxide results in an exponentially decreasing HbCO level that is most commonly referred to as "HbCO half-life." The HbCO half-life when breathing room air is approximately 5 hours, i.e., a 30% HbCO will be reduced to approximately 15% in 5 hours and approximately 7% in another 5 hours when breathing room air at one atmosphere.

Since oxygen competes with carbon monoxide for the same sites on the hemoglobin molecule, increased arterial oxygen tensions mean that increased numbers of dissolved oxygen molecules are competing for the hemoglobin sites occupied by carbon monoxide. This competitive factor of an increased arterial PO_2 is so significant that breathing 100% oxygen at one atmosphere will change the HbCO half-life to approximately 1 hour. Thus, *increasing the arterial PO_2 is the single most important factor in carbon monoxide elimination.* Severe cases of carbon monoxide poisoning, especially in the obtunded, unconscious, or chronic lung disease patient may require endotracheal intubation and mechanical ventilation to safely increase the arterial Po_2 maximally.

The use of the hyperbaric oxygen chamber is a useful therapeutic tool in the rapid elimination of carbon monoxide since arterial Po_2s greater than 1,500 mm Hg can be achieved.[11, 12] Its use remains controversial in circumstances that require hospital transfer or ambulance bypass of closer emergency medical care facilities. The use of a hyperbaric facility may be considered for the more severe cases of carbon monoxide poisoning or those cases that fail to respond appropriately to treatment; however, definitive evidence of an improved prognosis following the use of hyperbaric oxygenation is lacking.

Airway Injury

The efficient heat exchange and cooling mechanisms of the upper airway are highly protective of subglottic structures under most circumstances. An exception is the inhalation of hot steam which contains 4,000 times the heat capacity of air.[13] However, there is little or no protection for the glottis and supraglottic structures—explaining why the most immediate threat to life from thermal injury is typically tissue edema in the region of the hypopharynx. The presence of progressive hoarseness or stridor, especially when it appears in the first two hours, must be carefully evaluated and followed. Tissue edema may be further aggravated by the infusion of large volumes of resuscitative fluids required with large surface area burns. Burns of the tongue are particularly hazardous.

Early endotracheal intubation may be required to prevent a significant compromise of an obstructing airway. This should be accomplished as expeditiously and atraumatically as possible. It is important to contemplate the intervention well in advance before a life-threatening obstruction occurs. Emergency cricothyroidotomy or tracheostomy is best reserved for cases in which intubation is not possible because of hypopharyngeal edema or other factors.[14] Tracheostomy is best performed electively once control of the airway has been gained by placement of an endotracheal tube. In addition to thermal injury, the various gaseous and particulate products of combustion produce a wide range of chemical components that either separately or in combination cause airway irritability and obstructive symptoms (Table 6–2). Tissue reaction of the pulmonary mucosa results in impaired mucociliary action and cellular sloughing that creates an accumulation of epithelial debris and secretions. Inflammation, retained secretion, bronchospasm, and hemorrhage may combine and interact to compromise both central and peripheral airways.[15, 16]

TABLE 6–2.—TOXIC PRODUCTS OF COMBUSTION

SUBSTANCE BURNED	TOXIC PRODUCTS
Wood, cotton, paper	Acrolein, acetaldehyde, formaldehyde, acetic acid, formic acid
Petroleum products	Acrolein, acetic acid, formic acid
Melamine resins	Ammonia, hydrogen cyanide
Nitrocellulose film	Oxides of nitrogen, acetic acid, formic acid
Polyvinyl chloride	Hydrogen chloride, phosgene, chlorine
Polyurethane (nitrogen-containing compounds)	Isocyanate, hydrogen cyanide
Polyfluorocarbons	Octafluoroisobutylene

Lung Tissue Injury

The toxic constituents of smoke create a complex and still poorly understood series of interactions leading to profound tissue damage at the alveolar level. Modern office furnishings and construction materials include compounds capable of producing a wide range of toxic chemicals and gases upon combustion.[15, 20] A few of the various gases produced from combustion of modern synthetic polymers are hydrogencyanide, hydrochloric, sulfuric, acetic, and formic acids, phosgene, acrolein, and oxides of nitrogen and sulfur. These substances may directly destroy alveolar epithelium and indirectly damage capillary endothelium. Furthermore, the burn patient is susceptible to factors resulting in acute lung injury (see Chapter 12). The vigorous administration of resuscitative fluids required by the burn patient will increase water and colloid conductance across the capillaries due to increased permeability of the endothelium.[20, 21]

Fire-retardant materials are slow to ignite and burn, but they readily decompose in fires releasing gases of flourides, bromides, and iodides. These substances may actually produce sedative effects (bromides) and have anesthetic qualities that diminish the cough reflex and further allow corrosive acids and alkalies to invade the tracheobronchial tree.

LATE MANIFESTATIONS OF SMOKE INHALATION

The neurologic and behavioral complications of carbon monoxide poisoning are quite variable. A latent period of 1–9 days after apparent complete recovery may ensue before symptoms develop. Late sequelae of carbon monoxide poisoning are extensive and include mental retardation, personality changes, ataxia, parkinsonism, apraxia, dysphagia, and temporal-spatial forms of disorientation.

Bedside forced expiratory spirograms are useful as diagnostic aids in assessing obstructive and restrictive functions following smoke inhalation injury.[24, 25] Fiberoptic bronchoscopy affords a good evaluation of the cord structures, trachea, and large bronchi for erythema, hemorrhage, edema, soot, and ulceration, but it must be used with caution in the face of significant upper airway inflammation and edema.[25] Xenon perfusion-ventilation scanning may be useful in detecting early pulmonary damage subsequent to smoke inhalation several days before positive findings become apparent on the chest roentgenogram. False positive scans, especially in the face of preexisting lung disease, must be appreciated.[26, 27]

Pneumonias in the burn patient are usually secondary to nosocomial gram-negative bacteria and are often polymicrobial. Aspiration, hematogenous spread of bacteria from infected wounds, disruption of the normal tracheal muscosal protective barrier by introduction of endotracheal tubes or tracheostomy all provide portals of entry for opportunistic organisms. The compromised nutritional status and depression of the autoimmune system in the burn patient further aids the development of pneumonia and sepsis. The use of prophylactic antibiotics has not been shown to be beneficial in preventing bacterial pneumonias and may well "select out" drug resistant bacterial flora.[23]

Functional residual capacity may be increasingly compromised in burn patients by circumferential eschar formation and edema fluid about the thoracic and abdominal regions. Decompression by escharotomy will help improve functional residual capacity in these patients and guard against further restrictive pulmonary compromise. Some decompression may also be required because of chest wall edema developing within several days of the burn injury.

CASE STUDY

A 52-year-old building superintendent was brought to the emergency room at 10:45 a.m. as a result of a flash basement fire, which involved electrical insulating materials. He had been trapped in the basement for approximately 15 min prior to being rescued by the fire department. He was given oxygen on the scene and while being transferred to the hospital. He had a general history of good health except for occasional mild bronchitis. He smoked two packs of cigarettes a day for approximately 30 years.

Physical examination revealed a well developed, slightly obese, middle-aged white male. The patient appeared anxious and confused. His skin color was normal, but his face was covered with a sooty material. Vital signs showed a BP of 160/100 mm Hg, a pulse of 110/min, respirations 24/min, and a v_T of 400 ml. Auscultation of the patient's lungs demonstrated scattered rhonchi and occasional wheezes. His voice exhibited a mild degree of hoarseness, and no stridor was noted. Carbonaceous material was noted about his nasal passages and in his sputum. Superficial burns were present about the facial region. Indirect laryngoscopy revealed the pharyngeal mucosa to be erythematous and slightly edematous. The cords were not clearly visualized and no further attempts at instrumentation by other endoscopic techniques were carried out.

Laboratory data revealed normal serum electrolytes, a hemoglobin of 14.5 gm%, a hematocrit of 45%, and a WBC of 10,000/mm^{-3}. Arterial blood gases on 4 L/min of nasal oxygen showed a pH of 7.50, a P_{CO_2} of 22 mm Hg, a Pa_{O_2} of 90 mm Hg, a H_{CO_3} of 16.5 mEq/L, and a base deficit of -5 mEq/L. The Hb_{CO} level was 32% with a Hb_{O_2} of 66%. A "stat" chest x-ray was read as essentially normal with evidence of increased lung markings and some discoid atelectasis in the lower lobes. The ECG showed ST depression in leads II and V_{4-6}.

Discussion

A careful history to ascertain the nature and extent of the patient's exposure to smoke inhalation was appropriately attempted. Information as to the nature of confinement, intensity of exposure, and loss of consciousness are useful indicators of the extent of pulmonary injury. Unfortunately, initial accurate information is usually difficult to obtain owing to both the confusing nature of rescue activities and the often confused, obtunded, and otherwise impaired mental state of the victim.

Inspection of the facial area for evidence of burns or carbonaceous material about the nares, mouth, or oro-pharynx was carried out. The ventilatory pattern should be observed for regularity and ease of air movement and the chest auscultated for wheezes, rales, and rhonchi. Hoarseness of speech was noted and requires further scrutiny. This may be accomplished by repeated observation of airway status, indirect laryngoscopy, or direct laryngoscopy via fiberoptic laryngoscope or bronchoscope. A strong case may be made to avoid unnecessary instrumentation so that further tissue trauma is avoided.

The use of indirect laryngoscopy as carried out in this case may represent a reasonable compromise. Although it is difficult to clearly visualize the glottic structures with this technique, the hypopharynx can usually be well visualized with little risk of trauma. The decision not to proceed with further efforts to visualize the cords seems reasonable since significant oropharyngeal and posterior pharyngeal edema and mucosal damage is already present. The patient should be frequently examined for progressive airway compromise.

The Hb_{CO} of 32% confirms carbon monoxide poisoning. The arterial P_{O_2} of 90 mm Hg is inadequate treatment.

Case Study Continued

A #18 IV catheter was established in the left forearm and lactated Ringer's solution was administered. The patient was placed on a high flow oxygen system at an FI_{O_2} of 100%.

An arterial blood gas sample was obtained approximately one hour later and showed a pH of 7.46, a PCO_2 of 30 mm Hg, a PO_2 of 228 mm Hg, and a HbCO of 19%. The patient was more alert and better able to answer questions. He denied having lost consciousness at any time in the course of the fire.

Closer assessment of his upper airway demonstrated burned nasal hairs and slight oropharyngeal edema. The patient was transferred to the intensive care unit where an arterial line was established. A course of high dose steroids (Solumedrol 1 gm every 6 hours for 24 hours) was initiated. Respiratory therapy was begun and consisted of tapering oxygen therapy when the HbCO fell below 10% and using incentive spirometry and aerosolization therapy with racemic epinephrine every four hours. A gram stain of the sputum showed small carbon particles and polymorphonuclear leukocytes but no predominant organisms.

Throughout the first 24 hours the patient continued to cough up thin watery secretions. He complained of sore throat and continued to exhibit hoarseness without evidence of stridor or shortness of breath.

Discussion

The HbCO level responded as expected. The absence of progressive stridor and dyspnea is encouraging. Bronchodilators in parenteral or aerosolized form may prove useful in reducing bronchospasm. The use of agents such as racemic epinephrine in addition to bronchodilation may prove useful and effective as a mucosal decongestant and thereby relieve glottic edema early in the course of patient management. It should be realized that most commercially available inhalation bronchodilators do not contain decongestants. Humidification of inspired air by aerosol techniques such as ultrasonic rebulization may aid the patient by thinning inspissated mucoid secretions so he can cough them up.

The presence of a PaO_2 of 228 mm Hg on a high flow oxygen system at an FI_{O_2} of 100% may indicate the preexistence of pulmonary disease. This is certainly compatible with his history of heavy cigarette smoking. This must increase the concern for secondary complications such as bronchospasm, bronchitis and pneumonia. However, it must always be kept in mind that patients suffering from smoke inhalation often have a lowered arterial PaO_2 secondary to pulmonary injury and irritation due to the inhaled toxic constituents of smoke. This effect alone may account for or contribute to any and all of the above findings.

The use of prophylactic corticosteroids is controversial and is best reserved for specific indications such as glottic edema. Prophylactic antibiotics are not indicated (see Chapter 8 for further information on these topics).

Case Study Continued

After 24 hours in the intensive care unit, he still complained of throat soreness and difficulty swallowing. He was specifically examined for stridor on an hourly basis. Serial arterial blood gas measurements allowed for an initial reduction in his high flow oxygen therapy to an FI_{O_2} of 50%. At 24 hours post admission on an FI_{O_2} of 50%, he showed a pH of 7.44, a PCO_2 of 33 mm Hg, a PaO_2 of 140 mm Hg and a $HbCO$ of 3%. The FI_{O_2} was reduced to 30% with an arterial PO_2 of 80 mm Hg. Bedside spirometry was performed with his respiratory therapy treatments and showed a VT of 400 ml and a VC of 2.0 L. His mental status remained alert and orientated. His temperature was 97.3°F, pulse 82/min and regular, respirations 18/min, and BP 155/70 mm Hg.

Laboratory data showed his serum electrolytes to be within normal limits. His hematocrit was 46 and his WBC measured 12,700/mm^{-3}. Recorded fluids for the first 24 hours was 1,330 cc of fluid intake and 845 cc of output. His latest EKG showed resolution of the ST depression noted on admission.

The patient was discharged from the intensive care unit after 2 days and made an uneventful recovery.

REFERENCES

1. Gaston S.F., Schumann L.L.: Inhalation injury. *Am. J. Nurs.* p. 93, Jan. 1980.
2. Fein A., Leff A., Hopewell P.C.: Pathophysiology and management of the complications resulting from fire and the inhaled products of combustion: Review of the literature. *Crit. Care Med.* 8:94, 1980.
3. Kindwall E.P.: Carbon monoxide and cyanide poisoning, in Davis J.C., Hunt T.H. (eds.): *Hyperbaric Oxygen Therapy.* Bethesda, Undersea Medical Soc., 1977, chapter 13, pp. 177–190.
4. Chiodi H., Dill D.B., Consolagio F., et al.: Respiratory and circulatory responses to acute carbon monoxide poisoning. *Am. J. Physiol.* 134:683, 1941.
5. Beuhler J.H., et al.: Lactic acidosis from carboxyhemoglobinemia after smoke inhalation. *Ann. Intern. Med.* 82:803, 1975.
6. Goldbaum L.R., Ramirez R.G., Absalom K.B.: What is the mechanism of carbon monoxide toxicity? *Aviat. Space Environ. Med.* 46:1289–1291, 1975.
7. Chance B., Ericinisha M., Wagner M.: Mitochondrial responses to carbon monoxide toxicity. *Am. N.Y. Acad. Sci.* 174:193, 1970.
8. Garland H., Pearce J.: Neurological complications of carbon monoxide poisoning. *Q. J. Med.* 144:445–455, 1967.
9. Meigs J.W., Hughes J.P.W.: Acute carbon monoxide poisoning—an analysis of one hundred five cases. *Arch. Industa. Hyg. Occupatl. Med.* 6:344, 1952.
10. Plum F., Posner J.B., Hain R.F.: Delayed neurological deterioration after anoxia. *Arch. Intern. Med.* 110:18, 1962.
11. Myers R.A., Snyder S.K., Linberg S., Cowley R.A.: Volume of hyperbaric oxygen in suspected carbon monoxide poisoning. *J.A.M.A.* 246:2448–2480, 1981.
12. Smith G., Sharp G.R.: Treatment of carbon monoxide poisoning with oxygen under pressure. *Lancet* 1:905–906, 1960.
13. Phillips A.W., Tanner J.W., Cope O.: Burn therapy. IV. Respiratory tract damage (an account of the clinical x-ray and postmortem findings) and the meaning of restlessness. *Ann. Surg.* 158:799, 1963.
14. Echauser F.E., Billote J., Burke J.F., et al.: Tracheostomy complicating massive burn injury: A plea for conservatism. *Am. J. Surg.* 126:418, 1974.
15. Summer W., Haponik E.: Inhalation of irritant gases. *Clin. Chest Med.* 2:273–285, 1981.

16. Harrel L., Walker M.S., Charles G., et al.: Experimental inhalation injury in the goat. *J. Trauma* 21:962–964, 1981.
17. Proceedings: Consensus development conference supportive therapy in burn care, National Institute of General Medical Sciences. *J. Trauma.* No. 19 (Suppl. 11) p. 915, 1979.
18. Zawacki B.E., Jung R.C., Joyce J., et al.: Smoke, burns, and the natural history of inhalation injury in fire victims. *Ann. Surg.* 185:100–109, 1977.
19. Chu C.: New concepts of pulmonary burn injury. *J. Trauma* 21:958–961, 1981.
20. Eckhardt R.E., Hindin R.: The Health Hazards of Plastics. *J. Med.* 15:803–817, 1973.
21. Moncrief J.A.: Burns, in Schwartz S.I. (ed.): *Principles of Surgery*, ed. 2. New York, McGraw Hill Book Co., 1974, pp. 253–274.
22. Trunkey D.D.: Inhalation injury, symposium on burns. *Surg. Clin. North Am.* 58:1136, 1978.
23. Achauer B.M., Allyn P.A., Furmes D.W., et al.: Pulmonary complications of burns: The major threat to the burn patient. *Ann. Surg.* 177:311, 1973.
24. Whitener D.R., Whitener L.M., Robertson K.J., et al.: Pulmonary function measurements in patients with thermal injury and smoke inhalation. *Am. Rev. Respir. Dis.* 122:731–739, 1980.
25. Hunt J.L., Ager R.N., Pruitt B.A., Jr.: Fiberoptic bronchoscopy in acute inhalation injury. *J. Trauma* 15:641, 1975.
26. Petroff P.A., Hander E.W., Clayton W.H., et al.: Pulmonary function studies after smoke inhalation. *Am. J. Surg.* 132:346–351, 1976.
27. Schall G.L., McDonald H.D., Carr L.B., et al.: Xenon ventilation—perfusion lung scars. *J.A.M.A.* 240:2241–2445, 1978.

7 / Head Injury and Intracranial Hypertension

TOD SLOAN, M.D., PH.D.
ANTOUN KOHT, M.D.

ACCIDENTS are the leading cause of death in persons under age 45. Of the kinds of injuries incurred in accidents, head injury accounts for more than half the mortality.[1] Although more than 80% of persons who sustain head trauma experience no neurologic consequences,[2] more than 600,000 persons per year are admitted with severe head injury due to intracranial hematomas or cerebral lacerations.[3, 4] Three fourths of all motor vehicle accident fatalities are attributable to head injury,[5] and approximately 70% of all comatose head trauma admissions are accountable to highway accidents. Thus, accidental acute head injury represents a major challenge to the critical care physician.

MECHANISM OF INJURY

The bony skull forcefully collides with the brain gel substance at impact because each is accelerated and decelerated at different rates. These mechanical forces produce neuronal injury by several mechanisms (Table 7–1). Impact pressures as high as 4,000 mm Hg have been demonstrated in the animal model.[6–10] Pressure waves of 1,000–2,000 mm Hg cause transient loss of consciousness with apnea, although no neuronal damage can be demonstrated. Pressure waves greater than 2,000 mm Hg may produce disruption of larger blood vessels and subarachnoid hemorrhage.

Acceleration-deceleration within the brain tissue may lead to neuronal disruption with small vascular hemorrhages, i.e., brain contusion. It appears that the shift of the surface of the cortex is relatively greater than the shift of the deeper structures.[11–13] These shear forces often create the greatest damage on the side opposite the site of impact. Transient loss of consciousness and amnesia—concussion—is most commonly due to such cortical level damage, whereas brain stem injury or more severe cortical injury usually results in longer periods of unconsciousness.

TABLE 7–1.—MECHANISMS
OF NEURONAL INJURY

Primary factors
  Direct mechanical axonal injury
  Neurotransmitter failure
  Toxins
Secondary factors
  Ischemia
  Hemorrhage
  Edema

CASE STUDY

A 33-year-old man was brought to the emergency room at 10:00 P.M. following a motor vehicle accident. He was previously in good health with no known allergies. According to witnesses, he lost consciousness for about 5 minutes after striking his head on the windshield.

Paramedical personnel stated that when they arrived the patient was slightly confused and recalled none of the accident. On initial evaluation he complained of headache, neckache, and was slightly confused as to time and place. On physical examination he was slightly restless and had several scalp lacerations over the left parietal region and bilateral bloody nostrils. No other physical or neurologic abnormalities were noted. Vital signs were as follows: blood pressure (BP), 170/85 mm Hg; pulse, 55 beats per minute and regular; and respiratory rate, 15/minute and regular.

An intravenous (IV) line was started and blood specimens obtained for complete blood cell count, electrolyte level determination, crossmatching, and blood alcohol level determination. Skull, chest, and cervical spine x-ray studies were ordered.

Discussion

Initial information suggested mild intracranial injury (concussion). Since blood in the nostrils may be due to a basilar skull fracture or nasal trauma, skull x-ray studies and establishment of an IV line are indicated.

Preexisting metabolic disease such as diabetes mellitus or alcohol intoxication are known to worsen the neuronal injury secondary to trauma. Alcohol is present in up to 40% of head trauma victims,[14, 15] complicating the clinical evaluation as well as potentially worsening the brain injury.[16–18]

Secondary causes of neuronal damage must be considered as soon as possible (see Table 7–1). Ischemia is the common denominator of these secondary insults and may be due to hypotension, hypercarbia, hypoxia, or intracranial hypertension. Ensuring adequate ventilation and oxygenation is crucial.[19] Loss of airway patency and/or airway protective reflexes must be constantly evaluated. Since aspiration, atelectasis, and hypoventilation are common concomitants of head injury, hypoxemia is present in 30%–

50% of victims.[19-21] Although head trauma victims commonly present with hypotension,[22] this is seldom directly related to the cerebral injury[23] but rather is due to other injuries and blood loss.

Initial Neurologic Evaluation

Early quantification of head injury is crucial in determining appropriate therapy. The most widely accepted method for classification of head injury is the Glasgow Coma Scale (GCS), which is outlined in Table 7—2.[24] It must be noted that the GCS does not evaluate brain stem function, which is best evaluated by testing oculocephalic ("doll's eyes") and oculovestibular reflexes. In the latter, the eyes should tonically deviate away from the side of cold water infusion in the ear canal. Dysconjugate gaze suggests a brain stem lesion. Testing for doll's eyes is contraindicated when cervical spine injury is suspected; oculovestibular testing is contraindicated when inner ear damage is suspected.

Pontine damage is suggested when pinpoint pupils are observed in the absence of drug effects or by ocular bobbing (fast downward gaze followed by slow upward gaze).[25] Irregular, ataxic ventilation may also result from pontine damage.[19]

Medullary damage is suggested by loss of gag and cough response, bradycardia, and hypotension.[26] Hypotension in the patient with head trauma is a preterminal event when due to the brain injury.[23] However, shock is

TABLE 7–2.—THE GLASGOW COMA SCALE*

	POINTS
Eye opening	
Spontaneously	4
To speech	3
To pain	2
Never	1
Best verbal response	
Oriented	5
Confused	4
Inappropriate	3
Garbled	2
None	1
Best motor response	
Obeys commands	6
Localizes pain	5
Withdrawal	4
Abnormal flexion	3
Extension	2
None	1

*After evaluation of the patient, the points are summed. Severe head injury is often defined as a score below 8 for more than 6 hours.

usually due to other causes and must be aggressively evaluated and treated.

Transentorial herniation is suggested by pupil asymmetry (third cranial nerve palsy). The earliest sign of herniation is pupil dilatation due to loss of parasympathetic tone, on the same side of the mass causing the herniation (94% of cases).[27] Later signs include alteration of consciousness and asymmetric motor response, most commonly on the contralateral side of the mass causing the herniation.[27]

Case Study Continued

At 10:50 P.M., while in the radiology department, the patient developed mild right arm weakness that was followed by progressive obtundation over the next 15 minutes. At 11:20 P.M. he responded only to pain with incomprehensible utterances and normal flexor withdrawal of the left arm. The eyes opened in response to painful stimuli but the right arm and leg appeared paretic. BP was 180/90 mm Hg, pulse was 48/beats per minute, and respiratory rate was 24/minute and regular.

Chest x-ray was normal. Skull films revealed a linear skull fracture over the left parietal region. Cervical spine films showed no abnormality. Blood studies were normal.

Discussion

The patient's rapid deterioration suggests significant intracranial injury. Approximately 50% of deaths from head injury occur within 2 hours of injury,[28] often prior to arriving at a hospital. Initial evaluation and resuscitation are therefore of great importance. Many believe it is safest to assume that increased intracranial pressure (ICP) exists when the GCS is 7 or less, necessitating intubation and hyperventilation.[29] The justification for this approach is that the nervous system has less reserve than most organs and aggressive early therapy is the best way to avoid irreversible damage.

Case Study Continued

The trachea was orally intubated following the application by mask of 70% oxygen and the IV administration of 5 mg/kg of sodium pentothal, 1.5 mg/kg of lidocaine, and 1 mg/kg of succinyldicholine. The patient was hyperventilated and a subsequent arterial blood gas analysis revealed a pH of 7.52, a P_{CO_2} of 25 mm Hg, and a P_{O_2} of 250 mm Hg. BP was 135/70 mm Hg with a regular pulse of 73 beats per minute.

An emergency computerized tomographic (CT) scan was conducted at 11:50 P.M. During the scan the patient became restless and required IV pancuronium bromide (0.1 mg/kg). At the conclusion of the scan it was noted that the left pupil was dilated and unresponsive to light. The scan revealed a 7-mm midline shift to the right with a radiodense mass adjacent to the skull fracture over the left hemisphere.

Discussion

The intubation was accomplished orally to avoid intracerebral intubation through a possible basilar skull fracture. Care was taken to avoid neck movement despite the negative cervical spine films, as up to a 10% incidence of cervical spine injury has been reported with head trauma.[18, 30, 31] Succinylcholine was chosen to achieve prompt relaxation to facilitate intubation with rapid reversal of paralysis to allow further neurologic examination. Sodium pentothal and lidocaine were used to minimize the autonomic response to tracheal intubation, decrease intracranial pressure by direct vasoconstriction, and decrease metabolic rate. Sodium pentothal is a rapid and predictable sedative that allows neurologic examination within 15–20 minutes of administration. Obviously, the choice and dosage of drugs will depend on the cardiovascular status of the patient.

Pathophysiology of Increased ICP

The cerebrospinal fluid (CSF) compartment is normally maintained at a pressure of 0–10 mm Hg. Up to 40 ml of CSF can be acutely translocated to the dural sleeves of the spinal column to minimize increases in ICP. The venous pressure is normally maintained at 2–4 mm Hg above CSF pressure.[32] An additional 40 ml of venous blood can be acutely translocated outside the calvarium to minimize increases in ICP.

Brain perfusion is normally determined by the difference between the arterial pressure entering the skull (MAP) and the venous pressure leaving the skull (CVP). Intracranial hypertension raises the ICP above the venous pressure, necessitating the measurement of ICP to determine the cerebral perfusion pressure (CPP; MAP − ICP).

An increase in intracranial fluid volume will eventually exceed the volume capacity of the rigid cranium and result in increased ICP. This will eventually diminish cerebral blood flow and place pressure on brain tissue, which will ultimately result in cellular death.

Normally, a CPP above 50 mm Hg assures adequate intracranial blood flow. However, injured brain may require 90 mm Hg for adequate perfusion.[33] Obviously, as the ICP approaches MAP, blood flow will be seriously compromised, resulting in ischemia. Medullary ischemia may promote a systemic hypertension, which in turn promotes a reflex bradycardia, the combination—raised ICP, hypertension, and bradycardia—is known as Cushing's triad. Brain stem ischemia may result in abnormal ventilatory patterns. An irregular breathing pattern associated with Cushing's triad is known as Cushing's syndrome. These are severe and late signs of increased ICP and are not always present. It should be noted that patients with spinal cord trauma do not show the Cushing response.[21]

Emergency Management of Increased ICP

The neurologic deterioration in this patient is consistent with the CT findings of an expanding intracranial mass since the deterioration was too rapid to be attributed to cerebral edema. Increased ICP secondary to cerebral edema usually develops over a 12- to 24-hour period.

The patient exhibited hypertension on admission and had a consistently slow heart rate. All trauma patients with hypertension should be evaluated for increased ICP before treatment, especially before administration of vasodilators that might further raise the ICP.

The emergency management of increased ICP rests on the principle of decreasing intracranial fluid volume. This is readily accomplished by diminishing the venous and capillary blood volume. Elevation of the head in the neutral position promotes venous drainage. Airway obstruction or Valsalva maneuvers increase intrathoracic pressure and diminish venous drainage. Maintaining a clear airway, including endotracheal intubation when

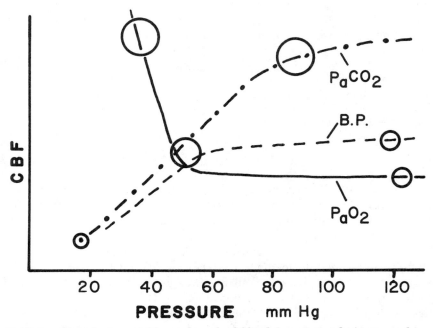

Fig 7–1.—*Physiologic variables and cerebral blood flow. Arterial oxygen, carbon dioxide, and blood pressure cause alterations in cerebral blood flow, as shown. These probably cause the alterations by causing vasoconstriction or vasodilation (depicted on the curves, open circles represent degree of vessel dilatation). Vessel dilation with rising flow will cause a proportionate rise in cerebral blood volume and therefore also will cause a corresponding rise in intracranial pressure.*

indicated, removes these factors and can thus help promote venous drainage from the head.

The cerebral blood volume (CBV) is responsive to arterial PCO_2 between 20 and 80 mm Hg (Fig 7–1). Rapid reduction in arterial PCO_2 results in diminished CBV and ICP. In a normal individual the cerebral vasoconstriction remains but the CSF production increases within 24 hours so that the effect of reducing CBV on ICP is diminished.

Adequate arterial oxygenation will prevent increases in CBV since an arterial PO_2 below 50 mm Hg promotes cerebral vasodilation (see Fig 7–1). It is essential that significant hypoxemia be immediately corrected in patients with increased ICP. Figure 7–1 also indicates that autoregulation of blood flow occurs in the normal individual at a MAP between 50 and 150 mm Hg. These limits shift upward in the patient with hypertension of 1 month's duration or more. Rapid changes in BP may have profound effects on CBF in the head-injured patient.

Brain tissue cannot be translocated. However, its fluid volume and extracellular water can be rapidly reduced with administration of an osmotic diuretic. Raising the osmotic pressure of the intravascular fluid rapidly reduces the excessive intravascular and extravascular fluid.

Case Study Continued

Mannitol (0.25 gm/kg) was administered IV preceded by furosemide (0.5 mg/kg). A Foley catheter was inserted and arrangements made for an emergency craniotomy.

Discussion: Intracranial Bleeding

Approximately 3% of patients with major head trauma have intracranial bleeding[34]; 40% of these are comatose on arrival at a hospital.[3] There are four major types of bleeding: extradural, subdural, infratentorial (posterior fossa), and intracerebral.

The injury may tear extradural veins (middle meningeal veins or venous sinuses) or the middle meningeal artery can be torn by fractures of the temporal or parietal bones. Skull fractures are associated with a 20-fold increased incidence of extradural hematomas.[35] These hematomas can manifest with otorrhagia (blood in the ear canal) or hematotympanum (blood behind the tympanic membrane). In the classic presentation of an intracranial bleed the patient has a lucid interval followed by deterioration, but only about one third of patients follow this pattern. Another one third are never unconscious, and the remaining are never conscious following the injury.[36]

Acute subdural hematomas are 2–3 times as common as epidural bleeds and have twice the mortality.[37] These are frequently due to arterial rupture on the cortical surface or to bleeding of the bridging veins on the surface of the cortex that form the normal venous drainage of the cortex. These vessels can be damaged by acceleration/deceleration injuries. Acute subdural hematoma can also be due to small vessel hemorrhage in a cortical contusion.[38] Patients with subdural hematomas may have a lucid interval (15%); however, the majority are never conscious (55%).[38] Mortality is markedly increased (60%–100%) if bilateral or multiple lesions occur.[38–41]

Subdural hematomas can develop very slowly (more than 24 hours) by the slow leakage from venous structures (so-called subacute hematoma), or they may develop at a later time (chronic subdural hematoma), as is often seen in the elderly or alcoholic patient. Posterior fossa hematomas are quite uncommon (2.5% of masses) and are highly lethal due to brain stem compression and upward herniation.[27]

Supratentorial mass lesions are common in patients with severe head injury and can be rapidly diagnosed by a shift of midline structures in the cerebrum. In one study of 200 head-injured patients with a GCS less than 8, 62% had a midline shift in excess of 1 cm.[42] Midline shift can be detected easily with CT scanning, but arteriograms and other tests that assess midline structures are acceptable alternatives.

When increased ICP is due to a mass lesion, the survival and morbidity depend on immediate operative intervention. The percentage of patients surviving mass lesions with a functional recovery has been reported as 60%–70% when surgery was conducted within 4 hours, but only 10% (with 3–4 times the total morbidity) when surgery was delayed beyond 4 hours.[37]

Case Study Continued

The patient was rushed to the operating room at 1:00 A.M. for evacuation of the hematoma and placement of an intraventricular pressure monitor. Anesthesia was maintained with narcotics (fentanyl citrate) supplemented with small concentrations of isoflurane and nitrous oxide in oxygen. Paralysis was supplemented with additional pancuronium bromide. A moderate-sized epidural hematoma was evacuated and the fractured bone flap realigned.

Following surgery the patient was transferred to the intensive care unit and a central venous catheter and oro-gastric tube were placed. His pupillary responses returned to normal. He was positioned with his head up 30 degrees and remained on full ventilatory support with P_{CO_2} ranging between 30 and 35 mm Hg. Inspired oxygen concentration was gradually tapered to 30% with Pa_{O_2} ranging between 70 and 80 mm Hg. Regular doses of Dilantin and nafcillin and sedation with phenobarbital were begun.

The ICP gradually rose to 20 mm Hg over the next 12 hours. By 4:00 P.M. on the day following admission (18 hours after injury), the ICP continually rose above 20 mm Hg. Concomitant with the ICP rise was a return of hypertension (160–180 mm Hg systolic) and restlessness. Right and left arm and leg motion were nearly identical in response to pain. Additional doses of mannitol (0.25 mg/kg) were given IV, which kept the ICP below 20 mm Hg except for transient rises during stimulation.

Discussion: Late Secondary Neurologic Damage

The prevention of late secondary neural insults rests primarily on maintenance of adequate cerebral perfusion. The intensive care of these patients must provide an optimal milieu for the survival of injured neural cells.

There are three general categories of brain cells in the injured patient. The first category comprises cells that are irreversibly damaged by the initial injury. Since neural cells do not regenerate, function will depend on collateral cell function, making salvage of the other categories of cells crucial. In the second category are cells that have not been damaged and will survive unless subsequent insult occurs. In the third category are cells that are surviving on the thinnest of margins. These cells have sufficient energy to meet the minimal needs for basal metabolism but insufficient energy for normal metabolism and electrical function. These cells are in a so-called ischemic penumbra, where small decreases in oxygen delivery can cause irreversible cell death.

One method of considering the factors involved in the survival of these marginal cells is the concept of energy balance. As depicted in Figure 7–2, the supply of nutrients (notably oxygen and glucose) is balanced against energy demands. Any factors that favorably influence the balance (i.e., reduce demands relative to the supply) should favor the repair and survival of the cells.

Factors that should favorably reduce the consumption of oxygen are those that depress metabolism. Seizure activity will markedly increase oxygen consumption so that seizure prevention is paramount. Patients with subdural hematomas, dural tears from skull fractures, or penetrating injuries are at high risk for developing subsequent seizure foci. The use of Dilantin to suppress seizures can be very useful.[43]

Head positioning 10–30 degrees upward (in the absence of a cervical spine injury) and oxygenation in excess of 90% hemoglobin saturation (Pa_{O_2} >60 mm Hg) are mandatory. Eucapneic ventilation (Pco_2 35–40 mm Hg) or slight hyperventilation (Pco_2 30–35 mm Hg) are desirable if ICP is well controlled. A Pco_2 of 25–30 mm Hg may help control ICP. Arterial Pco_2 below 20 mm Hg may threaten adequate brain perfusion by producing excessive vasoconstriction. In patients with a focus of ischemia, continued hyperventilation appears to be of value because the ischemic focus adds

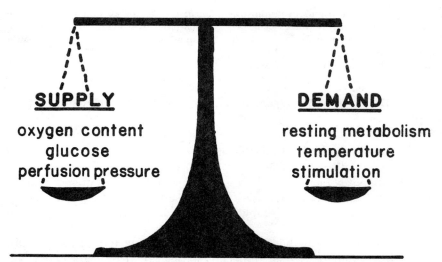

Fig 7–2.—*Balance of nutrient supply and demand in neural tissue. The survival of injured neural tissue depends on the relative amount of oxygen available for tissue survival and repair versus the demand for this oxygen. If the demand exceeds the supply, the tissue will be ischemic and sustain further injury.*

lactic acid to the CSF and prevents metabolic compensation of CSF pH. This appears to promote continued reduction in CBF.[44, 45]

The patient should receive adequate sedation and/or paralysis to reduce the transient rises in ICP that occur from stimuli such as tracheal suctioning. BP control is important since local autoregulation in the area of injury is probably abnormal[46–48] and transient hypertension may contribute to edema formation. The differential diagnosis of hypertension in these patients includes (1) raised ICP pressure; (2) underlying, preexisting hypertensive disorder, and (3) pain from surgery or associated injuries (e.g., bony fractures). It is important to note that if hypertension is due to raised ICP, the ICP must be treated first. Hypertension itself should be treated with drugs that are not cerebral vasodilators (e.g., trimethaphan rather than sodium nitroprusside).

Hyperthermia should be prevented since it increases metabolic rate and oxygen demand. Hypervolemia must be avoided; however, fluid volume should not be restricted to the point of compromising adequate perfusion.

Case Study Continued

At 4:30 P.M. the fluctuations in ICP with ventilation and arterial pulsation became exaggerated and the mean ICP gradually rose to over 30 mm Hg de-

spite additional furosemide administration. Periodic pressure waves of 35–40
mm Hg occurred and lasted for 10–20
minutes. An infusion of pentobarbital
was begun and adjusted to keep the

mean ICP below 20 mm Hg. Fluid administration was decreased to the minimum utilizing the central venous catheter as a guide.

Discussion: Management of Intracranial Hypertension

Monitoring

ICP monitoring can be a valuable adjunct to management of the severely
head-injured patient. Over 50%–88%[3, 49, 50] of patients who require operative treatment of head injury have postoperative ICP rises greater than 20
mm Hg.[51] Elevations in ICP were found in 30% of head-injured patients
who were unable to follow simple commands and in 69% when a cerebral
contusion was present.[3, 49, 50]

There are several methods available for monitoring ICP. The two most
common techniques used in the acute setting are the subarachnoid bolt
and the intraventricular catheter. The subarachnoid bolt can be inserted in
the intensive care area, emergency room, or operating room. The intraventricular catheter must be placed in the operating room. The normal ICP
varies between 0 and 10 mm Hg, with occasional fluctuations up to 15 mm
Hg. Elevations above 20 mm Hg sustained over 1 minute are definitely
abnormal.[52, 53]

Intracranial monitoring is particularly valuable when the patient's mental
status cannot be assessed due to coma or pharmacologic therapy. Clinical
experience suggests that neurologic abnormalities are consistently observed
with an ICP above 40 mm Hg[54] and in some patients with an ICP above
25–30 mm Hg. For this reason, a majority of clinicians aggressively treat
ICP rises over 15–20 mm Hg. The importance of ICP in outcome is emphasized by the correlation of mortality with raised ICP. If the ICP is sustained over 60 mm Hg, the result is uniformly fatal in adults (children are
generally more tolerant of higher pressures). Elevations above 40 mm Hg
correlate with a 40%–62% mortality, whereas levels over 20 mm Hg correlate with a 26% mortality. The mortality falls to 14% when the ICP remains below 20 mm Hg.[49, 51] In general, raised ICP is thought to be the
principal cause of death in half of the deaths due to head trauma.[50]

The normal ICP trace includes variations with arterial pulsations (the so-
called C waves) and breathing (the so-called B waves of Lundberg).[53] These
waves probably represent the increase in ICP associated respectively with
rises in arterial blood volume and with increases in intrathoracic pressure
and an associated rise in cerebral venous volume.

When the tracing becomes abnormal, intracranial compliance is reduced. As depicted in Figure 7–3, when the volume in the cranium rises, compensatory mechanisms are exhausted and ICP will rise exponentially. Although the absolute ICP is helpful in understanding the patient's location on the curve, intracranial compliance testing is more specific. Small volumes of saline (0.5–2 ml) are injected through the ventricular catheter and the pressure response is noted. With the intraventricular catheter, small amounts of CSF can be removed if necessary to reduce ICP. With the subarachnoid bolt, compliance testing must be done cautiously with very small amounts of saline (e.g., 0.1 ml) since fluid cannot be removed.

EEG monitoring in the absence of drug effects can be quite useful in ascertaining general neural function as well as identifying hazardous seizure activity. Evoked potentials can be specifically useful in ascertaining the functioning of particular neural pathways but are not a good index of global function.[55] The use of multiple evoked potential tests in a multimodality battery is, however, emerging as a valuable tool.[54]

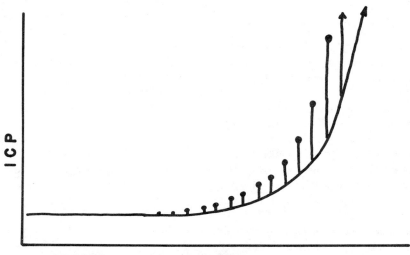

INTRACRANIAL VOLUME

Fig 7–3.—Intracranial compliance curve. As volume is acutely added to the intracranial vault, the pressure remains relatively unchanged until the compensatory mechanisms are exhausted. From this point, the pressure begins an exponentially increasing climb. If small volumes are intermittently added to the curve, the small pressure rise also exponentially increases (the response to a small volume injection is shown by the vertical lines on the basic curve). Thus, both the absolute ICP value and the compliance response to a small injected volume can be used to assess the placement of the patient on the curve.

Pharmacologic Therapy

A variety of pharmacologic maneuvers are available for reducing ICP and oxygen consumption. Mannitol is the standard osmotic diuretic. The recommended dose of mannitol ranges from 0.25 to 0.5 gm/kg and works well for 2–3 hours. Higher doses are associated with a high incidence of serum hyperosmolarity. Other osmotic agents such as urea and glycerol can be used but may produce rebound intracranial hypertension (urea) and hemolysis (glycerol).

The loop diuretics are useful for their dehydrating effects as well as their specific actions. Ethacrynic acid has a specific effect on cerebral edema,[56] but its usefulness is limited by overall fluid balance problems at doses where this effect occurs. Furosemide has a specific effect on CSF production by inhibiting sodium transport[57] and inhibiting carbonic anhydrase.[58] The inhibition of sodium transport also inhibits water uptake in edematous brain.[59, 60]

Corticosteroids are currently used because of demonstrated efficacy in edema related to metastatic tumors[61, 62] and possible value at higher doses for trauma.[62, 63] However, definitive efficacy in trauma has not been shown.[64-66] The steroids presumably help by restoring normal vascular permeability but can exacerbate diabetes mellitus, increase the chances of infection, delay healing, and promote gastrointestinal bleeding.

Barbiturates are of value in reducing ICP in patients with head trauma[67, 68] by reducing CBV via vasoconstriction. This improves CPP and oxygen delivery. The efficacy of barbiturates in favorably affecting the balance of oxygen supply and demand rests on their ability to reduce oxygen consumption[69] to 25%–30% of the awake value. This effect occurs when the EEG is flat, and no additional value is gained by the use of larger doses. Furthermore, these drugs appear to act by free radical scavenging to reduce lipid membrane damage.[70-73] Their efficacy in improving outcome due to the control of ICP is well substantiated; however, the use of very deep levels of barbiturate coma has failed to produce clear improvement in outcome in head injury.

Lidocaine has a vasoconstrictor action which reduces ICP and, by interrupting sodium and potassium flux in the cells, may reduce cellular metabolism.

Therapy of Disputed Value

Hyperbaric oxygen has been successful in treating cerebral ischemia. However, in trauma patients, transient improvement is limited to the duration of the treatment.[74] This mode of therapy is presumably helpful via reduction of ICP by the weak vasoconstrictor action of oxygen at high pressures (the effect is about one third as potent as a reduction in Pa_{CO_2}).[75]

Hypothermia, by virtue of its ability to reduce cerebral metabolism beyond barbiturate effect, has been used in coma. At 32° C, the rate of oxygen consumption as well as the CBV are decreased 40%–50%. Thus, both oxygen demand and edema formation[76, 77] are decreased with a relative increase in delivery compared to demand. Problems associated with hypothermia are mainly due to the development of cardiovascular abnormalities at temperatures below 28° C.

Hemodilution has been suggested as a means of improving cerebral blood flow by reducing blood viscosity.[78, 79] However, good studies in head trauma are lacking.

Dimethyl sulfoxide (DMSO) is currently under investigation and clear efficacy in head trauma remains to be shown. The effects of DMSO include an osmotic effect to reduce edema,[80] stabilization of mitochondria,[81] and favorable alterations in prostaglandin synthesis.[82]

Surgical resection of the cortex or closure of the head in the absence of a bone flap would also theoretically help ICP,[83] but data supporting the value of these approaches in improving outcome are lacking.

Case Study Continued

Due to the progressive deterioration, the patient underwent a repeated CT scan at 6:00 P.M. that revealed edema in the region of the cortex adjacent to the site of the hematoma. Neurologic examination revealed eye opening and appropriate motor withdrawal from pain, but no verbal response. The EEG showed mild generalized slowing with no spike activity. Evoked potential studies revealed a slightly delayed right median nerve response but normal brain stem auditory evoked response. Therapy as outlined above was continued.

Discussion: Cerebral Edema

Cerebral edema is a major problem in the head-injured patient. There are three general patterns of swelling: swelling that occurs adjacent to a contusion or hematoma, swelling of the ipsilateral hemisphere after removal of a mass lesion, and diffuse bilateral swelling due to global ischemia.[84, 85]

The formation of edema is postulated to occur by several mechanisms, but the most important is related to transient blood-brain barrier malfunction that occurs at the time of impact.[86, 87] Such focal disruption of vascular integrity results in leakage of water through the vessel walls—so-called vasogenic edema.[88] The major increase in edema occurs 24–72 hours after injury.[89] Hypertension can contribute to edema formation.[88]

Other mechanisms of edema formation include metabolic factors such as membrane transport mechanisms, cytotoxic injury to the cells with cellular water uptake, and interstitial edema. Also postulated, but poorly substantiated, are edema formation by neurogenic mechanisms[90] or the production of edemagenic factors (free radicals, serotonin, prostaglandins).[91-94] Sodium levels below 120 mEq/L can cause a rise in cellular water and promote edema. Thus, the regulation of fluids and electrolytes is important.

Case Study Continued

The patient remained stable, and about 72 hours following admission the pentobarbital infusion was gradually discontinued and the ICP remained 10–15 mm Hg. The serum sodium level gradually fell until it reached 128 mEq/L. Fluid restriction and careful maintenance of fluid balance reversed the hyponatremic trend.

Discussion: Noncerebral Complications

A variety of noncerebral sequelae can arise in the head-injured patient. One of the more common problems is fluid and electrolyte imbalance resulting from endocrine disturbance or simply due to diuretic therapy and incorrect IV fluid administration.

Endocrine dysfunction, including anterior pituitary dysfunction[95, 96] and posterior pituitary dysfunction, can occur. Inappropriate secretion of antidiuretic hormone (SIADH) is common with head trauma[97] and can result in hyponatremia due to decreased free water secretion by the kidneys. Diabetes insipidus with deficiency of ADH is also common and can lead to an unexplained polyuria. With the use of diuretics and the potential abnormalities in ADH, careful monitoring of fluid and electrolyte balance is important.

Pulmonary consequences are common and include noncardiac pulmonary edema (see Chap. 12). The etiology of this so-called neurogenic pulmonary edema may be increased sympathetic tone[98, 99] with subsequent pulmonary capillary leakage.[100-103]

Cardiac sequelae from head injury include ECG abnormalities. The ECG may exhibit varied effects (decreased rate, decreased QT intervals, nodal rhythm, and ST-T abnormalities).[95] Cardiac arrest and atrial fibrillation have been reported.[45, 104, 105] The etiology of these effects may be vagal from central autonomic stimulation.[93, 106, 107]

Coagulation defects, both hypercoagulability and hypocoagulability (including disseminated intravascular coagulation), have been reported.[108]

Case Study Continued

After 5 days, the patient began to show increasingly normal response to stimulation. By 10 days, he was able to walk and converse with the staff. Reha-bilitation of residual arm weakness was undertaken, and he progressively im-proved, to be discharged after 35 days of hospitalization.

Conclusion

The final outcome for the patient with head injury rests on the ability of the critical care physician to manage the acute sequelae of the trauma and produce a favorable milieu for neuronal recovery. It is useful to reflect on this case in order to compare the outcome with the factors influencing out-come with head injury. These are: (1) Progressively increasing mortality when the GCS is below 8, especially when it is below 5. (2) Marked cor-relation of mortality with abnormal motor responses, with mortality of 0%–52% with normal motor responses and 23%–90% with abnormal re-sponses.[109–111] (3) The presence of mass lesions, notably with midline shift of greater than 5 mm. (4) Abnormal pupillary responses. (5) Hypotension with systolic pressures less than 90 mm Hg. (6) Age over 60 years. (7) Elevated ICP.

The outcome of serious head injury is often dismal, with 15%–20% of patients dying. However, 50% of patients can make a meaningful recovery. Since the magnitude of the initial insult cannot be altered after the fact, the real challenge to the critical care physician is management of the sub-sequent physiologic derangements (notably ischemia and raised ICP), which are potentially reversible and markedly influence outcome.

REFERENCES

1. Baker C.C., Oppenheimer L., Stephens B., et al.: Epidemiology of trauma deaths. Am. J. Surg. 140:144–150, 1980.
2. Galbraith S.L.: Age distribution of extradural hemorrhage without skull fracture. Lancet 1:1217–1218, 1973.
3. Becker D.P., Miller J.D., Ward J.D., et al.: The outcome from severe head injury with early diagnosis and intensive management. J. Neurosurg. 47:491–502, 1977.
4. Caveness W.F.: Incidence of craniocerebral trauma in the United States with trend from 1970–1975, in Thompson R.A., Green J.R. (eds.): Complications of Central Nervous System Trauma. Adv. Neurol. 22:1–3, 1979.
5. Gissane W.: The nature and causation of road injuries. Lancet 2:695, 1963.
6. Lindgren S., and Rinder L.: Experimental studies in head injury. Biophysik 2:320–329, 1965.
7. Sullivan H.G., Martinez A.J., Becker D.P., et al.: Fluid percussion model of mechanical brain injury in the cat. J. Neurosurg. 45:520–534, 1976.
8. Bremer A.M., Yamada K., West C.R.: Ischemic cerebral edema in primates: Effects of acetazolamide, phenytoin, sorbitol, dexamethasone and methylprednisone on brain wa-ter and electrolytes. Neurosurgery 6:149–154, 1980.

9. Saunders M.L., Miller J.D., Stablein D., et al.: The effects of graded experimental trauma on cerebral blood flow and responsiveness to CO_2. *J. Neurosurg.* 51:18–26, 1979.
10. Wei E.P., Dietrich D.W., Povlishock J.T., et al.: Functional morphologic and metabolic abnormalities of the cerebral microcirculation after concussive brain injury in cats. *Circ. Res.* 48:95–103, 1981.
11. Holbourn A.H.S.: Mechanisms of head injuries. *Lancet* 2:438–441, 1943.
12. Pudenz R.H., Shelden C.H.: Lucite calvarium: Method for direct observation of the brain, cerebral trauma and brain movement. *J. Neurosurg.* 3:487–505, 1946.
13. Strich S.J.: Shearing of nerve fibers as a cause of brain damage due to head injury: A pathological study of twenty cases. *Lancet* 2:443–448, 1961.
14. Jennett B.: Some medicolegal aspects of the management of acute head injury. *Br. Med. J.* 1:1383–1385, 1976.
15. Patel A.R., Jennett B., Galbraith S.L.: Alcohol and head injury. *Lancet* 1:1369–1370, 1977.
16. Flamm E.S., Demopoulos H.B., Seligman M.L., et al.: Ethanol potentiation of central nervous system trauma. *J. Neurosurg.* 46:328–335, 1977.
17. Galbraith S.L.: Misdiagnosis and delayed diagnosis in traumatic intracranial hematoma. *Br. Med. J.* 1:1438–1439, 1976.
18. Trowbridge A., and Giesecke A.H.: Multiple injuries. *Clin. Anesth.* 11:79–84, 1976.
19. North J.B., Jennett S.: Abnormal breathing patterns associated with acute brain damage. *Arch. Neurol.* 31:338–344, 1974.
20. Katsurada K., Yamada R., Sugimoto R.: Respiratory insufficiency in patients with severe head injury. *Surgery* 73:191–199, 1973.
21. Sinha R.P., Ducker T.B., Perot P.L.: Arterial oxygenation: Findings and its significance in central nervous system trauma patients. *JAMA* 224:1258–1260, 1973.
22. Frowein R.A., Steinmann H.W., auf der Harr K., et al.: Limits to classification and prognosis of severe head injury. *Adv. Neurosurg.* 5:16–26, 1978.
23. Illingworth G., Jennett W.B.: The shocked head injury. *Lancet* 2:511–514, 1965.
24. Teasdale G., Jennett B.: Assessment of coma and impaired consciousness: A practical scale. *Lancet* 2:81–84, 1974.
25. Fisher C.M.: Ocular bobbing. *Arch. Neurol.* 11:543–546, 1964.
26. van der Ark G.D.: Cardiovascular changes with acute subdural hematoma. *Surg. Neurol.* 3:305–308, 1975.
27. Pitts L.: Neurological evaluation of the head injury patient. *Clin. Neurosurg.* 29:203–224, 1982.
28. Sevitt S.: Fatal road accidents in Birmingham: Times of death and their course. *Injury* 4:281–293, 1973.
29. Cooper P.R.: Resuscitation of the multiply injured patient. *Clin. Neurosurg.* 29:225–239, 1982.
30. Beck G.P., Neill L.W.: Anesthesia for associated trauma in patients with head injuries. *Anesth. Analg.* 42:687–695, 1963.
31. Crighton H.C., Giesecke A.H.: One year's experience in the anesthetic management of trauma. *Anesth. Analg.* 45:835–842, 1966.
32. Johnston I.H., and Rowan J.O.: Raised intracranial pressure and cerebral blood flow: Venous outflow tract pressures and vascular resistances in experimental intracranial hypertension. *J. Neurol. Neurosurg. Psychiatry* 37:392–402, 1974.
33. Miller J.D.: Physiology of trauma. *Clin. Neurosurg.* 29:103–130, 1982.
34. Kalsbeek W.D., McLaurin R.L., Harris B.S.H., et al.: The national head and spinal cord injury survey: Major findings. *J. Neurosurg.* 53 (suppl.):S19–31, 1980.
35. Jennett B., Teasdale G.: *Management of Head Injuries.* Philadelphia, F.A. Davis Co., Contemporary Neurology Series No. 20, 1981, p. 101.
36. Jamieson K.G., Yelland J.D.N.: Extradural hematoma: Report of 167 cases. *J. Neurosurg.* 29:13, 1968.
37. Seelig J.M., Becker D.P., Miller J.D., et al.: Traumatic acute subdural hematoma: Major mortality reduction in comatose patients treated within four hours. *N. Engl. J. Med.* 304:1511–1518, 1981.

38. Jamieson K.G., Yelland J.D.N.: Surgically treated traumatic subdural hematomas. *J. Neurosurg.* 37:137, 1972.
39. Fell D.A., Fitzgerald S., Moiel R.H., et al.: Acute subdural hematomas: Review of 144 cases. *J. Neurosurg.* 42:37, 1975.
40. Moiel R.H., Caram P.C.: Acute subdural hematoma: A review of 84 cases. A six-year evaluation. *J. Trauma* 7:660, 1967.
41. Talalla A., Morin M.A.: Acute traumatic subdural hematoma: A review of 100 consecutive cases. *J. Trauma* 11:771, 1971.
42. Frost E.A.M., Arancibia C.U., Shulman K.: Pulmonary shunt as a prognostic indicator in head injury. *J. Neurosurg.* 50:768–772, 1979.
43. Martin M.: Pharmacologic therapeutic modalities: Phenytoin, dimethyl sulfoxide and calcium channel blockers. *Crit. Care Q.* 5:72–81, 1983.
44. Katsurada K., Sugimoto T., Onji Y.: Significance of cerebrospinal fluid bicarbonate ions in the management of patients with cerebral injury. *J. Trauma* 9:799–805, 1969.
45. McLaurin R.L., King L.R.: Recognition and treatment of metabolic disorders after head injuries. *Clin. Neurosurg.* 19:281–300, 1972.
46. Langfitt T.W., Kassell N.F., Weinstein J.D.: Cerebral blood flow with intracranial hypertension. *Neurology* 15:761–773, 1965.
47. Langfitt T.W., Weinstein J.D., Kassell N.F.: Vascular factors in head injury: Contribution to brain swelling and intracranial hypertension, in Caveness W.F., Walker A.E. (eds.): *Head Injury: Conference Proceedings.* Philadelphia, J.B. Lippincott Co., 1966, pp. 172–194.
48. Lewelt W., Jenkins L.W., Miller J.D.: Autoregulation of cerebral blood flow after experimental percussion injury of the brain. *J. Neurosurg.* 53:500–511, 1980.
49. Miller J.D.: Disorders of cerebral blood flow and intracranial pressure after head injury. *Clin. Neurosurg.* 29:162–173, 1982.
50. Miller J.D., Becker D.P., Ward J.D., et al.: Significance of intracranial hypertension in severe head injury. *J. Neurosurg.* 47:503–516, 1977.
51. Miller, J.D., Butterworth J.F., Gudeman S.K., et al.: Further experience in the management of severe head injury. *J. Neurosurg.* 54:289–299, 1981.
52. Langfitt T.W.: The incidence and importance of intracranial hypertension in head injured patients, in Beks J.F.W., Bosch D.A., Brock M. (eds.): *Intracerebral Pressure.* Berlin, Springer–Verlag, 1976, vol. 3, pp. 58–62.
53. Lundberg N.: Continuous recording and control of ventricular fluid pressure in neurosurgical practice. *Acta Psychiatr. Neurol. Scand.* 36 (suppl. 149):1–193, 1960.
54. Greenberg R.P., Mayer D.J., Becker D.P.: Correlation in man on intracranial pressure and neuroelectric activity determined by multimodality evoked potentials, in Beks J.F.W., Bosch D.A., Brock M. (eds.): *Intracerebral Pressure.* Berlin, Springer–Verlag, 1976, vol. 3.
55. Kish G., Kozloff L., Joseph W.L., et al.: Indications for early thoracotomy in the management of chest trauma. *J. Thorac. Surg.* 22:23–28, 1976.
56. Bourke R.S., Kimelberg K.H., Daze M.A., et al.: Studies on the formation of astroglal swelling and its inhibition by clinically useful agents, in Popp A.J., et al. (eds.): *Neural Trauma.* New York, Raven Press, 1979.
57. Canadian Cooperative Study: Randomized trial of aspirin and sulfinpyrazone in threatened stroke. *N. Engl. J. Med.* 299:53, 1978.
58. Gilman A.G., Goodman L.S., Gilman A.: *Goodman and Gilman's The Pharmacological Basis of Therapeutics,* ed. 6. New York, Macmillan Publishing Co., Inc., 1980, pp. 90–97.
59. Burhley L.E., Reed D.J.: The effect of furosemide on sodium–22 uptake into cerebrospinal fluid and brain. *Exp. Brain Res.* 14:503–510, 1972.
60. Tutt H.P., Pappius H.M.: Studies on the mechanism of actions of steroids in traumatized brain, in Reulen H.J., Schurmann, K. (eds.): *Steroids and Brain Edema.* New York, Springer–Verlag, 1972, pp. 147–151.
61. Faupel G., Reulen J.H., Miller D.J., et al.: Double blind study on the effects of steroids on severe closed head injury, in Pappius H.M., Feindel W. (eds.): *Dynamics of Brain Edema.* Berlin, Springer–Verlag, 1976, pp. 337–343.

62. Gobiet W., Bock W.J., Liesegang J., et al.: Treatment of acute cerebral edema with high doses of dexamethasone, in Beks J.F.W., Bosch D.A., Brock M., (eds.): *Intracerebral Pressure*. Berlin, Springer–Verlag, 1976, vol. 3, p. 232.

63. Faupel G., Reulen H.J., Miller D.J., et al.: Double blind study on the effects of dexamethasone on severe closed head injury, in Pappius H., et al. (eds.): *Dynamics of Brain Edema*. Berlin, Springer–Verlag, 1976.

64. Cooper P.R., Moody S., Clark W.K., et al.: Dexamethasone and severe head injury: A prospective study. *J. Neurosurg.* 51:306–316, 1979.

65. Gudeman S.K., Miller J.D., Becker D.P.: Failure of high–dose steroid therapy to influence intracranial pressure in patients with severe head injury. *J. Neurosurg.* 51:301–306, 1979.

66. Pitts L.H., Kaktis J.V.: Effects of megadose steroids on outcome following severe head injury, in *Proceedings of the American Association of Neurological Surgeons' National Meeting*. Los Angeles, 1979.

67. Marshall L.F., Smith R.W., Shapiro H.M.: The outcome with aggressive treatment in severe head injuries: Part I. The significance of intracranial pressure monitoring. *J. Neurosurg.* 50:20, 1979.

68. Marshall L.F., Smith R.W., Shapiro H.M.: The outcome with aggressive treatment in severe head injuries: Part II. Acute and chronic barbiturate administration in the management of head injury. *J. Neurosurg.* 50:26, 1979.

69. Brodersen P., Jorgensen E.O.: Cerebral blood flow and oxygen uptake and cerebrospinal fluid chemistry in severe coma. *J. Neurol. Neurosurg. Psychiatry* 37:384–391, 1974.

70. Demopoulos H.B., Flamm E.S., Seligman M.L., et al.: Antioxidant effects of barbiturates in model membranes undergoing free radical damage, in Ingvar D.H., Lassen N.A. (eds.): *Cerebral Functions, Metabolism and Circulation*. Copenhagen, Munksgaard, 1977.

71. Flamm E.S., Demopoulos H.B., Seligman M.L., et al.: Free radicals in cerebral ischemia. *Stroke* 9:445–447, 1978.

72. Flamm E.S., Demopoulos H.B., Seligman M.L., et al.: Possible molecular mechanisms of barbiturate–medicated protection in regional cerebral ischemia, in Ingvar D.H., Lassen N.A. (eds.): *Cerebral Functions, Metabolism and Circulation*. Copenhagen, Munksgaard, 1977.

73. Nordstrom C.H., Rehncrona S., Siesjo B.K.: Effects of phenobarbital in cerebral ischemia: Part II. Restitution of cerebral energy state, as well as of glycolytic metabolites, citric acid cycle intermediates, and associated amino acids after pronounced incomplete ischemia. *Stroke* 9:335–343, 1978.

74. Mogami H., Hayakawa T., Kanai N., et al.: Clinical applications of hyperbaric oxygenation in the treatment of acute cerebral damage. *J. Neurosurg.* 31:636–643, 1969.

75. Miller J.D., Ledingham I.M.: Reduction of increased intracranial pressure: Comparison between hyperbaric oxygen and hyperventilation. *Arch. Neurol.* 24:210–216, 1971.

76. Clasen R.A., Pandolfi S., Russell J., et al.: Hypothermia and hypotension in experimental cerebral edema. *Arch. Neurol.* 19:472–486, 1968.

77. Lakowski E.J., Klatzo I., Baldwin M.: Experimental study of the effects of hypothermia on local brain injury. *Neurology* 10:499–505, 1960.

78. Johannssen H., Siesjo B.K.: Blood flow and oxygen consumption in the rat brain in dilutional anemia. *Acta Physiol. Scand.* 91:136–138, 1974.

79. Massmer K., Gomandt L., Jesch F., et al.: Oxygen transport and tissue oxygenation during hemodilution with dextran, in Bruley D.F., Bicker H.J. (eds.): *Oxygen Transport in Tissue*. New York, Plenum Press, 1973, pp. 669–680.

80. Ruinckel D.N., Swanson J.R.: Effect of dimethyl sulfoxide on serum osmolarity. *Clin. Chem.* 26:1745–1747, 1980.

81. The effect of DMSO on the calcium paradox. *The DMSO Report* 1:1–8, 1972.

82. DMSO mechanism in edema and stroke. *The DMSO Report* 1:4, 1981.

83. Clark K., Nash T.M., Hutchinson G.C.: The failure of circumferential craniotomy in acute traumatic cerebral swelling. *J. Neurosurg.* 29:367–371, 1968.

84. Bruce D.A., Alvi A., Bilanuik L., et al.: Diffuse cerebral swelling following head injuries in children: The syndrome of "malignant brain edema." *J. Neurosurg.* 54:170–178, 1981.

85. Zimmerman R.A., Bilanuik L.T., Bruce D.A., et al.: Computed tomography of pediatric head trauma: Acute general cerebral swelling. *Radiology* 126:403–408, 1978.
86. Povlishock J.T., Becker D.P., Sullivan H.A., et al.: Vascular permeability alterations to horseradish peroxidases in experimental brain injury. *Brain Res.* 1533:223–239, 1978.
87. Povlishock J.T., Becker D.P., Miller J.D., et al.: The morphopathologic substrates of concussion. *Acta Neuropathol.* 47:1–11, 1979.
88. Klatzo I.: Presidential address: Neuropathological aspects of brain edema. *J. Neuropathol. Exp. Neurol.* 26:1–14, 1967.
89. Klatzo I.: Pathophysiological aspects of brain edema, in Reulen H.J., Schurman K. (eds.): *Steroids and Brain Edema.* Berlin, Springer–Verlag, 1972, pp. 1–8.
90. Long D.M.: Traumatic brain edema. *Clin. Neurosurg.* 29:174–202, 1982.
91. Costa J.L., Ito U., Spatz M., et al.: 5–Hydroxytryptamine accumulation in cerebrovascular injury. *Nature* 248:135–136, 1974.
92. Demopoloulos H.B., Flamm E.S., Seligman M.L., et al.: Membrane pertubations in central nervous system injury: Theoretical basis for free radical damage and a review of the experimental data, in Popp A.J., et al. (eds.): *Neural Trauma.* New York, Raven Press, 1979.
93. Fenske A., Sinterhauf K., Reulen H.J.: The role of monoamines in the development of cold–induced edema, in Pappius H.M., Feindel W. (eds.): *Dynamics of Brain Edema.* Berlin, Springer-Verlag, 1976, pp. 150–154.
94. Flamm E.S., Demopoulos H.B., Seligman M.L., et al.: Barbiturates and free radicals, in Popp A.J., et al. (eds.): *Neural Trauma.* New York, Raven Press, 1979.
95. Jacobsen S.A., Danufsky P.: Marked electrocardiographic changes produced by experimental head trauma. *J. Neuropathol. Exp. Neurol.* 13:462–466, 1954.
96. Dzur, J., Winternitz W.W.: Posttraumatic hypopituitarism: Anterior pituitary insufficiency secondary to head trauma. *South. Med. J.* 69:1377–1379, 1976.
97. Becker F.C., Schwartz W.B.: Increased antidiuretic hormone production after trauma to the craniofacial complex. *J. Trauma* 13:112–115, 1973.
98. Mackay E.M.: Experimental pulmonary edema: IV. Pulmonary edema accompanying trauma to the brain. *Proc. Soc. Exp. Biol.* 74:695, 1950.
99. Millen J.E., Glauser F.L., Zimmerman M.: Physiologic effects of controlled concussive head trauma. *J. Appl. Physiol.* 49:856–862, 1980.
100. Bowers R.E., McKeen C.R., Park B.E., et al.: Increased pulmonary vascular permeability follows intracranial hypertension in sheep. *Am. Rev. Respir. Dis.* 119:637–641, 1979.
101. Greenberg J., Alve A., Reivich M.: Local cerebral blood volume response to carbon dioxide in man. *Circ. Res.* 43:324–331, 1978.
102. Robin, E.D., Gary L.C., Grenvick A., et al.: Capillary leak syndrome in pulmonary edema. *Arch. Intern. Med.* 130:66–71, 1972.
103. van der Zee H., Malik A.B., Lee B.C., et al.: Lung fluid and protein exchange during intracranial hypertension and role of sympathetic mechanisms. *J. Appl. Physiol.* 48:273–280, 1980.
104. Marks J.: Central nervous system influence in the genesis of atrial fibrillation. *Ohio State Med. J.* 52:1054–1055, 1956.
105. Marshall A.J.: Transient atrial fibrillation after minor head injury. *Br. Heart J.* 38:984–985, 1976.
106. Hersch C.: Electrocardiographic changes in head injuries. *Circulation* 23:853–860, 1961.
107. Weinberg S.J., Fuster J.M.: Electrocardiographic changes produced by localized hypothalamic stimulations. *Ann. Intern. Med.* 53:332–341, 1960.
108. String T., Robinson A.J., Blaisdell F.W.: Massive trauma: Effect of intravascular coagulation on prognosis. *Arch. Surg.* 102:406–410, 1971.
109. Baratham G., Dennyson W.G.: Delayed traumatic intracerebral hemorrhage. *J. Neurol. Neurosurg. Psychiatry* 35:698–706, 1972.
110. Bricolo A., Trazzi S., Alexandre A., et al.: Decerebrate rigidity in acute head injury. *J. Neurosurg.* 47:680–698, 1977.
111. Bruce D.A., Raphaely R.C., Goldberg A.I., et al.: The pathophysiology, treatment, and outcome following severe head injury in children. *Childs Brain* 5:174–191, 1979.

8 / Pulmonary Aspiration

JEFFREY VENDER, M.D.
BARRY A. SHAPIRO, M.D.

THE GREEK POET, Anacreon, was believed to have died in 475 B.C. after aspirating a grape seed,[1] and death by aspiration has frequently appeared in the literature ever since. Aspiration is a commonly described cause of morbidity and mortality, from the earliest recorded medical literature to this day. Following Mendelson's classic description of postpartum aspiration pneumonitis,[2] clinical and laboratory research has established the existence of a broad spectrum of "pulmonary syndromes" resulting from aspiration of various materials under many conditions. Aspiration pneumonitis usually refers to the inflammation resulting from aspirated material and does not necessarily imply infection.

INCIDENCE AND DIAGNOSIS OF ASPIRATION

Aspiration is a major cause of anesthetic mortality,[3-5] a common cause of pulmonary disease in the hospitalized patient,[6, 7] and believed to be a major cause of morbidity and mortality in critically ill patients.[7, 8] The incidence of pulmonary aspiration is difficult to establish because it most commonly occurs when the airway protective reflexes (swallow, gag, laryngospasm, and cough) are obtunded so that the patient shows little or no distress. Furthermore, healthy, sleeping individuals often aspirate oral contents without any resulting pulmonary dysfunction.[9]

Pulmonary aspiration is most often a presumptive and/or retrospective diagnosis based on both the assumption of compromised airway defense mechanisms at the time of aspiration and pulmonary pathology attributable to the aspiration. Airway defense mechanisms are often deficient in altered states of consciousness, gastrointestinal disorders, and following therapeutic interventions.

114

Altered Neurologic States

The neurologically intact and awake individual has airway protective reflexes, coughing and laryngospasm, which greatly reduce the likelihood of clinically significant aspiration. Clinical evaluation of pharyngeal (gag and swallow) and tracheal (cough) reflexes are often helpful, although 10%–15% of the normal population has diminished or absent gag responses, and these reflexes tend to be diminished in the geriatric patient.[10]

Obtundation is usually associated with depression of airway protective reflexes. This altered neurologic state is commonly associated with cerebrovascular accidents, drug overdose, alcohol intoxication, postictal states, sedative administration, general anesthesia, cardiopulmonary resuscitation, and severe debilitation, as well as numerous specific CNS disorders.[11-13] Comatose patients must be assumed to have depressed airway protective reflexes and often require intubation for airway protection.

Gastrointestinal Disorders

Increased gastric pressure secondary to intestinal obstruction or diminished gastric emptying time increases the potential for pulmonary aspiration.[14] Esophageal disorders such as achalasia, stricture or spasm, pharyngoesophageal diverticulae, and hiatal hernia have been associated with an increased incidence of pulmonary aspiration.[15-17] Neurologic dysphagias have been shown to enhance the potential for pulmonary aspiration.[18]

Iatrogenic Factors

Mechanical disruption of airway defense mechanisms is common in critically ill patients. Nasogastric tubes may disrupt the cardiac sphincter and allow reflux in the presence of gastric dilation or obstruction.[19] Although properly inflated balloon cuffs on tracheal tubes offer significant protection from massive aspiration, small amounts of pharyngeal fluid may enter the trachea around the inflated cuff.[20-22] Although the clinical significance of this phenomenon is not clear, it indicates that precautions are necessary, despite the presence of a tracheal balloon cuff.

Tracheostomy tubes often prevent adequate glottic protection during swallowing by limiting the ability of the pharyngeal muscles to elevate the larynx.[23] This often requires an inflated cuff during oral feedings despite intact protective reflexes.

Nasogastric tube feedings frequently result in high residual volumes in the stomach that increase the risk of aspiration. Many drugs may prolong gastric emptying time, resulting in larger gastric residual volumes and an increased possibility of aspiration.

PATHOPHYSIOLOGY FOLLOWING ASPIRATION

Pulmonary aspiration leads to a pathologic spectrum determined by numerous patient- and non-patient-related factors. The introduction of a foreign inoculum into the pulmonary tree is the common denominator in all aspiration syndromes. The clinical presentation, pathophysiology, and therapeutic approach will be greatly influenced by the nature, volume, frequency, and distribution of the aspirated inoculum.[32] Three distinct classifications of inocula exist: toxic, nontoxic, and bacterial.

Toxic Inocula

Toxic fluids of clinical significance include acids, alcohols, volatile hydrocarbons, oils, and animal fats. The severity of pulmonary damage is influenced by the acidity, volume, and composition of the aspirate.[33] The most common and best studied of this group is the chemical pneumonitis resulting from gastric acid aspiration (Mendelson's syndrome).[2] Pulmonary damage from toxic fluids may be immediate or may appear within a few hours.[33, 34] Gross changes include edema, necrosis, and atelectasis. Microscopic changes include degeneration of bronchial epithelium, peribronchial hemorrhage and exudate, necrosis of alveolar epithelium, and alveolar infiltration of polymorphonuclear cells.

The most important factor in toxic fluid aspiration appears to be acidity.[35] A small volume (0.3 ml/kg) of pH 1 fluid introduced into dog tracheas results in significant pulmonary reaction.[34] Available data suggest that toxic fluids with a pH less than 2.5 consistently result in pulmonary pathology, whereas fluids with a pH greater than 2.5 seldom result in significant pathology.[8, 36–38] The acidity is neutralized within seconds after contact with the pulmonary mucosa, leaving little validity to the concept of tracheal lavage following toxic fluid aspiration.[3, 8, 33, 39]

With 0.1N HCl (pH 1) solutions, the volume of aspirate appears to play a secondary role.[40] Volume may be significant when the pH of the aspirate is between 1.5 and 3.0,[8, 34, 41] since it appears that aspirated volumes of such fluids must exceed 0.3–0.4 ml/kg to produce significant effects.[42, 43] Evidence in man indicates that the greater the volume and pulmonary distribution of toxic fluid aspirate, the higher the morbidity and mortality.[6, 8, 34] This influence of the aspirate composition in man is demonstrated by the near 100% mortality following fecal-gastric fluid aspiration.[35, 44]

Clinical Presentation

Following significant toxic fluid aspiration the patient may manifest dyspnea, wheezing, rales, rhonchi, cough, fever, tachycardia, hypotension, and cyanosis. Initial findings may vary, and any or all may not be present for as long as 6 hours after the aspiration. The damage to bronchial epithelium can produce bronchospasm and a massive mucosal exudation that results in pink, frothy airway fluid, dyspnea, and wheezing, which are easily mistaken for cardiogenic pulmonary edema.[8, 34] The intravascular volume loss secondary to exudation can be quite significant.

X-ray studies commonly show patchy alveolar infiltrates limited to segments of lung that were gravity-dependent at the time of aspiration.[3, 42, 45, 46] However, 25%–40% of patients have diffuse bilateral infiltrates.[32, 47] Radiologic findings may be delayed 4–8 hours.[3]

A decreased arterial Po_2 is an early finding consistent with chemical pneumonitis and does not necessarily correlate with either the clinical or radiologic findings.[3] The etiology of the arterial hypoxemia is partly attributable to venous admixture secondary to bronchospasm and inflammation that is initially responsive to oxygen therapy. However, severe chemical pneumonitis involves significant true shunting[48] from factors such as reflex airway closure,[49, 50] altered surfactant activity,[32, 34, 51] and alveolar-capillary leak.[32, 52–54] High Fi_{O_2} as well as positive end-expiratory pressure (PEEP) therapy may be required to maintain adequate arterial oxygenation.

Although the work of breathing is increased secondary to diminished pulmonary compliance,[51] alveolar ventilation is usually adequate (arterial Pco_2 <40 mm Hg). The potential for prolonged respiratory derangement has been reported[8] and the need for ventilatory assistance must be continuously evaluated.

Secondary Bacterial Infection

The pulmonary pathology present in the first 24 hours following toxic fluid aspiration cannot be attributed to bacterial pneumonitis.[33, 35, 40] However, secondary bacterial pneumonitis (bacterial superinfection) has been reported to occur in 20%–50% of patients within 24–72 hours following toxic fluid aspiration.[2, 55, 56] Chemical pneumonitis appears to leave the lung more vulnerable to infection.[57]

The pathogenic organisms of secondary bacterial pneumonia are almost always representative of the patient's oropharyngeal flora. Hospitalized patients have a progressive increase in *Staphylococcus aureus* and gram-negative bacilli colonizing the oropharynx[33, 58–61] due to the hospital environment, nutritional and immunologic factors, and therapeutic factors such as steroids and antibiotics. This explains the higher incidence of staphylococcal and gram-negative pneumonias following toxic fluid aspiration in the hospitalized patient. Although some evidence exists for administration of prophylactic penicillin in patients who aspirate toxic fluid outside the hospital,[56, 62, 63] there is no evidence that prophylactic antibiotics reduce the incidence of bacterial superinfection in the hospitalized patient.[6, 40, 55]

Adult Respiratory Distress Syndrome (ARDS)

This severe form of lung endothelial and epithelial damage is believed to be the result of severe systemic or pulmonary insult (see Chap. 12). Although definitive data are lacking, certain insults (sepsis, disseminated intravascular coagulation, multiple trauma, fat embolism) are associated with a high incidence of ARDS. Some studies suggest that ARDS is a frequent sequela to toxic fluid aspiration.[32, 33, 64]

Nontoxic Inocula

Aspiration of nontoxic materials can be separated into two distinct categories: aspiration of nontoxic fluids (water, saline, milk, blood, barium, gastric fluid with pH >7.3) and aspiration of particulate matter. The degree of pulmonary dysfunction due to such aspiration is primarily determined by the volume and/or composition of the aspirate.[33] These events do not cause chemical pneumonitis but may result in secondary bacterial infection.

Nontoxic Fluid Aspiration

Aspiration of small amounts of nontoxic fluid usually provokes an acute nonspecific reaction such as coughing and breath-holding. This is usually reversible and self-limited. There are no characteristic radiographic findings and seldom significant sequelae unless the hypoxemia and intrathoracic pressure variations of the acute reaction precipitate cardiovascular events. Near-drowning is a common example of massive aspiration of nontoxic fluid.

Near-Drowning

Near-drowning may be defined as water submersion after which the victim is in a potentially salvageable condition. Approximately 15% of near-drowning victims develop laryngospasm that prevents water aspiration.[65] Such "dry" drowning is a true asphyxiation without direct pulmonary damage.

Eighty-five percent of near-drowning victims have significant water aspiration. Most of these will survive with appropriate therapy if they are rescued before hypoxic brain damage occurs.[66] Cold water submersion produces hypothermia that results in metabolic and cardiovascular changes that make resuscitation possible even after 30 minutes of submersion.[67]

Largely determined by the volume and tonicity[68, 69] of the fluid aspirated, early pathophysiologic events in human near-drowning are hypoxemia, hypotension, and pulmonary edema. Salt water drowning is associated with a high incidence of hypovolemic shock and hemoconcentration. Fresh water drowning is associated with hypervolemia, hemodilution, and occasionally hemolysis. Both salt and fresh water near-drowning can alter electrolyte balance. Pulmonary edema associated with salt water near-drowning is largely the result of the hypertonicity of the aspirated fluid, whereas in fresh water near-drowning the edema is mainly attributable to hypervolemia.[37, 70]

A post-immersion syndrome may occur within 24–48 hours and will manifest with respiratory distress or apnea, hypoxemia, pulmonary edema, fever, and leukocytosis.[37] This usually occurs after the patient has been clinically stable and apparently unaffected by the near-drowning incident. Many near-drownings are associated with alcohol and drug ingestion which may have obtunded airway protective reflexes; therefore, the possibility of concomitant toxic gastric fluid aspiration must be entertained.

Particulate Aspiration

Small particles (foodstuffs) are often associated with gastric content aspiration. These cause partial obstruction and produce inflammation with granulomatous resolution but are seldom a significant problem.[36, 37, 71]

Large particulate (foreign body) aspiration produces symptoms dependent on the size of the aspirate and its location within the pulmonary tree.[72] Large particulate aspiration is most common in the pediatric age group.[73] Total obstruction of the proximal airway results in asphyxiation, while partial obstruction may present with dyspnea, hoarseness, stridor, cough, and cyanosis.[37, 74] A peripheral total obstruction causes atelectasis, while a partial obstruction may cause either atelectasis or a distal emphysema ("ball valve obstruction").[37] In general, the more peripheral the obstruction, the smaller the amount of functional lung occluded, and therefore the less life-threatening the event. After appropriate supportive therapy, definitive treatment requires removal of the foreign body by bronchoscopy. If the obstructing object is not removed, the probability of a distal pneumonitis developing is great.[40, 75]

Bacterial Inocula

Primary bacterial aspiration is the most common type of pulmonary aspiration. It is a difficult diagnosis that is often made in retrospect or by exclusion. Unlike the usually observed toxic and nontoxic aspiration associated with factors such as cough, choking, and laryngospasm, aspiration of bacteria usually involves a small volume and is relatively unnoticed. It is heralded by the onset of symptoms of bacterial pneumonia at least 24 hours after the aspiration. With repeated aspiration the presenting symptoms may be due to lung abscess, empyema, or necrotizing pneumonia 1–3 weeks after the initial insult. In patients with factors predisposing to aspiration, the appearance of new pulmonary infiltrates on chest x-ray films raises the possibility of primary bacterial aspiration.

The bacteria most frequently responsible are those present in the patient's oropharyngeal secretions.[58] Factors such as gingivodental disease and sinusitis significantly influence the virulence and number of oropharyngeal bacteria.[76, 77] Primary bacterial aspiration pneumonia typically involves polymicrobial isolates, including anaerobes.[58, 78] Host defense capabilities are important, since normal people are known to occasionally aspirate pharyngeal secretions during sleep without sequelae.[9]

Reasonable criteria for making the diagnosis of primary bacterial aspiration include (1) a clinical status predisposing the patient to aspiration, (2) clinical evidence of bacterial pneumonitis, including chest x-ray infiltrate, and (3) bacteriologic evaluation of pulmonary secretions.

MANAGEMENT OF ASPIRATION

The overall success of management depends on the early recognition of aspiration and institution of therapy to ensure adequate pulmonary gas exchange and limit pulmonary damage. Specific therapy includes (1) oxygen therapy, (2) airway protection and tracheobronchial hygiene, (3) airway pressure therapy [PEEP, continuous positive airway pressure (CPAP), positive pressure ventilation], (4) drug therapy (bronchodilators, corticosteroids, antibiotics), and (5) bronchoscopy.

PREVENTION OF ASPIRATION

Aspiration must be viewed as a preventable phenomenon that occurs frequently and can add considerably to morbidity and mortality in critically ill patients. Every reasonable effort must be made to minimize the incidence of aspiration in the susceptible population. Anticipation and prevention are more effective that postaspiration therapy!

Patient position is important, since gravity plays a crucial role in the regurgitation process. Although the supine or reverse Trendelenburg (head-up) position may diminish the incidence of passive regurgitation, it also encourages aspiration of pharyngeal contents. The ideal position to prevent both regurgitation and aspiration is the lateral Trendelenburg, which encourages oropharyngeal pooling and ready access for suctioning.[19, 24] However, factors such as intracranial disease and gastric motility disturbances commonly require a head-up position. When in doubt, the airway should be protected by intubation with a cuffed tube.

Care must be taken when using drugs such as muscle relaxants, anesthetics, narcotics, tranquilizers, and sedatives, as these can diminish the protective airway reflexes as well as prolong gastric emptying time.[24] A nasogastric tube does not ensure an empty stomach, even when continuous suction is applied. Nasogastric feedings are best administered in small amounts in the head-up position.

A great deal of data exist concerning the alteration of gastric fluid pH to diminish the pulmonary injury if aspiration occurs.[25] *Oral antacids* are effective in maintaining acceptable gastric pH but are associated with increased gastric volume.[26] Some antacid formulas are associated with precipitate formation in gastric contents, which, if aspirated, may cause pulmonary damage.[27–29] Sodium citrate is presently preferred since no precipitate is formed. Cimetidine, an H_2-receptor antagonist, increases gastric pH while reducing the volume of gastric secretions.[30, 31] Cimetidine is associated with a number of side effects; however, new H_2-receptor antagonists are being developed that have fewer side effects and are longer acting.[31] It has been suggested that a combination of antacid therapy and cimetidine provides the greatest protection in reducing acid aspiration in susceptible patients.

CASE STUDY

A 72-year-old man was brought to the emergency room after suffering a "seizure" at home. His wife reported that he vomited a significant quantity of yellowish liquid during the seizure. Past history revealed the presence of organic brain syndrome, hiatal hernia, and a mild "stroke" 1 year previously.

On admission the patient's sensorium appeared depressed. Vomitus was noted on his clothing. Blood pressure (BP) was 122/90 mm Hg, pulse rate was 124 beats per minute and regular, respiratory rate was 42/minute and unlabored, and temperature was 97.2° F. Residual vomitus was noted in the oropharynx and severe periodontal disease was present. On chest examination· bilateral rales were

heard with mild expiratory wheezing. No cardiac or abdominal abnormalities were noted. The patient was arousable but somnolent when undisturbed.

Initial laboratory tests revealed a hemoglobin concentration of 14 gm dl and a WBC count of $9,800/mm^{-3}$ with a mild leftward shift. An electrocardiogram revealed sinus tachycardia with occasional premature atrial contractions and nonspecific ST segment and T wave abnormalities. Chest x-ray studies revealed mild bilateral patchy alveolar infiltrates greatest at the right base, and arterial blood gas analysis showed a pH of 7.49, a P_{CO_2} of 31 mm Hg, and a P_{O_2} of 46 mm Hg on room air.

Discussion

Toxic fluid aspiration must be assumed. A history of vomiting during seizure (unprotected airway), the x-ray findings, and the arterial blood gas values are all compatible and suggest the diagnosis. Decisions must be made pertaining to airway management, oxygen therapy, and steroid and antibiotic therapy.

Airway Management

The oropharynx should be suctioned immediately to help clear the airway, stimulate coughing, and confirm the diagnosis. Airway protective reflexes must be evaluated and the advisability of intubation considered. A nasotracheal intubation with only topical anesthesia would be ideal, since central drug depression could be avoided and the nasal tube would be best tolerated as the patient's level of consciousness improved. Bronchoscopy does not appear necessary since no particulate matter is suspected in the aspirate.

Pulmonary lavage with a neutral or alkaline solution has been recommended by some following intubation. There appear to be little or no data to support this procedure, since the acid media is neutralized within seconds of contact with pulmonary mucosa. Furthermore, studies have demonstrated an increase in the area of lung injury and altered pulmonary compliance following pulmonary lavage with alkaline solutions.[39, 79, 80] Present recommendations support only the instillation of small aliquots of sterile saline (5–10 ml) in an effort to stimulate coughing and enhance pulmonary toilet.[42]

Oxygen Therapy

Hypoxemia is a common result of aspiration and can contribute to tachypnea and tachycardia. The early pulmonary insults lead to hypoxemia that is relatively responsive to oxygen therapy (venous admixture). Thirty to fifty percent inspired oxygen concentrations should result in an acceptable arterial PO_2 and often a decrease in respiratory rate. Oxygen therapy is indicated, with or without the placement of an endotracheal tube. Mechanical ventilation is not required unless the patient is in acute or impending ventilatory failure. Early institution of PEEP/CPAP may be considered as it can restore pulmonary function to nearly normal within 24–48 hours by increasing functional residual capacity and improving the ventilation-perfusion relationships.[30]

Corticosteroids

Since toxic fluid aspiration results in a pulmonary inflammatory response, steroids have been recommended to reduce the degree of inflammation.[35, 42, 80, 81] Studies demonstrating stabilization of lysosomal membranes and prevention of leukocyte and platelet agglutination in the lungs have been cited as further rationale for early administration of steroids following aspiration.[79, 82, 83]

Despite a plethora of studies, the information on corticosteroids remains conflicting, anecdotal, uncontrolled, and controversial.[32, 84, 85] If steroids are indicated at all, they must be administered within "minutes" of the insult to have a significant effect.[32, 47] Although large doses administered for less than 36 hours do not appear to alter defense mechanisms or enhance colonization, some animal studies suggest that steroid therapy interferes with lung healing and promotes granuloma and abscess formation.[71]

Justification for steroid therapy following aspiration is entirely theoretical and must be weighed against the potential harm to each patient.[33, 86, 87] Indiscriminate use of steroids is probably best avoided until well-controlled experimental data are available to support their use.[55]

Antibiotics

Although the evidence supporting the use of prophylactic antibiotics following toxic and nontoxic fluid aspiration is scanty, many physicians continue the practice. In the critically ill patient population this practice appears to be ineffective[55] and potentially harmful because it may increase the incidence of antibiotic-resistant, gram-negative organisms responsible for the secondary bacterial pneumonia and expose the patient to the risk of drug reactions.[3, 47, 60, 88] Antibiotics can potentially eliminate from the oropharyngeal flora Streptococcus viridans, which normally inhibits the colonization of more virulent gram-negative bacilli and staphylococci.[2] One exception to this general rule is aspiration of intestinal fluid with a high bacterial count, which demands immediate administration of the appropriate antibiotics.

A logical approach is to anticipate a secondary bacterial infection and serially monitor the tracheobronchial secretions, chest x-ray findings, and clinical condition. Evidence of pulmonary infection 24 hours after aspiration should be specifically treated based on microbiologic evidence of colonization of tracheal secretions. The avoidance of antibiotic therapy in the first 24–48 hours limits the potential risks of inappropriate antibiotics and provides the framework for rational antibiotic therapy.[3] If prophylactic antibiotics are to be employed, both aerobic and anaerobic coverage should be included.

Case Study Continued

The patient was given 40% oxygen by air entrainment mask. Assessment of the patient's airway revealed obtundation of airway protective reflexes. Following administration of topical anesthesia to the right nostril and nasopharynx with 10% cocaine and breathing an aerosol mist of 2% lidocaine for 5 minutes, an 8-mm endotracheal tube was placed via the nasal route without difficulty. Following manual ventilation and preoxygenation, the trachea was repeatedly suctioned until the return was clear. The patient's condition stabilized with a BP of 118/85 mm Hg, heart rate of 118 beats per minute, and respiratory rate of 32/minute. Arterial blood gas analysis with the patient breathing 40% oxygen revealed a pH of 7.46, a P_{CO_2} of 32 mm Hg, and a P_{O_2} of 88 mm Hg.

Approximately 3 hours after admission the patient had frothy pink sputum and complained of increasing shortness of breath. BP was 108/58 mm Hg, pulse was 128 beats per minute, and respiratory rate was 44/minute. Diffuse rhonchi were heard bilaterally and the chest x-ray film revealed a diffuse pulmonary edema pattern. Heart tones were normal without an S_3 or S_4. Arterial blood gas analysis with an $F_{I_{O_2}}$ of 0.4 revealed a pH of 7.44, a P_{CO_2} of 32 mm Hg, and a P_{O_2} of 52 mm Hg.

Discussion

Although cardiogenic edema must be considered and ruled out, a more likely diagnosis is noncardiogenic edema secondary to toxic fluid aspiration. The significant deterioration in arterial oxygenation on 40% supplemental oxygen (88 to 52 mm Hg) suggests increasing right-to-left shunting (true shunting). This is most likely secondary to factors such as surfactant destruction, dilution, or alteration by the aspirated acid with consequent alveolar collapse and alveolar edema.[30] Since this process can be expected to worsen over the next several hours, there is little chance that increasing the $F_{I_{O_2}}$ will ensure adequate arterial oxygenation.

Airway Pressure Therapy

There is no reason to institute mechanical assistance of ventilation at this point. However, this may become a reasonable alternative if other measures do not improve the patient's complaint of dyspnea. CPAP/PEEP has therapeutic value in the management of noncardiogenic edema, and some investigators contend that early application can lessen the severity of the disease process.[89, 90] Bronchodilator therapy should be considered.

Fluid Therapy

The development of noncardiogenic edema secondary to increased endothelial permeability makes the lung sensitive to small increases in vascular pressure. There is controversy concerning the ideal fluid to use in patients with endothelial cell damage. The use of various osmotic agents has been recommended but may be deleterious.[42, 91] A balance between a vascular volume sufficient for organ perfusion and a vascular pressure that will not promote further fluid extravasation into the interstitium must be achieved. In patients with preexisting cardiac disease or unstable fluid balance, a pulmonary artery catheter should be employed to evaluate vascular pressure and measure cardiac output. Ideally, the pulmonary artery occluded pressure should be maintained at the lowest value compatible with an acceptable cardiac and urine output.

Case Study Continued

The patient was placed on 10 cm H_2O PEEP and 450 ml of crystalloid solution was administered intravenously (IV). BP was 115/78 mm Hg, pulse was 115 beats per minute, and respiratory rate was 28/minute without complaint of shortness of breath. Arterial blood gas values at an F_{IO_2} of 0.35 were as follows: pH, 7.44; P_{CO_2}, 35 mm Hg; and P_{O_2}, 70 mm Hg.

Over the next 2 days the pulmonary edema pattern on x-ray studies improved and the CPAP was decreased to 5 cm H_2O with an F_{IO_2} of 0.28. Arterial blood gas analysis showed a pH of 7.41, a P_{CO_2} of 38 mm Hg, and a P_{O_2} of 72 mm Hg. BP was 122/80 mm Hg, pulse

was 105 beats per minute, and respiratory rate was 20/minute. The patient's sensorium was markedly improved. He was extubated without event and maintained the same vital signs and blood gas values at an oxygen flow of 2 L/minute via nasal cannula.

Eighteen hours after extubation (3½ days after aspiration) the patient had a spiking temperature of 102.8°F rectally. WBC count rose from 11,000 to 17,000/mm^3 and the chest x-ray film showed a new infiltrate in the right lower lobe. Heart rate and respiratory rate had trended upward. Arterial P_{O_2} had declined to 55 mm Hg with oxygen delivered via the nasal cannula.

Discussion

All evidence suggests the appearance of a secondary bacterial pneumonia. Predicted on sputum specimens previously obtained for culture and sensitivity, specific antibiotic therapy was instituted. The patient was placed on a 35% air entrainment mask and his ability to cough and breathe deeply was assessed frequently. Antipyretic agents were administered.

Case Study Continued

Within 12 hours the patient's temperature was below 100° F without antipyretics. His pneumonia resolved

without incident and he was able to cough up secretions with some assistance and encouragement.

REFERENCES

1. Broe P.J., Toung T.J.K., Cameron J.L.: Aspiration pneumonia. *Surg. Clin. North Am.* 60:1551–1564, 1980.
2. Mendelson C.L.: The aspiration of stomach contents into the lungs during obstetric anesthesia. *Am. J. Obstet. Gynecol.* 52:191–205, 1946.
3. Little J.W.: Pulmonary aspiration. *West. J. Med.* 131:122–129, 1979.
4. Bannister W.K., Sahilaro A.J.: Vomiting and aspiration during anesthesia. *Anesthesiology* 23:251–264, 1962.
5. Edwards G., Morton H.J.V., Pask E.A., et al.: Deaths associated with anesthesia: Report of 1,000 cases. *Anesthesia* 11:194–220, 1956.
6. Cameron J.L., Mitchell W.H., Zvidema G.D.: Aspiration pneumonia: Clinical outcome following documented aspiration. *Arch. Surg.* 106:49, 1973.
7. Cameron J.L., Zvidema G.D.: Aspiration pneumonia: Magnitude and frequency of the problem. *JAMA* 219:1194, 1972.
8. Awe W.L., Fletcher W.S., Jacob S.W.: The pathophysiology of aspiration pneumonitis. *Surgery* 60:232–239, 1966.
9. Huxley E.J., Vinoslav J., Gray W.R., et al.: Pharyngeal aspiration in normal adults and patients with depressed consciousness. *Am. J. Med.* 64:564–568, 1978.
10. Pontoppidan H., Beeche H.K.: Progressive loss of protective reflexes in the airway with the advance of age. *JAMA* 174:2209–2213, 1960.
11. Greenberg H.G.: Aspiration pneumonia after cardiac arrest and resuscitation. *J. Am. Geriatr. Soc.* 15(2):48–52, 1967.
12. Brown M., Glassenberg M.: Mortality factors in patients with acute stroke. *JAMA* 224:1493–1495, 1973.
13. Mrazek S.A.: Bronchopneumonia in terminally ill patients. *J. Am. Geriatr. Soc.* 17:969–973, 1969.
14. Chase H.F: Role of delayed gastric emptying time in the etiology of aspiration pneumonia. *Am. J. Obstet. Gynecol.* 56:673–679, 1948.
15. Belsey R.H.: Pulmonary complications of esophageal disease and their treatment. *Br. J. Dis. Chest* 54:342–348, 1960.
16. Cohen S.: Motor disorders of the esophagus. *N. Engl. J. Med.* 301:184–192, 1979.
17. Chernow B., Johnson L.F., Janowitz W.R., et al.: Pulmonary aspiration as a consequence of gastroesophageal reflux. *Dig. Dis. Sci.* 24:839–844, 1979.
18. Smith R.A., Norris F.H.: Symptomatic care of patients with amyotrophic lateral sclerosis. *JAMA* 234:715–717, 1975.
19. Cameron J.L., Zvidema G.D.: Aspiration pneumonia: Magnitude and frequency of the problem. *JAMA* 219:1194–1196, 1972.
20. Culver G.A., Makel H.P., Beecher H.K.: Frequency of aspiration of gastric contents of the lungs during anesthesia and surgery. *Ann. Surg.* 133:289–292, 1951.
21. Spray S.B., Zvidema G.D., Cameron J.L.: Aspiration pneumonia: Incidence of aspiration with endotracheal tubes. *Am. J. Surg.* 131:701–703, 1976.
22. Pavlin E.G., Van Nimwegan D., Hornbein T.F.: Failure of high compliance low pressure cuff to prevent aspiration. *Anesthesiology* 42:216–219, 1975.
23. Cameron J.L., Reynolds J., Zvidema G.D.: Aspiration in patients with tracheostomies. *Surg. Gynecol. Obstet.* 136:68–70, 1973.
24. Turndorf H., Rodis I.D., Clark T.S.: Silent regurgitation during general anesthesia. *Anesth. Analg.* 53:700–703, 1974.
25. Taylor G., Pryse–Davies J.: The prophylactic use of antacids in the prevention of the acid aspiration syndrome. *Lancet* 1:288–297, 1965.
26. Stoelting R.K.: Response to atropine, glycopyrrolate, and Riepan of gastric pH and volume of adult patients. *Anesthesiology* 48:367–369, 1978.
27. Kuchling A., Joyce T.H., Cooke S.: The pulmonary lesion of antacid aspiration, abstracted, in *Proceedings of the Annual Meeting of the American Society of Anesthesiologists*, 1975, p. 281.

28. Gibb C.P., Schwartz D.J., Wynne J.W., et al.: Antacid pulmonary aspiration in the dog. *Anesthesiology* 51:380–385, 1979.
29. Bond V.K., Stoelting R.K., Gupta C.D.: Pulmonary aspiration syndrome after inhalation of gastric fluid containing antacids. *Anesthesiology* 51:452–453, 1979.
30. Stoelting R.K.: Gastric fluid pH in patients receiving cimetadine. *Anesth. Analg.* 57:675–677, 1978.
31. Manchikanti L., Kraus J.W., Edds S.P.: Cimetadine and related drugs in anesthesia. *Anesth. Analg.* 61:595–608, 1982.
32. Stewardson R.H., Nyhus L.M.: Pulmonary aspiration. *Arch. Surg.* 12:1192–1197, 1977.
33. Wynne J.W., Modell J.H.: Respiratory aspiration of stomach contents. *Ann. Intern. Med.* 87:466–474, 1977.
34. Greenfield L.J., Singleton R.P., McCaffree D.R., et al.: Pulmonary effects of experimental graded aspiration of hydrochloric acid. *Ann. Surg.* 170:74–86, 1969.
35. Hamelberg W., Bosomworth P.P.: Aspiration pneumonitis: Experimental and clinical observations. *Anesth. Analg.* 43:669–677, 1964.
36. Teabeaut J.H.: Aspiration of gastric contents: An experimental study. *Am. J. Pathol.* 28:51–67, 1952.
37. Ribaudo C.A., Grace W.J.: Pulmonary aspiration. *Am. J. Med.* 50:510–520, 1971.
38. Schwartz D.J., Wynne J.W., Gibbs C.P., et al.: The pulmonary consequences of aspiration of gastric contents at pH values greater than 2.5. *Am. Rev. Respir. Dis.* 121:119–126, 1980.
39. Wamberg K., Zeskov B.: Experimental studies on the course and treatment of aspiration pneumonia. *Anesth. Analg.* 45:230–236, 1966.
40. Bartlett J.G., Gonbach S.L.: The triple threat of aspiration pneumonia. *Chest* 68:560–566, 1975.
41. Cameron J.L., Caldini P., Toung J.K., et al.: Aspiration pneumonia: Physiologic data following experimental aspiration. *Surgery* 72:238–245, 1972.
42. Broe P.J., Toung T.J.K., Cameron J.L.: Aspiration pneumonia. *Surg. Clin. North Am.* 60:1551–1564, 1980.
43. Hupp J.R., Peterson L.J.: Aspiration pneumonitis: Etiology, therapy, and prevention. *J. Oral Surg.* 39:430–435, 1981.
44. Vilinskas J., Schweizer R.T., Foster J.H.: Experimental studies on aspiration of contents of obstructed intestines. *Surg. Gynecol. Obstet.* 135:568–570, 1972.
45. Kross D.E., Effman E.L., Putman C.E.: Adult aspiration pneumonia. *A.F.P.* 22:73–78, 1980.
46. Wilkins R.A., DeLacey G.J., Flor R., et al.: Radiology in Mendelson's syndrome. *Clin. Radiol.* 27:81–85, 1976.
47. LeFrock J.L., Clark T.S., Davies B., et al.: Aspiration pneumonia: A ten year review. *Am. Surg.* 45:305–313, 1979.
48. Moseley R.V., Doty R.B.: Physiologic changes due to aspiration pneumonitis. *Ann. Surg.* 171:73–76, 1970.
49. Halmagyi D.F.J., Colebatch J.H.J., Starzecki B.: Inhalation of blood, saliva, and alcohol: Consequences, mechanism, and treatment. *Thorax* 17:244–250, 1962.
50. Colebatch H.J.H., Halmagyi D.F.J.: Reflex airway reaction to fluid aspiration. *J. Appl. Physiol.* 17:787–794, 1962.
51. Cameron J.L., Caldini P., Toung J.K., et al.: Aspiration pneumonia: Physiologic data following experimental aspiration. *Surgery* 72:238–245, 1972.
52. Glausen F.L., Millen J.E., Falls R.: Effects of acid aspiration on pulmonary alveolar epithelial membrane permeability. *Chest* 76:201–205, 1979.
53. Brigham K.L.: Factors affecting lung vascular permeability. *Am. Rev. Respir. Dis.* 115:165–169, 1977.
54. Jones J.G., Grossman R.F., Slavin M.B., et al.: Alveolar–capillary membrane permeability: Correlation with functional, radiographic, and postmortem changes after fluid aspiration. *Am. Rev. Respir. Dis.* 120:399–410, 1979.
55. Bynum L.J., Pierce A.K.: Pulmonary aspiration of gastric contents. *Am. Rev. Respir. Dis.* 114:1129–1136, 1976.

56. Arms R.A., Dines D.E., Tinstman T.C.: Aspiration pneumonia. *Chest* 65:136–139, 1974.
57. Johanson W.G., Jay S.J., Pierce A.K.: Bacterial growth in vivo: An important determinant of the pulmonary clearance of *Diplococcus pneumoniae* in rats. *J. Clin. Invest.* 53:1320–1325, 1974.
58. Bartlett J.G., Gorbach S.L., Finegold S.M.: The bacteriology of aspiration pneumonia. *Am. J. Med.* 56:202–207, 1974.
59. Wolfe J.E., Bone R.C., Ruth W.E.: Effects of corticosteroids in the treatment of patients with gastric aspiration. *Am. J. Med.* 63:719–722, 1977.
60. Johanson W.G., Pierce A.K., Sanford J.P.: Changing pharyngeal bacterial flora of hospitalized patients: Emergence of gram–negative bacilli. *N. Engl. J. Med.* 281:1137–1140, 1969.
61. Johanson W.G., Pierce A.K., Sanford J.P.: Nosocomial respiratory infections with gram–negative bacilli: The significance of colonization of the respiratory tract. *Ann. Intern. Med.* 77:701–706, 1972.
62. Bartlett J.G.: Aspiration pneumonia: Clinical notes. *Resp. Dis.* 18(4):3–8, 1980.
63. Murray H.W.: Antimicrobial therapy in pulmonary aspiration. *Am. J. Med.* 66:188–190, 1979.
64. Horovitz J.H., Carrico C.J., Shires G.T.: Pulmonary response to major injury. *Arch. Surg.* 108:349–355, 1974.
65. Spitz W.O., Blanke R.V.: Mechanism of death in fresh water drowning. *Arch. Pathol.* 71:661–668, 1961.
66. Redding J.S., Cozine R.A., Voight C., et al.: Resuscitation from drowning. *JAMA* 178:1136–1139, 1961.
67. Siebke H., Breiver H., Rod T., et al.: Survival after a 40 minute submersion without cerebral sequelae. *Lancet* 1:1275–1277, 1975.
68. Kylstra J.A.: Survival of submerged mammals. *N. Engl. J. Med.* 272:198–200, 1965.
69. Donald K.W.: Drowning. *Br. Med. J.* 2:155–160, 1955.
70. Modell J.H., Graves S.A., Ketover A.: Clinical course of 91 consecutive near–drowning victims. *Chest* 70:231–238, 1976.
71. Wynne J.W., Reynolds J.L., Hood I.C., et al.: Steroid therapy for pneumonitis induced in rabbits by aspiration of foodstuff. *Anesthesiology* 51:11–19, 1979.
72. Brooks J.W.: Foreign bodies in the air and food passages. *Ann. Surg.* 175:720–732, 1972.
73. Kim I.G., Brummett W.M., Humphrey A., et al.: Foreign body in the airway: A review of 202 cases. *Laryngoscope* 83:347–354, 1973.
74. Haugen R.K.: The cafe coronary: Sudden deaths in restaurants. *JAMA* 186:142–143, 1963.
75. Lansing A.M., Jamieson W.G.: Mechanisms of fever in pulmonary atelectasis. *Arch. Surg.* 87:184–192, 1963.
76. Lorber B., Swenson R.M.: Bacteriology of aspiration pneumonia. *Ann. Intern. Med.* 81:329–331, 1974.
77. Bartlett J.G., Finegold S.M.: Anaerobic infections of the lung and pleural space. *Am. Rev. Respir. Dis.* 110:56–77, 1974.
78. Johanson W.G., Harris G.D.: Aspiration pneumonia, anaerobic infection, and lung abscess. *Med. Clin. North Am.* 64:385–394, 1980.
79. Lewinski A.: Evaluation of methods employed in the treatment of the chemical pneumonitis of aspiration. *Anesthesiology* 26:37–44, 1965.
80. Bosomworth P.P., Hamelberg W.: Etiologic and therapeutic aspects of aspiration pneumonitis. *Surg. Forum* 13:158–159, 1962.
81. Dines D.E., Titus J.L., Sessler A.D.: Aspiration pneumonitis. *Mayo Clin. Proc.* 45:347–360, 1970.
82. Starling J.R., Rudolf L.E., Ferguson W., et al.: Benefits of methylprednisolone in the isolated perfused organ. *Ann. Surg.* 177:566–571, 1973,
83. Wilson J.W.: Treatment and prevention of pulmonary cellular damage with pharmacologic doses of corticosteroid. *Surg. Gynecol. Obstet.* 134:675–681, 1972.
84. Chapman R.L., Downs J.B., Modell J.H., et al.: The ineffectiveness of steroid therapy in treating aspiration of hydrochloric acid. *Arch. Surg.* 108:858–861, 1974.

85. Downs J.B., Chapman R.L., Modell J.H., et al.: An evaluation of steroid therapy in aspiration pneumonitis. *Anesthesiology* 40:129–135, 1974.
86. Lowrey L.D., Anderson M., Calhoun T., et al.: Failure of corticosteroid therapy for experimental acid aspiration. *J. Surg. Res.* 32:168–172, 1982.
87. Lee M., Sukumavan M., Berger H.W., et al.: Influence of corticosteroid treatment on pulmonary function after recovery from aspiration of gastric contents. *Mt. Sinai J. Med.* 47:341–346, 1980.
88. Sprunt K., Leidy G.A., Redman W.: Prevention of bacterial overgrowth. *J. Infect. Dis.* 123:1–10, 1971.
89. Schmidt G.B.: Prophylaxis of pulmonary complications following abdominal surgery, including atelectasis, ARDS, and pulmonary embolism. *Ann. Surg.* 9:29–73, 1977.
90. Chapman R.L., Modell J.H., Ruiz B.C., et al.: Effect of continuous positive pressure, ventilation, and steroids on aspiration of hydrochloric acid in dogs. *Anesth. Analg.* 53:556–562, 1974.
91. Toung T.J., Cameron J.L., Kimura T., et al.: Aspiration pneumonia: Treatment with osmotically active agents. *Surgery* 89:588–593, 1981.

9 / Acute Renal Failure

FRANK A. KRUMLOVSKY, M.D.
NAUMAN QURESHI, M.D.

ACUTE RENAL FAILURE (ARF) can be defined as an acute deterioration in renal function. This may occur over hours, days, or even weeks. Prompt recognition and management of ARF are of critical importance, since the severity and duration of failure and the ultimate degree of recovery depend largely on prompt institution of appropriate therapy, which in turn depends on determination of etiology and understanding of pathophysiologic mechanisms.

CLASSIFICATION

ARF is most appropriately divided into prerenal, postrenal, and intrarenal types. As indicated above, it is of critical importance to classify a given case of ARF by etiology and pathogenesis as promptly as possible, since success in modifying the severity or reversing the cause depends on appropriate therapy based on pathophysiologic mechanisms.[1]

Prerenal azotemia, probably the most common type of ARF, is due to renal hypoperfusion as a result of decreased effective renal blood flow; this in turn is almost invariably secondary to hypotension, intravascular hypovolemia, or poor cardiac output. Hypotension is relative and is related to preexisting blood pressure (BP), age, and preexisting status of the renal macrovasculature and microvasculature. Thus, an apparently normal BP may in fact represent hypotension in an elderly or previously hypertensive patient. Intravascular hypovolemia is most commonly due to acute blood loss, third space losses, sepsis, overdiuresis, gastrointestinal losses (vomiting, diarrhea, nasogastric suction) or hypoalbuminemia. A continuous spectrum exists between prerenal azotemia secondary to renal hypoperfusion and ischemic acute tubular necrosis (ATN); thus, prompt recognition and appropriate management of prerenal status can abort progression to ischemic ATN, or minimize its severity and duration should it occur.

Postrenal azotemia refers to complete or incomplete obstruction of the urinary tract at any point along its course. It must be emphasized that a normal urine output does not rule out obstructive uropathy. ARF secondary to incomplete obstruction may manifest with severe azotemia and normal urine volume. Thus, obstruction must be ruled out in all patients with ARF who do not respond promptly and completely to correction of prerenal factors.[2-4]

ATN is the most common type of intrarenal ARF and can be subclassified into ischemic and nephrotoxic types. Ischemic ATN represents a progression of prerenal azotemia in which prolonged or severe renal hypoperfusion has resulted in structural renal damage. Nephrotoxic ARF is less common but of great importance, since withdrawal of the offending agent may permit prompt recovery. Just as in the case of incomplete obstruction, ATN may present in a nonoliguric form, in which worsening azotemia and eventually the full-blown uremic syndrome may be seen in the presence of a normal urine output. A partial listing of commonly encountered nephrotoxic drugs is given in Table 9–1.[5-8] Many drugs, especially the aminoglycoside antibiotics, are direct tubular toxins and toxicity is dose-related. Heme pigments are also direct tubular toxins; thus, intravascular hemolysis or rhabdomyolysis with myoglobinuria may produce ATN. Other agents may cause an allergic interstitial hypersensitivity nephritis, which is not

TABLE 9–1.—NEPHROTOXIC DRUGS (PARTIAL LISTING)

Allopurinol†	Methoxyflurane*‡
Aminoglycosides*	Mitomycin*
Amphotericin*	Nonsteroidal anti-inflammatory drugs†§‖
Azathioprine†	Para-amino-salicylic acid†
Captopril‖	Paramethadione‖
Cephalosporins*†	Penicillamine‖
Cimetedine†	Penicillins†‖
cis-Platinum*	Penthrane‡
Clofibrate†	Phenindione†
Colistin*	Phenytoin†
Diphenylhydantoin†	Phenylbutazone†
Enflurane*‡	Polymyxin*
Furosemide‡	Rifampin†
Gold†‖	Sulfonamides†
Heroin‖	Tetracyclines*†
Iodinated contrast media*‡	Thiazides†
Mercury*‖	Trimethadione‖
Mesantoin‖	Vancomycin†
Methotrexate‡	

*Direct tubular toxin.
†Acute allergic interstitial nephritis.
‡Obstructive crystalluria.
§Prostaglandin inhibition.
‖Glomerulonephritis, nephrotic syndrome, or tubular basement membrane disease.

dose-related (see Table 9–1).[8] Drug-induced hypersensitivity nephritis may be recognized by the findings of eosinophilia, eosinophiluria, fever, and/or skin rash, although at times none of these is present. ARF secondary to iodinated contrast media is commonly seen[9] and results from the direct tubular toxic effects of an agent and/or its uricosuric effects. Patients with preexisting renal insufficiency, renal hypoperfusion from any cause [dehydration, congestive heart failure (CHF), diabetes mellitus, multiple myeloma, or recent iodinated contrast studies] are at increased risk for contrast-induced ARF. ARF related to administration of nonsteroidal antiinflammatory drugs is being seen with increasing frequency.[10–13] These agents are prostaglandin inhibitors and decrease renal blood flow. In a setting of preexisting renal hypoperfusion, they are likely to further decrease renal blood flow, since in this situation maintenance of renal perfusion is increasingly dependent on the vasodilator prostaglandins. These agents are also apparently capable of causing acute and chronic interstitial nephritis, the nephrotic syndrome, and ATN.

Space permits only brief mention of other less commonly encountered causes of intrarenal ARF.[14] ARF secondary to acute glomerulonephritis or systemic vasculitis can usually be recognized by active urine sediment (RBCs, RBC casts, and/or proteinuria), which is not typical of ATN. The hepatorenal syndrome appears to be related to intrarenal arteriolar vasoconstriction and resembles severe prerenal azotemia in many respects, although it does not respond well to appropriate therapeutic measures for prerenal azotemia; a Le Veen shunt may be helpful in some cases. Intratubular precipitation of sulfonamides, myeloma protein, or urates represent variants of intrarenal obstruction. Acute cortical necrosis may result from disseminated intravascular coagulation (DIC) secondary to gram-negative sepsis or obstetric accidents. Presumably, the clotting mechanism is activated as part of a generalized Shwartzman-like reaction as a result of sepsis and bacterial endotoxemia or by release of thromboplastin, as may occur in abruptio placentae. The patient is usually severely oliguric or anuric. ARF may also occur secondary to thrombotic microangiopathy (hemolytic-uremic syndrome, thrombotic thrombocytopenic purpura, idiopathic postpartum ARF).

DIFFERENTIAL DIAGNOSIS

The first steps in establishing the differential diagnosis (Fig 9–1) are history and physical examination. In the case of prerenal azotemia, the latter will usually reveal signs of intravascular hypovolemia [orthostatic hypotension and/or tachycardia, flat neck veins and/or low central venous pressure (CVP) or pulmonary artery occluded pressure (PAOP)], hypotension (rela-

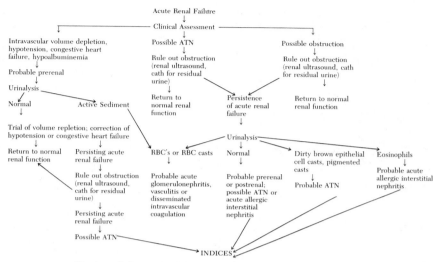

Fig 9–1.—Differential diagnosis of acute renal failure.

tive to the patient's usual blood pressure), or evidence of CHF. The history will provide clues as to possible recent hypotensive insults (trauma, surgery, sepsis, myocardial infarction), recent or current exposure to nephrotoxic drugs, or the presence of symptoms or conditions indicative or causative of urinary tract obstruction.

The urine should next be examined.[15] In prerenal or postrenal azotemia, the urinalysis findings are characteristically within normal limits. In ATN, dirty brown epithelial cell casts may be seen, although the urinalysis may at times be normal. The presence of an active sediment (macroscopic or microscopic hematuria, RBC casts, and/or proteinuria) argues against prerenal or postrenal azotemia or ATN and suggests glomerulonephritis, systemic vasculitis, or DIC. The presence of eosinophiluria raises the question of acute allergic interstitial nephritis, although the urinalysis is often normal in this condition.

Concurrently with the urinalysis, renal ultrasound should be performed routinely to rule out obstruction and evaluate gross renal anatomy in all patients who have not responded promptly to correction of prerenal factors.[2-4] If there is any question of vascular trauma or occlusion, renal isotope scans should be obtained as well.

At the same time, it is appropriate to review the urinary indices. (Table 9–2).[15-21] These must be determined, if possible, prior to any therapeutic intervention, since results may be made uninterpretable following many therapeutic measures, such as administration of mannitol or furosemide. A

TABLE 9–2.—URINARY INDICES IN ACUTE RENAL FAILURE

INDEX	VALUE	
Urine Na (mEq/L)	< 20–30	> 30–40
Urine specific gravity	> 1.108	< 1.018
Urine osmolality	> 400	< 400
Urine/plasma osmolality ratio	1.2–3.0	0.9–1.2
Urine/plasma creatinine ratio	> 30–40	< 20–30
Renal failure index*	< 1	> 1
Fractional excretion of sodium†	< 1	> 1
Serum BUN:creatinine ratio	> 10:1 ↓	~10:1 ↓
	Probably prerenal—treat with optimization of intravascular volume; if no immediate response, mannitol, dopamine, and/or furosemide, (see text on treatment of early ATN).	Probably established ATN, possibly chronic obstruction, acute interstitial nephritis— treat as for prerenal or early ATN initially; if no response, treat as established renal failure (see text).

$$*\text{Renal failure index} = \frac{\text{Urine Na}}{\text{Urine/plasma creatinine}}$$

$$†\text{Fractional excretion of sodium} = \frac{\text{Urine Na/Plasma Na}}{\text{Urine Cr/Plasma Cr}} \times 100.$$

random sample of urine will provide data of comparable validity to a longer timed collection and results can be made available almost immediately. In prerenal azotemia, results will be consistent with renal hypoperfusion with well-preserved tubular function (high urine specific gravity and osmolality, high urine/plasma osmolality and creatinine ratios, low renal failure index, low fractional excretion of sodium, and high BUN/creatinine ratio). Conversely, in ATN, ability to conserve sodium and water is decreased because of tubular damage, resulting in lower urine specific gravity and osmolality, low urine/plasma osmolality and creatinine ratios, high renal failure index, high fractional excretion of sodium, and normal BUN/creatinine ratio. The renal failure index and fractional excretion of sodium appear to be the most reliable and discriminatory of these tests. Urinary indices in other types of ARF are less characteristic. Values in obstructive uropathy, especially if chronic, resemble those seen in ATN, but acute obstruction may manifest with a prerenal picture. Cortical necrosis and hepatorenal syndrome typically are associated with prerenal indices. Recent reports have indicated that some types of ATN, especially those due to iodinated contrast media or myoglobinuria, as well as some cases of nonoliguric ATN may manifest with prerenal indices.[17, 18, 21] The reason for this is not totally clear, but may relate to a patchy process in which most of the glomerular filtrate is formed in nephrons with intact tubules, or possibly to intrarenal (intratubular) obstruction or to contrast-induced vasoconstriction, which may precede the development of ATN. Indices may not be totally diagnostic or even internally consistent in every case[19]; in the majority of cases, however, urinary indices provide a valuable guide to etiology, pathophysiology, and appropriate management in patients with ARF.

PATHOPHYSIOLOGY OF ATN

Space does not permit adequate discussion of this complex topic. Suffice it to say that considerable evidence exists supporting the role of both tubular obstruction and renal arteriolar vasoconstriction in the pathophysiology of the oliguria of ATN.[22, 23] Therapeutic efforts are directed toward both of these mechanisms.

THERAPY

In the case of obstructive uropathy, management is simple and obvious; the obstruction must be relieved. For this reason, obstruction must be ruled out in all cases of ARF which do not respond promptly and completely to correction of prerenal factors. Obstruction is usually ruled out most easily by renal ultrasound. Occasionally, if renal ultrasound is nondiagnostic or the index of suspicion is high, more invasive measures with a higher degree of risk, such as the drip infusion nephrotomogram retrograde pyelography, will be necessary.

In the case of prerenal azotemia, initial management consists of optimizing intravascular volume and BP so as to maximize renal perfusion. Adequacy of intravascular volume status can usually be evaluated clinically (absence of orthostatic hypotension or tachycardia, neck veins filling from below to estimated CVP of 5–6 cm H_2O); but not infrequently, especially in the critically ill patient, insertion of a CVP line or Swan-Ganz catheter will be required to ensure optimal filling pressures. Cardiac output, if low, should be optimized as well. When evidence of volume depletion is unequivocal, normal saline or colloid should be administered to correct the problem.

The most critical point in management of ARF is the situation when prerenal azotemia is progressing along its continuous spectrum leading toward ATN, or early ATN is developing but has not yet become established. Here, therapeutic interventions are of greatest potential value. Optimizing intravascular volume and cardiac output has already been mentioned. If intravascular volume status permits, mannitol, 12.5 gm IV initially, followed by 12.5 gm IV q2-4h until a total of 50 gm has been given or until CVP or PAOP have become optimized or until signs of adequate intravascular volume, as outlined above, are present, may be of benefit via several mechanisms. It may cause a solute diuresis, increasing intratubular pressure and flow rate, which may relieve or prevent tubular obstruction[24, 25]; it may also decrease glomerular afferent arteriolar and endothelial cell swelling, thus potentially improving renal blood flow; finally, it may help correct intravascular volume depletion. Unfortunately, the use of mannitol is often limited by increased intravascular volume or elevated left atrial filling pressures.

Dopamine has been shown to produce renal cortical vasodilation and increased renal cortical blood flow in experimental hemorrhagic shock, and in dopaminergic doses (2–5 μg/kg/minute) may be of great benefit in the management of early ischemic ATN.[26]

Loop diuretics, furosemide in particular, may be of benefit in several ways. The solute diuresis resulting from their use may result in increased intratubular pressure and flow, thus relieving or minimizing the tubular obstructive component of early ATN.[24, 25] Loop diuretics may also convert some cases of oliguric ATN to nonoliguric ATN[27]; this facilitates clinical management but probably does not alter the eventual course of ATN. Obviously, diuretics should not be administered in the setting of intravascular volume depletion until the latter has been corrected.

Dopamine (3 μg/kg/minute) and furosemide used together have been shown to have a synergistic protective effect in experimental ARF in normotensive, normovolemic animals.[28] Possible mechanisms include blockade of glomerulotubular feedback with decreased renal renin release, renal vasodilation secondary to furosemide-induced prostaglandin release, and induction of a solute diuresis. We have used this combination with considerable success in the early stage of clinical ATN.

Other modalities of intervention in early ATN are less generally accepted. There is recent evidence that calcium transport across the tubular cell may play a role in the genesis of ATN, and verapamil has been used to diminish the severity of ATN in the experimental animal.[15] Angiotensin-converting enzyme inhibitors have likewise been shown to modify the course of ATN if given early enough in the course. To date, none of these latter modalities has found general acceptance in the clinical situation.

Once ARF becomes established, management consists primarily of conservative fluid, electrolyte and nutritional management, with dialysis if necessary, until renal function improves. Care must be taken to avoid volume overload. Urine electrolytes must be quantitated, as well as electrolyte composition of other fluid losses (nasogastric suction, ostomy losses, etc.), and replaced appropriately to avoid hyponatremia or hypernatremia. Serum potassium must be monitored closely, and high potassium treated appropriately with Kayexalate or dialysis, using calcium gluconate, sodium bicarbonate, or glucose and insulin acutely if necessary.[29, 30] Serum bicarbonate levels should be maintained at 15 mEq/L or higher by means of exogenous bicarbonate administration. At least 100 gm of glucose and 30–40 gm of high biologic value protein should be administered daily to minimize endogenous catabolism and encourage positive nitrogen balance. Hyperphosphatemia and hypocalcemia should be treated with aluminum hydroxide and calcium gluconate administration, respectively, as indicated. Indications for dialysis include volume overload, hyperkalemia, or metabolic acidosis that cannot be controlled by conservative management. Uremic pericarditis or uremic gastroenteritis with hemorrhage constitute almost absolute indications for dialysis. We prefer to dialyze patients with ARF aggressively and early (BUN, approximately 100 mg/dl) to attempt to avoid these serious complications.

Dosage adjustments of many drugs are required in renal failure. Excellent comprehensive guides for alteration of drug dosages in renal failure are available.[31]

CASE STUDY: DAYS 1–3

A 42-year-old white man was brought to the emergency room because of multiple traumas sustained after a 20-foot fall from a cliff. He was discovered about 30 minutes later in a nearby creek. He had previously been in good health, except for some vague problems with high BP for which he had never been treated.

On admission he was obese, weighing 195 lb. The skin was cyanotic, pale and cold. BP was 78/40 mm Hg, pulse was 132 beats per minute, respirations were 38/minute and shallow, and temperature was 94° F rectally. He was disoriented and confused. Bony deformities were obvious in the right shin and left thigh. He was diffusely tender to touch, more so over the left chest. The insertion of a Foley catheter was difficult and revealed gross hematuria.

Laboratory tests revealed the following values: hemoglobin, 12.2 gm/dl; hematocrit, 37%; and WBC, 11,200/mm³.

Urinalysis revealed a pH of 6, a specific gravity of 1.018, 4+ occult blood, 1+ protein, and RBCs too numerous to count. Chest x-ray studies showed multiple rib fractures on the left with a 30%–40% pneumothorax. Heart size was normal. An electrocardiogram (ECG) showed left ventricular hypertrophy and a J spike. Serum electrolyte and amylase levels were normal. Arterial blood gas analysis showed a pH of 7.52, a P_{CO_2} of 26 mm Hg, and a P_{O_2} of 71 mm Hg on 3 L of oxygen by nasal cannula. Fractures were confirmed in the shafts of the left femur and right tibia and fibula by x-rays. He also had fractures of the pubic rami with gross displacement.

He was treated with warmed blankets, 2 units of packed RBCs, and 4 L of saline. BP came up to 112/68 mm Hg and rectal temperature to 96.5° F. Urine output was 55 ml over the next 90 minutes.

After a chest tube was placed on the

left, an IV pyelogram was obtained which showed delayed visualization of the collecting system bilaterally, but no parenchymal defect. A computerized tomographic (CT) scan of the head with contrast infusion was normal. CT scan of the abdomen showed some ascitic fluid and a probable hematoma of the spleen. Abdominal paracentesis revealed gross blood. An aortogram with celiac angiogram revealed leakage of contrast material from the splenic artery, but was otherwise normal. The abdomen was explored and a lacerated spleen was removed. No other source for the liter of blood in the peritoneal cavity could be identified. During the operation the patient required 4 additional units of blood.

For the next 3 days urine output averaged 40–50 ml/hour and mean arterial pressure (MAP) was 60–80 mm Hg. The patient was alert and communicative. The color of his urine became gradually lighter; however, the BUN rose to 65 mg/dl with a serum creatinine value of 4.5 mg/dl. Urinalysis showed a pH of 5.5, specific gravity of 1.011, 4+ occult blood with more than 100 RBCs per high power field, and numerous dirty brown granular casts, epithelial cells, and cellular debris. Other laboratory tests revealed the following values: serum calcium, 6.2 mg/dl; phosphorus, 8.2 mg/dl; uric acid, 13.2 mg/dl; lactic dehydrogenase (LDH), 473 IU; alkaline phosphatase, 360 IU; SGOT, 156 units/ml; CPK, 12,000 IU. Urine Na^+ was 42 mEq/L; K^+, 31 mEq/L; Cl^-, 30 mEq/L; urine creatinine, 52 mg/dl; and urine osmolality, 370 mOsm/kg. During this period the patient underwent internal fixation of the lower extremity fractures and wiring of the pelvis.

The renal service was consulted because of increasing BUN and creatinine levels.

Discussion

The patient had evidence of ARF with a BUN of 65 mg/dl and a serum creatinine level of 4.5 mg/dl. The renal failure had developed in the setting of good urine volumes and a normal serum potassium level.

There are several potential causes for ARF in this setting, as described below.

1. Urinary obstruction is a distinct possibility in a patient with multiple trauma; disruption of the urethra, compression of the ureters by pelvic or retroperitoneal hematoma, or ureteral obstruction from blood clots are all possibilities to be considered. A good urine volume does not exclude obstruction, since obstruction could be partial or intermittent. Another related possibility is leakage of urine into neighboring structures (pelvis, peritoneum, or groin). Obstruction can be easily and reliably excluded by renal ultrasound,[2] an excellent screening test for obstruction since it does not rely on renal function for visualization[3] and avoids the risks of a dye load. Urinary tract obstruction as a cause of ARF must always be excluded because it can so readily be diagnosed and treated and because it may, if missed, result in irreversible loss of renal function. Ordering an ultrasound scan in ARF should be as automatic as doing a urinalysis.[4]

2. Physical damage to the renal tissue or its vasculature secondary to trauma was excluded by the angiogram. In every patient with ARF following abdominal trauma, the renal arteries and veins should be evaluated promptly. Any delay in the diagnosis of renal artery thrombosis may result in irreversible total loss of renal function.[32, 33]

3. ATN is the commonest cause of an acute deterioration in renal function. In this particular patient, contributory factors, alone or in any combination, include (1) hypotension with ischemia of the kidneys (prerenal azotemia which has progressed to ATN, especially likely in the setting of preexisting hypertension by history and ECG); (2) pigment nephropathy due to myoglobinuria or hemoglobinuria; (3) radiocontrast dye toxicity; and (4) other toxins, such as methoxyflurane during general anesthesia.

The absence of oliguria is totally compatible with the diagnosis of ATN. In a recent series of 92 prospectively studied patients with ATN, 59 had a nonoliguric picture.[27] This subgroup is characterized by lower morbidity and mortality and a less frequent need for dialysis. Others have also published similar results.[34, 35]

The urine sodium level of 43 mEq/L and fractional excretion of sodium (FeNa) of 2.8% are typical of ATN.[15-20] However, these findings are also compatible with obstruction of the urinary tract.

Pigment nephropathy is a very likely possibility. The evidence for rhabdomyolysis and myoglobinuria in this patient includes extensive muscle trauma in a male with large muscle mass, hypothermia, possible compartmental syndrome in the legs, bruises and generalized muscle tenderness, impressive elevation of CPK as well as other enzymes, hyperphosphatemia, and hypocalcemia.[36] The classic finding on urinalysis is 3–4+ occult blood with no or few RBCs on microscopy. This was not seen here, probably due to coincident trauma to, and bleeding from, the urinary tract. Some further diagnostic studies to reinforce the diagnosis of myoglobinuria include (1) centrifugation of the urine and then detecting occult blood in the supernatant, and (2) testing urine for myoglobin and serum for aldolase and creatinine. The problem with myoglobin measurements, however, is that present techniques are not specific in the presence of hemoglobin. In our experience myoglobinuria severe enough to result in ATN is usually associated with CPK values in excess of 10,000 IU. Hemoglobinuria due to a transfusion reaction is also a possibility.[37] The citrated blood would also explain the low serum calcium value. However, hemoglobin, because of its molecular weight of 68,000 daltons and its binding in the serum to hepatoglobin, is not freely filtered at the renal glomerulus, in contrast to myoglobin, which has a molecular weight of only 17,000. In general, if a patient has enough hemoglobin in the serum to cause ATN, one should see pink discoloration of serum due to hemoglobinemia, which was not observed here.

Iodinated contrast toxicity is a major cause of ATN.[8, 38, 39] Predisposing risk factors in this patient include volume depletion, hyperuricemia, and the large dose of contrast material required for multiple procedures (angiography, IV pyelography, CT scan).[8, 38, 39]

Anesthesia records must be reviewed to see if methoxyflurane was employed. ATN with large urine volumes is the classic presentation.[40] However, with the increasing awareness of its nephrotoxic potential, this agent has now been almost abandoned. Also, the urinalysis report did not mention oxalate crystals.

4. Acute uric acid nephropathy, another contributing factor to ATN, is possible but unlikely because of the low serum level.[41] To exclude this possibility, a spot sample of urine should be sent for uric acid and creatinine analysis. Whenever the uric acid:creatinine ratio exceeds 1.0, uric acid nephropathy is likely.[42]

Case Study Continued: Days 4–10

Based on the assumption that the patient had ATN due to a combination of hypotensive ischemia, myoglobinuria, and contrast nephropathy, a forced alkaline diuresis with acetazolamide, IV sodium bicarbonate, and mannitol was started. Over the next 5 days the patient continued to improve and BUN and creatinine levels declined. The urine pH was consistently above 7.

Ten days after admission his BP again dropped to 90/48 mm Hg and urine output decreased. Temperature was 99° F and pulse was 122 beats per minute; weight was 198 lb. He was confused and somewhat agitated. The axillae and tongue were dry. The neck veins were flat at 30°, and at 60° the BP dropped to 60/palpable. Generalized abdominal distention and tenderness were noted and were more marked on the left. The abdominal wound looked clean and no drainage was visible. Bowel sounds were generally hypoactive. The Foley catheter was draining small amounts of light-colored urine, with almost no in-

crease after administration of furosemide, 40 mg IV.

Laboratory studies revealed the following values: WBCs, 12,200/mm³, with 64% segmented neutrophils and 12% band forms. Serum sodium was 130 mEq/L; chloride, 95 mEq/L; bicarbonate, 18 mEq/L; potassium, 6.5 mEq/L; BUN, 38 mg/dl; glucose, 195 mg/dl; serum creatinine, 1.4 mg/dl; CPK, 7,000 IU; and calcium, 7.8 mg/dl. Arterial blood gas analysis on room air showed a pH of 7.28; a PCO_2 of 29 mm Hg, and a PO_2 of 66 mm Hg. Urinalysis revealed a pH of 7.8, a specific gravity of 1.023, 2+ occult blood, 2–5 RBCs and 15–20 WBCs per high power field, a few dirty brown granular casts, and 3+ bacteria. A chest film showed blunting of the left costophrenic angle and atelectasis in the left lower lung field. An ECG showed an increase in amplitude of T waves in leads V_2 to V_4.

The patient was given 50 mEq of IV sodium bicarbonate, 50 ml of 50% dextrose in water, and 300 ml of normal saline. An hour later BP remained at 84/ 45 mm Hg and pulse was 135 beats per minute with occasional premature atrial contractions. Temperature rose to 101° F. Urine output continued to be poor ($<$ 20 ml/hour). Urine sodium concentration was 43 mEq/L, chloride, 16 mEq/L; potassium, 32 mEq/L, and creatinine, 25 mg/dl. FeNa was 1.9%.

Discussion

Oliguria and hyperkalemia have complicated an otherwise uneventful recovery from ATN. Whenever this occurs one must reevaluate the patient as one would a new case of ARF, with particular consideration of obstruction, renal hypoperfusion, or superimposed drug nephrotoxicity.

In this case the lower supine BP with a further orthostatic drop, poor skin turgor, recent forced diuresis, and elevated BUN:creatinine ratio all suggest renal hypoperfusion. However, the fact that the patient had gained 3 lb since admission, as well as the urine Na^+ of 44 mEq/L and the FeNa of 1.9%, contradict this; the latter are usually strong arguments against renal hypoperfusion. We must, however, remember that the patient had recently received furosemide, and this makes urinary indices uninterpretable.

A saline challenge was given with negligible response, also arguing against intravascular volume depletion. Since the patient was now oliguric, further fluids could have precipitated pulmonary edema. On the other hand he was in shock, and therefore his intravascular volume may have become severely depleted and required replacement. Thus, faced with conflicting data, a critical decision must be made regarding volume status and volume repletion. Additional data, namely, central filling pressures, become imperative.

The explanation for the hyperkalemia at this point is probably multifactorial: (1) an increased load from tissue breakdown after trauma and rhabdomyolysis, (2) efflux of potassium from cells in response to acidosis, and (3) inability of the kidneys to excrete the excess load of potassium due to decrease in urine volume. If all other variables remain constant, urinary potassium excretion varies in direct proportion to urine volume. This is because distal tubular potassium secretion is dependent on the potassium concentration gradient between the intracellular fluid in the distal tubular cell and the lumen. Large urine volumes and flow rates past the distal tubular cell maintain a steep potassium gradient and promote kaliuresis.[43] The appropriate immediate therapy for hyperkalemia was employed.[29, 30] Since ECG changes were not significant and patient's cardiographic status was not being monitored, calcium was not given. Potassium ion exchange resins do not have an immediate effect. However, they are superior to the other modalities employed here, in that the potassium load is removed, not merely transferred into the cell to present a problem later.

A point worth mentioning in the management of this and other cases of ARF is the advisability of removing indwelling bladder catheters as soon as possible to minimize the risk of infection.[44] In this patient this should have been done after the pelvis was wired.

Case Study Continued: Days 10–12

The patient was transferred to the intensive care unit and a flow-directed balloon-tipped catheter (Swan-Ganz) was floated into the pulmonary artery. Recorded pressures were as follows: pulmonary artery, 26/6 mm Hg; PAOP, 5 mm Hg; cardiac output, 10.2 L/minute; cardiac index, 4.9 L/minute; total systemic resistance, 670 dynes/sec/cm^{-5}; and $A - Vo_2$ difference, 7.3. Serum lactate was 35 mg/dl. Therapy with IV fluids, clindamycin, tobramycin, and ampicillin was begun. Eight hours later the MAP was 80 mm Hg, PAOP was 11 mm Hg, and cardiac output was 12.4 L/minute. Urine sodium now was 5 mEq/L; chloride, 3 mEq/L; and potassium, 18 mEq/L. The creatinine level in urine was 65 mg/dl and in serum was 2.4 mg/dl. The serum sodium was 142 mEq/L, and FeNa was 0.13%.

The next day the patient appeared better oriented. However, he complained of abdominal bloating. Examination revealed a distended abdomen with tenderness and guarding in the area of the splenectomy wound. No rebound tenderness or rigidity could be elicited. Bowel sounds were hypoactive. Flat plate of the abdomen did not show free air in the abdomen; however, there were dilated loops of bowel suggesting an ileus. Fever, tachypnea, and low urine output persisted. Ultrasound of the abdomen revealed multiple cystic echoes in the left upper quadrant. The

kidneys were normal in size and without hydronephrosis. Urine sodium concentration at this time was 18 mg/dl and serum creatinine was 4.2 mg/dl. An exploratory laparotomy revealed 500 cc of pus in the splenic bed. Gram stain of the fluid revealed numerous gram-negative rods.

During the day following surgery the patient's course was complicated by hypoxemia and a diffuse bilateral infiltrate was noted on chest x-ray. Mechanical ventilation was instituted. He also developed a picture consistent with DIC.

Cultures of blood, pleural fluid, urine, and abdominal drainage all yielded gram-negative rods sensitive to ampicillin. Anaerobic cultures were negative and so the patient was continued on ampicillin alone. A random serum level of tobramycin before it was stopped was reported as 6.5 μg/ml.

Subsequently, the patient became normotensive with a MAP of 80 mm Hg and a urine output of 20–25 ml/hour. Mental status remained poor. Rales up to the mid lung fields and asterixis were noted.

Laboratory tests revealed the following values: serum sodium, 130 mEq/L; chloride, 98 mEq/L; bicarbonate, 13 mEq/L; potassium, 6.5 mEq/L; BUN, 165 mg/dl; glucose, 210 mg/dl; calcium, 7.2 mg/dl; albumin, 3.4 gm/dl; creatinine, 7.2 mg/dl; urine sodium concentration, 62 mEq/L; urine creatinine, 52 mg/dl; and calculated FeNa, 6.45%.

Discussion

The events that transpired between days 10 and 12 were primarily related to sepsis due to an intra-abdominal abscess, accompanied by an adynamic ileus and sequestration of fluid in the bowel. The hypotension and renal hypoperfusion that followed were reflected in the low urine sodium, chloride, and FeNa values. Earlier the furosemide masked this picture. The measurement of PAOP was very helpful in determining the correct fluid management. Appropriate therapy with antibiotics and drainage of the abscess resulted in general improvement. However, adult respiratory distress syndrome, DIC, and toxic tobramycin levels were noted. Due to the multiple insults of sepsis, hypotension, and probable aminoglycoside toxicity, full-blown ATN with overt uremia developed, as reflected in the most recent laboratory data.

Could this have been prevented? To some extent, yes. If the sequestration of fluid in the bowel with intravascular volume depletion and hypoperfusion had been recognized earlier and managed appropriately with volume repletion instead of furosemide, the progression of prerenal azotemia to ATN might have been prevented.

Tobramycin toxicity undoubtedly contributed to the development of ATN. In ARF, after the usual loading dose of aminoglycoside has been administered, the subsequent maintenance doses should be based not on the serum creatinine value, but instead initially on the assumption that the patient is anephric. For example, even when the serum creatinine level is only 2.0 mg/dl (and rising) in a patient with ATN, the glomerular filtration rate, and hence the ability to excrete aminoglycosides, may be essentially zero. With continuing renal failure, the serum creatinine level will eventually rise, but so will the serum drug levels, unless due care with dosing is taken early on. Frequent 2-hour measurements of creatinine clearance rates are helpful in estimating drug dosages in patients with ARF who are not functionally anephric.

At this point the therapeutic decision is simple. The patient has established ATN with clinical uremia, as manifested by fluid overload, a wide anion gap metabolic acidosis, hyperkalemia, and mental obtundation.[45]

Case Study Continued: Days 12–36

Hemodialysis through a subclavian catheter was instituted. Narcotic analgesics were discontinued. Three days later, after daily dialysis therapy, the patient was breathing comfortably at a rate of 18/minute. The lungs were clear on examination and urine output had increased progressively. His serum chemistries subsequently improved, and 3 weeks later he was discharged from the hospital with normal BUN and creatinine values.

Discussion

Indications for dialysis in ARF have already been discussed. The acidosis and hyperkalemia could have been managed without dialysis; however, administration of sodium bicarbonate and potassium ion exchange resins would have been required, both of which present a significant sodium load, which would have further jeopardized the patient's ventilatory status. Also, the deterioration in mental status was probably a result of uremia.[45] Furthermore, risks of pericarditis and gastrointestinal bleeding secondary to uremia can be minimized by early dialysis. The diuretic phase sometimes seen during recovery from ATN is conspicuously absent here. This is probably due to the fact that the osmoles (urea, creatinine, etc.) that accumulate during the oliguric phase of ATN had in this case been largely removed through dialysis. In the absence of osmoles, the osmolar diuresis that contributes to the polyuric phase is absent. Narcotics were withheld, since they can contribute to mental deterioration. Also, narcotics may cause a drop in BP, which can create problems on hemodialysis. It should be remembered that normeperedine, the metabolite of meperedine (Demerol), can accumulate in renal failure and cause seizures. If narcotics are needed, morphine is preferred. This patient's complicated hospital course emphasizes the transitions in renal pathophysiology that can occur from one day to the next. Only an appreciation of this fact and the meticulous medical attention that it demands will optimize management in this group of critically ill patients.[46, 47]

REFERENCES

1. Krumlovsky F.A., Conn J.: Acute renal failure, in Beal J.M. (ed.): *Critical Care for Surgical Patients.* New York, Macmillan Publishing Co., 1981, pp. 508–518.
2. Sanders R.C., Berman S.: B-scan ultrasound in the diagnosis of hydronephrosis. *Radiology* 108:375–382, 1973.
3. Sanders R.C.: The place of diagnostic ultrasound in the examination of kidneys not seen on excretory urography. *J. Urol.* 114:813–821, 1975.
4. Qureshi N.: Obstructive uropathy, in Earle D.P.: *Manual of Clinical Nephrology.* Philadelphia, W.B. Saunders Co., 1982, pp. 467–477.
5. Humes H.D., Weinberg J.M.: Drug–induced nephrotoxicity. *DM* 28(5):1–81, 1982.
6. Linton A.L., Lindsay R.M.: Drug–induced acute interstitial nephritis. *Kidney* 15:1–4, 1982.
7. Fillastre J.P., Mery J.L., Godin M.: Drug-induced glomerulonephritis. *Dial. Transplant.* 10:716–736, 1981.
8. van Ypersele de Strithou C.: Acute oliguric interstitial nephritis. *Kidney Int.* 16:751–765, 1979.
9. Krumlovsky F.A., Simon N.M., Santhanam S., et al.: Acute renal failure associated with administration of radiographic contrast material. *JAMA* 239:125–127, 1978.
10. Quigley M.R., Ritchfield M., Krumlovsky F.A., et al.: Concurrent naproxyn and penicillamine-induced renal disease in rheumatoid arthritis. *Arthritis Rheum.* 25:1016–1019, 1982.

11. Zawada E.T.: Renal consequences of nonsteroidal anti-inflammatory drugs. *Postgrad. Med.* 71:223–230, 1982.
12. McCarthy J.T., Schwartz G.L., Blair T.J., et al.: Reversible nonoliguric acute renal failure associated with zomepirac therapy. *Mayo Clin. Proc.* 57:351–354, 1982.
13. Torres V.E.: Present and future of the nonsteroidal anti-inflammatory drugs in nephrology, editorial. *Mayo Clin. Proc.* 57:389–393, 1982.
14. Levinsky N.G., Alexander E.A.: Acute renal failure, in Brenner B., Rector F.C. (eds.): *The Kidney.* Philadelphia, W.B. Saunders Co., 1976.
15. Schrier R.W.: Acute renal failure. *JAMA* 247:2518–2525, 1982.
16. Miller T.R., Anderson R.J., Linas S.L., et al.: Urinary diagnostic indices in acute renal failure. *Ann. Intern. Med.* 89:47–50, 1978.
17. Steiner R.W.: Low fractional excretion of sodium in myoglobinuric renal failure. *Arch. Intern. Med.* 142:1216–1217, 1982.
18. Fang L.S.T., Sirota R.A., Ebert T.H., et al.: Fractional excretion of sodium with contrast media induced acute renal failure. *Arch. Intern. Med.* 140:531–533, 1980.
19. Oken D.E.: On the differential diagnosis of acute renal failure. *Am. J. Med.* 71:916–920, 1981.
20. Espinel C.H., Gregory A.W.: Differential diagnosis of acute renal failure. *Clin. Nephrol.* 13:73–77, 1980.
21. Diamond J.R., Yoburn D.C.: Nonoliguric acute renal failure associated with a low fractional excretion of sodium. *Ann. Intern. Med.* 96:597–600, 1982.
22. Levinsky N.G.: Pathophysiology of acute renal failure. *N. Engl. J. Med.* 296:1453–1458, 1977.
23. Schrier R.W., Conger J.D.: Acute renal failure: Pathogenesis, diagnosis, and management, in *Renal and Electrolyte Disorders.* Boston, Little, Brown & Co., 1976, pp. 289–318.
24. Cronin R.E., de Torrente A., Miller P.D., et al.: Pathogenetic mechanisms in early norepinephrine-induced acute renal failure: Functional and histologic correlates of protection. *Kidney Int.* 14:115–125, 1978.
25. Patak R.R., Fadem S.Z., Lifschultz M.D., et al.: Study of factors which modify the development of norepinephrine-induced acute renal failure in the dog. *Kidney Int.* 15:227–237, 1979.
26. Nerberger R.E., Passmore J.C.: Effects of dopamine on canine intrarenal blood flow distribution during hemorrhage. *Kidney Int.* 15:219–226, 1979.
27. Anderson R.J., Linas S.L., Berns A.S., et al.: Nonoliguric acute renal failure. *N. Engl. J. Med.* 296:1134–1138, 1977.
28. Lindner A., Cutler R.E., Goodman W.C.: Synergism of dopamine plus furosemide in preventing acute renal failure in the dog. *Kidney Int.* 16:158–166, 1979.
29. Kunis K.L., Lowenstein J.: The emergency treatment of hyperkalemia. *Med. Clin. North Am.* 65:165–176, 1981.
30. Cox M., Sterns R.H., Singer I.: The defense against hyperkalemia: The roles of insulin and aldosterone. *N. Engl. J. Med.* 299:525–531, 1978.
31. Bennett W.M., Muther R.S., Parker R.A., et al.: Drug therapy in renal failure, dosing guidelines for adults. *Ann. Intern. Med.* 93:62–89, 286–325, 1980.
32. Stables D.P., Fouche R.F., Niekerk D.P., et al.: Traumatic renal artery occlusion: 21 cases. *J. Urol.* 115:229–233, 1976.
33. Magilligan J.D. Jr., DeWeese J.A., May A.G., et al.: The occluded renal artery. *Surgery* 78:730–738, 1975.
34. Myers C., Roxe D.M., Hano J.E.: The clinical course of nonoliguric acute renal failure. *Cardiovasc. Med.* 2:669–672, 1977.
35. Vertel R.M., Knochel J.: Nonoliguric acute renal failure. *JAMA* 200:598–602, 1967.
36. Oivero J., Ayus J.C.: Rhabdomyolysis and acute myoglobinuric renal failure. *Arch. Intern. Med.* 138:1548–1549, 1978.
37. Schmidt P.J., Holland P.V.: Pathogenesis of acute renal failure associated with incompatible transfusion. *Lancet* 2:1169–1172, 1967.

38. Hanaway J., Black J.: Renal failure from contrast injection following computerized tomography. *JAMA* 238:2056–2057, 1977.
39. Weinrauch L.A., Robertson W.S., D'Elia J.A.: Contrast media induced acute renal failure. *JAMA* 239:2018–2019, 1978.
40. Mazze R.I., Shne G.L., Jackson S.H.: Renal dysfunction association with methoxyflurane anesthesia. *JAMA* 216:278–288, 1971
41. Kjellstrand C.M., Campbell D.C., VonHartitzsch B., et al.: Hyperuricemic acute renal failure. *Arch. Intern. Med.* 133:349–359, 1974.
42. Kelton J., Kelby W.N., Holmes E.W.: A rapid method for the diagnosis of acute uric acid nephropathy. *Arch. Intern. Med.* 138:612–615, 1978.
43. Good D.W., Wright F.S.: Luminal influences on potassium secretion: Sodium concentration and fluid flow rate. *Am. J. Physiol.* 236(S):F192–F205, 1979.
44. Montgomerie J.Z., Kalmanson G.M., Guze L.B.: Renal failure and infection. *Medicine* 47:1–32, 1968.
45. Cooper J.D., Lazarowitz V.C., Arieff A.J.: Neurodiagnostic abnormalities in patients with acute renal failure. *J. Clin. Invest.* 61:1448–1455, 1978.
46. Lewers D.T., Maher J.F., Schreiner G., et al.: Long-term follow-up of renal function and histology after acute tubular necrosis. *Ann. Intern. Med.* 73:523–529, 1970.
47. Briggs J.D., Kennedy A.C., Young L.N., et al.: Renal function after acute tubular necrosis. *Br. Med. J.* 3:513–516, 1967.

10 / Cardiogenic Shock

KERRY KAPLAN, M.D.
RICHARD DAVISON, M.D.

CARDIOGENIC SHOCK may occur as the end stage of any form of heart disease but most often follows an acute myocardial infarction (MI). Since the advent of coronary care units and vigorous treatment of arrhythmias, cardiogenic shock has become the most frequent cause of mortality following MI. Cardiogenic shock occurs when enough myocardial contracting function is lost to result in a cardiac output which is inadequate to meet the body's needs and causes a reduction of blood flow to vital organs.

Approximately 50% of patients who develop cardiogenic shock following MI do so within 24 hours.[1] In other patients, up to a week's delay in the onset of cardiogenic shock may reflect ongoing myocardial ischemia and infarction.[1, 2] Cardiogenic shock occurs more frequently with anterior than with inferior infarcts, probably because anterior infarcts tend to involve more left ventricular muscle.[3] Autopsy studies confirm that the severity of heart failure increases with the size of the infarct, and that if 40% of the left ventricular muscle is lost, cardiogenic shock will result.[4] If circulatory support is not instituted, cardiogenic shock is usually fatal within a short time (55%–85% mortality within 24 hours).[1, 5, 6]

Cardiogenic shock is diagnosed when the clinical manifestations of shock are present (hypotension, oliguria, altered sensorium, cool clammy skin) in the absence of significant persistent pain, arrhythmias, or diminished left ventricular filling pressure.

Hemodynamic monitoring is necessary to make the diagnosis and to appropriately treat the patient. Intra-arterial pressure monitoring is advocated because blood pressure (BP) determined with the cuff method underestimates the true pressure in patients with shock and high systemic vascular resistance.[7] It also allows easy access for frequent blood tests and arterial blood gas determinations. Insertion of a flow-directed pulmonary catheter is necessary to exclude inadequate left ventricular filling and to monitor the results of therapy. In cardiogenic shock the cardiac index (CI) is decreased while the left ventricular filling pressure is increased. Patients with a CI less than 2.0 L/minute/m^2 and a left ventricular filling pressure (left ventricular end-diastolic pressure or pulmonary arterial end-diastolic pressure) greater than 15 mm Hg have a very high mortality.[8] Pulmonary artery end-diastolic pressure has been shown to correlate closely with left ventricular end-diastolic pressure in patients in shock.[9]

Although cardiogenic shock in the setting of MI most commonly develops secondary to loss of myocardial function, there are other causes. It may be related to mechanical factors such as rupture of the ventricular septum or papillary muscle. Infarction of the right ventricle may result in inadequate filling of the left ventricle and is treated by expanding the intravascular volume.[10] Pharmacologic agents such as β-receptor blockers or calcium channel blockers may cause shock which reverses over time when the drug is stopped.

The goal of therapy in patients with cardiogenic shock is to maximize cardiac output at a minimum left ventricular filling pressure while maintaining a positive balance between myocardial oxygen supply and demand. The major determinants of cardiac output and myocardial oxygen demand are the same: they both increase with increases in heart rate, contractility, and left ventricular filling pressure. Oxygen consumption increases and cardiac output falls as BP rises. Therefore, balance between oxygen supply and demand must be considered during any therapeutic intervention in patients with MI.

CASE STUDY 1: DAY 1

A 62-year-old white man with no previous history of heart disease presented to the emergency room after 4 hours of severe substernal chest pressure radiating to the left arm and shoulder and associated with shortness of breath and diaphoresis. His vital signs were as follows: pulse rate, 110 beats per minute, respirations, 24/minute and unlabored; BP, 110/70 mm Hg; and oral temperature, 97.5° F. He appeared anxious and was diaphoretic. Auscultation of the lungs revealed rales in both bases. On cardiac examination a gallop rhythm was heard.

The patient was given three sublingual nitroglycerin tablets in 10 minutes without relief. Three 2-mg doses of morphine sulfate were administered intravenously (IV) over 10 minutes and the pain abated. Arterial blood gas values determined on room air were as follows: pH, 7.47; Pco$_2$, 38 mm Hg; Po$_2$, 60 mm Hg; and O$_2$ saturation, 88%. After 2 L of oxygen by nasal cannula was begun, arterial blood gases were again measured, as follows: pH, 7.43; Pco$_2$, 41 mm Hg; Po$_2$, 82 mm Hg; and O$_2$ saturation, 96%. A portable upright anteroposterior chest x-ray film showed a normal-sized heart and no signs of pulmonary edema. The electrocardiogram (ECG) showed 2–3-mm ST-segment elevation in leads I, aV$_L$, and V$_{2-5}$. Orders were written for bed rest with commode privileges and a liquid diet. Serum creatinine phosphokinase (CPK), lactate dehydrogenase (LDH), glutamic oxaloacetate (SGOT), as well as CPK and LDH isoenzyme values were determined on admission, every 8 hours for the first 24 hours, and again at 48 and 72 hours.

Discussion

Even though an MI cannot be diagnosed with certainty until serial ECGs and enzyme values are evaluated, all patients with a suspected MI should be treated as if they had one until the diagnosis can be excluded. Morphine sulfate is frequently necessary to relieve the pain of an acute MI. In addition to its analgesic and sedative effects, it is a powerful venodilator and thus reduces oxygen consumption by decreasing venous return and left ventricular wall tension. Because of its parasympathomimetic action it should be used with caution in patients with significant bradyarrhythmias. IV meperidine (Demerol), which has parasympatholytic effects, may be substituted.[11] The dose of the drug is titrated for clinical effect. The starting dose of IV morphine sulfate is 2–3 mg, and this dose may be repeated as often as every 3–5 minutes. Small doses of IV promethazine (Phenergan) or diazepam (Valium) seem to potentiate the analgesic effects of morphine and may help reduce the total dose of narcotic required.

Morphine may cause nausea or vomiting, which can be treated with promethazine IV. Occasionally an indwelling bladder catheter is necessary to relieve narcotic-induced urinary retention.[11]

A major goal in the treatment of acute MI is to minimize the amount of myocardium damaged. Arterial oxygenation has a direct effect on myocardial oxygen supply. Therefore, reasonable practice is to maintain arterial oxygen saturation at 90% or greater.[12]

Oxygen demands are reduced by placing the patient at bed rest and supplying an easily digested meal. Hemodynamically stable patients are allowed to use a bedside commode because it is less strenuous, less likely to cause vagal stimulation, and associated with a milder Valsalva effect than the use of a bed pan.[11]

Case Study 1 Continued: Day 2

During the night the patient had three separate episodes of moderate substernal chest pressure at rest, in each case relieved within 5 minutes by one nitroglycerin tablet taken sublingually. An ECG obtained during the first episode revealed an additional 2 mm of ST-segment elevation in the anterior leads. Another ECG obtained 15 minutes after the pain abated showed regression of the acute changes. After the first episode of pain, nitroglycerin ointment, 1 inch topically every 4 hours, was started. After the second episode it was increased to 3 inches every 4 hours, and after the third episode, isosorbide dinitrate, 40 mg orally every 6 hours, was begun.

An ECG obtained on the second day showed persistence of the ST-segment elevation in the anterior leads and new Q waves in leads I, aV_L and V_{2-3}. The enzyme levels were diagnostic of an MI and included a total CPK peaking at 6 times the upper limit of normal, 11% CPK myocardial fraction (CPK-MB), and an LDH value 4 times the upper limit of normal, with the LDH 1 fraction equal to the LDH 2 fraction.

Vital signs at this time were as follows: pulse rate, 95 beats per minute; respirations, 18/minute; and BP, 100/70 mm Hg. Bibasilar rales and an S_3 gallop were present.

During the day the patient had another episode of severe substernal chest pressure lasting 45 minutes. It was unrelieved by three tablets of sublingual nitroglycerin and required 8 mg of morphine sulfate IV before the pain abated. A continuous infusion of IV nitroglycerin was begun at 25 µg/minute and increased by 25 µg/minute every 5 minutes following a check of the BP until a dosage of 100 µg/minute was reached.

Discussion

Recurrent myocardial ischemia following infarction is a bad prognostic sign. It should be treated vigorously to prevent infarct extension. A stepwise increase in topical and/or long-acting nitrates is suggested as the first therapeutic measure. Depending on the frequency and severity of the symptoms, IV nitroglycerin can be used. It offers several advantages over the topical and oral forms of nitrates, including ease of administration, high bioavailability, and ability for rapid titration. IV nitroglycerin infusions are started at 25 µg/minute and increased by 25 µg/minute every 5 minutes if no side effects occur. The initial goal is a dose of 100–200 µg/minute, and the infusion is then titrated for clinical response. The major potential adverse reaction is a decrease in BP; however, with close attention to volume status, most patients tolerate the drug well. Nitrates work by increasing venous capacitance, decreasing venous return to the heart, and thus decreasing left ventricular wall tension. They also increase coronary artery blood flow, although the clinical significance of this effect is uncertain. It is possible that by relaxing vascular smooth muscle, IV nitroglycerin prevents the occurrence of coronary artery spasm.[13]

Case Study 1 Continued: Day 3

On the third day the patient had a 45-minute episode of severe substernal pressure relieved by 10 mg of morphine sulfate. The IV nitroglycerin dosage was increased to 200 µg/minute. One hour later he was found to be confused and agitated and trying to pull out his IV line. His pulses were thready and the systolic BP was palpable at 70 mm Hg. Respirations were 28/minute and mildly labored, and pulse rate was 120 beats per minute and regular. The skin was cold and clammy. Neck veins were visible 2 cm above the suprasternal notch at 30°. Lung fields had rales halfway up posteriorly. The heart tones were distant, but a definite gallop sound could be heard. Arterial blood gas determination showed a pH of 7.48, a P_{CO_2} of 32 mm Hg, a P_{O_2} of 54 mm Hg, and an O_2 saturation of 88%. The patient was placed in soft restraints; indwelling bladder and intra-arterial catheters were inserted, and oxygen administration was changed to a high-flow system with an $F_{I_{O_2}}$ of 40%. A flow-directed intrapulmonary catheter was inserted and hemodynamic variables were measured (Table 10–1, column headed "Baseline"). Volume loading was done with 100-cc boluses of normal saline every 10 minutes, with hemodynamic variables checked for response. When the PAOP reached 20 mm Hg and remained there for 15 minutes, hemodynamic parameters were again measured (see Table 10–1, column headed "Following Volume Loading"). At this time the patient was still confused and disoriented. His pulses and respiratory rate were unchanged. The urine output over the previous hour had been 10 cc. A dopamine infusion was started at 1 µg/kg/minute and increased to 5 µg/kg/minute over the next 4 hours. Hemodynamic parameters were again measured (see Table 10–1, column headed "Following Dopamine") and the urine output remained between 30 and 40 cc/hour.

TABLE 10–1.—HEMODYNAMIC MEASUREMENTS

PARAMETER	BASELINE	FOLLOWING VOLUME LOADING	FOLLOWING DOPAMINE
Right atrium (mm Hg)	8	9	9
Pulmonary artery (mm Hg)	40/18	38/22	40/20
Pulmonary artery occluded (mm Hg)	14	20	18
Cardiac index (L/min/m²)	1.4	1.6	1.9
A − Vo₂ difference (vol%)	9.8	8.4	7.2
Mean arterial pressure (mm Hg)	60	64	68

Discussion

When an acute change in mental status occurs in the days following an infarct, drug toxicity, hypoxia, and inadequate cerebral perfusion must be considered. Hypoxia may be very difficult to judge clinically and, if suspected, should be confirmed by determination of arterial blood gas values. Patients with decreased cerebral blood flow will usually have associated signs of poor perfusion.

A rapid examination revealed signs of decreased tissue perfusion, and invasive monitoring was instituted to follow intra-arterial and pulmonary artery pressure and cardiac outputs. Initial values showed a decreased CI and an increased A − Vo₂ difference with a PAOP of 14 mm Hg.

The patient had clinical and hemodynamic evidence of shock—more specifically, of cardiogenic shock complicating acute MI. The initial approach should be directed toward detection and correction of contributing factors that can be specifically treated (Table 10–2).

Discussion

Although a PAOP of 14 mm Hg would be considered adequate in a patient without heart disease, increasing the PAOP to the 18–20 mm Hg range following an MI results in increased cardiac output in the majority

TABLE 10–2.—Reversible Causes of
Hypotension Following Myocardial
Infarction

Myocardial ischemia
Bradyarrhythmia or tachyarrhythmia
Increased vagal tone
Hypoxemia
Acidosis
Drug toxicity
Surgically correctable lesions (PMR, VSR)*
Pericardial tamponade
Hypovolemia

*PMR, papillary muscle rupture; VSR, ventricular
septal rupture.

of patients.[14] If an optimal left ventricular filling pressure is reached (defined as no increase in cardiac output as PAOP is increased) and tissue perfusion is still inadequate, pharmacologic intervention is necessary to increase cardiac output and, one hopes, perfusion.

If the mean arterial pressure (MAP) is greater than 70–80 mm Hg and the systemic vascular resistance is increased, a vasodilator such as nitroprusside (see chapter 3) would be the first agent used. With a lower BP, sympathomimetic agents such as dopamine, dobutamine, or norepinephrine should be used.

Following volume loading the patient had a PAOP of 20 mm Hg and a CI of 1.6 L/minute/m^2; his clinical status revealed an underperfused state (oliguria, confusion). Because the MAP was in the 60s, dopamine infusion was initiated. Repeated hemodynamic measurements revealed an increase in CI along with a narrowing of the $A - Vo_2$ difference. However, of more significance, the urine output (reflecting renal tissue perfusion) increased and the patient was noted to be oriented and cooperative.

Dopamine is the metabolic precursor of norepinephrine. Its pharmacologic effects are dose related. At infusion rates of 1–2 µg/kg/minute it causes renal and splanchnic artery vasodilation (dopaminergic effects). As the infusion rate is increased to 2–10 µg/kg/minute, β-adrenergic effects predominate, with increased heart rate and contractility. At levels above 10–12 µg/kg/minute, α-adrenergic (vasoconstrictive) effects predominate. The infusion rates at which the various effects predominate vary from patient to patient and can be assessed by direct hemodynamic measurements in any patient. In general the initial dosage should be low (1–2 µg/kg/minute) and the rate increased as the clinical response indicates. Major complications from the use of dopamine are rare; they include tachycardia, ventricular arrhythmias, and hypotension.[15]

Dobutamine is a synthetic catecholamine that acts predominantly to increase cardiac contractility without causing marked tachycardia or a decrease in peripheral vascular resistance. Like dopamine, it must be given by continuous infusion because its serum half-life is approximately 2 minutes. The initial dosage is 2.5 μg/kg/minute, and the infusion may be increased to 10–15 μg/kg/minute, depending on the clinical response. At higher doses tachycardia and decreased systemic vascular resistance may become evident. Unlike dopamine, dobutamine does not directly dilate the renal arteries. The major complication is precipitation of ventricular arrhythmias.[16]

Norepinephrine stimulates both α- and β-adrenergic receptors. At low doses it stimulates predominantly β-adrenergic receptors in the heart, while at higher doses α-adrenergic effects become evident. Infusion should be started at 1 μg/kg/minute and titrated to the desired clinical response.[17]

Case Study 1 Continued: Day 4

The patient remained hemodynamically stable overnight with urine outputs of 30–50 cc/hour, a MAP of 65–75 mm Hg, and cardiac indices of 1.9–2.2 L/minute/m^2.

Early in the morning he had a 30-minute episode of severe substernal pressure that was relieved by 12 mg of morphine sulfate IV. Over the next several hours his urine output was only 10–15 cc/hour and he became more con-fused and developed a mild metabolic acidosis. Hemodynamic evaluation at that time revealed a MAP of 60 mm Hg, a PAOP of 24 mm Hg, a CI of 1.4, and an A−Vo$_2$ difference of 9.4. Intra-aortic balloon counterpulsation was instituted via a percutaneous approach to the right femoral artery. Hemodynamic variables returned to the range of the day before.

Discussion

The patient remained stable until another episode of myocardial ischemia occurred and was followed by signs of worsening tissue perfusion. The MAP was too low to allow the use of vasodilators. Pressors could have been increased in hopes of improving cardiac output; however, this would have resulted in an increase in myocardial oxygen demands. Instead, it was decided to initiate intra-aortic balloon counterpulsation.

Counterpulsation improves myocardial function by reducing afterload and increasing coronary blood flow. An intra-aortic balloon may be inserted in the femoral artery either by a cutdown or by a percutaneous approach using the Seldinger technique. A 30–40cc balloon is passed up the aorta and secured just distal to the origin of the left subclavian artery. It is timed to an ECG impulse or an arterial pulse tracing to inflate at the onset of diastole (anacrotic notch of the arterial pulse tracing). When it is caused to deflate just prior to myocardial contraction, the afterload of the left ventricle is reduced by the creation of a potential space and the initiation of blood flow in a centrifugal direction. Diastolic inflation of the balloon propels blood toward the heart and coronary arteries, although it is controversial whether blood flow to ischemic myocardium is actually increased.

In patients with a low output state or cardiogenic shock, counterpulsation may improve the hemodynamic status and allow consideration of cardiac surgery. The majority of patients cannot be weaned from an intraaortic balloon without myocardial revascularization. The timing of cardiac surgery in patients with cardiogenic shock is controversial: some authorities suggest immediate surgery and some prefer to wait at least a week after MI. Intra-aortic balloon insertion is followed by a high rate of complications, including thrombosis, ischemia, embolism, hemorrhage, and infection.[18]

Case Study 1 Continued

Despite intra-aortic counterpulsation, the patient continued to have two to three episodes daily of substernal pressure associated with 1–2 mm of ST-segment depression in leads II, III, and aV_F. Cardiac catheterization was done on the seventh hospital day and revealed a left ventricular end-diastolic pressure of 20 mm Hg. The anterior and anterolateral walls were akinetic and the posterior wall was hypokinetic. The ejection fraction was 23%. There was total occlusion of the left anterior descending artery just distal to the first septal perforator, an area of 70% luminal narrowing in the midcircumflex artery, and an area of 95% luminal narrowing in the proximal right coronary artery.

Despite poor left ventricular function and the recent MI, it was felt that urgent coronary artery revascularization was indicated because of the continuing myocardial ischemia despite maximal medical support. A two-vessel coronary artery bypass was done, but despite massive support with pressor agents, the patient could not be removed from cardiopulmonary bypass without hemodynamic decompensation and was declared dead in the recovery room.

CASE STUDY 2: DAY 1

A 52-year-old white woman was admitted to the coronary care unit after three episodes of substernal chest pain radiating to the left shoulder, each lasting 20 minutes and associated with shortness of breath and lightheadedness. She had suffered an anterior, non-Q wave MI 8 months previously but had had no cardiac complaints since. She was taking no medication.

On physical examination the BP was 90/60 mm Hg, the pulse was 54 beats per minute and regular, and respirations were 24/minute and mildly labored. Jugular venous distention was noted 2 cm above the clavicle at 30°. Fine end-inspiratory rales were audible in both bases. S_1 and S_2 were normal in intensity and splitting. An S_3 was present at the apex and left lower sternal border. No murmurs were audible. The patient's abdomen was soft, nontender, and without organomegaly. All pulses were present and symmetric. No pitting edema was present.

An ECG revealed a sinus rhythm at a rate of 50 per minute and 3 mm of ST-segment elevation in leads II, III, and aV_F and 2 mm of ST-segment depression in leads V_{2-4}. A chest x-ray film showed a normal-sized heart without signs of pulmonary venous congestion.

Arterial blood gas determination on room air disclosed a pH of 7.47, a P_{CO_2} of 34, a P_{O_2} of 72, and an O_2 saturation of 92%.

The pulse remained in the 50s while the patient was awake and fell to the low 40s when she was asleep. She had no further chest pain, shortness of breath, or lightheadedness.

Discussion

Although the patient had no prolonged episodes of chest pain, her presentation was consistent with an acute MI. The initial ECG picture was consistent with this diagnosis and localized the infarct to the inferior wall. Bradyarrhythmias are common following inferior wall MI. They most commonly reflect increased vagal tone and usually respond to atropine. Attempts to speed the heart rate should be made only if the patient becomes symptomatic. Signs of lowered cardiac output (cold clammy skin, decreased cerebral perfusion, decreased urine output), pulmonary edema, or refractory ventricular ectopy are indications for intervention. Atropine can be given in 0.4–0.5 mg boluses every 3–5 minutes to a total dose of 1.5 mg, depending on the response.

Because of the difficulty in closely controlling the heart rate with atropine and because of its side effects, a temporary pacemaker is preferable to control heart rate. In experienced hands, insertion of a temporary transvenous pacemaker can be accomplished safely, although ventricular fibrillation requiring cardioversion may occur in patients with right ventricular infarction.[19]

Case Study Continued: Day 2

She rested comfortably and had no complaints. The BP was 100/70 mm Hg, the pulse was 66 beats per minute and regular, and respirations were 20/minute and unlabored. Jugular venous distention was evident 1½ cm above the clavicle. Rales were heard over one third of the posterior thorax. A grade 1-2/6 late systolic decrescendo murmur was heard along the lower left sternal border. An S_3 was audible at the apex. There was no peripheral edema. Evaluation of the cardiac enzymes revealed a CPK rise to 4 times the upper limits of normal, an LDH rise to 3 times normal, and a CPK-MB value of 10%. The LDH 1 fraction was less than the LDH 2 fraction. An ECG revealed Q waves in leads II, III, and aV_F and a return of the ST segments to baseline. A repeat chest x-ray showed no cardiomegaly or pulmonary vascular redistribution.

The patient was allowed to sit at her bedside to take meals and the oxygen was continued.

Discussion

The ECG and enzyme changes are consistent with an acute Q wave inferior wall MI. Over one half of MI patients will develop a soft, high-pitched, apical systolic decrescendo or holosystolic murmur due to papillary muscle dysfunction in the first several days. These murmurs occur more often with inferior than with anterior infarcts and are caused by the failure of a papillary muscle or its supporting ventricular muscle to shorten appropriately as the left ventricle contracts.[20]

The pulmonary rales and S_3 were suggestive of congestive heart failure (CHF) and raise the issue of treatment with diuretics or digitalis. An acute MI causes a localized area of left ventricular dysfunction which, if large enough, necessitates high left ventricular diastolic filling pressures to maintain an adequate cardiac output. Rales, which reflect the increased filling pressure, are not an uncommon finding in the first several days following an MI. Diuretic agents are indicated only if increased pulmonary water causes hypoxemia or increased work of breathing. As an infarct heals, left ventricular compliance decreases, which allows lower filling pressures, and rales frequently disappear over the next several days.

In the past, physicians were concerned with the hemodynamic, metabolic, and arrhythmogenic effects of digitalis in the setting of an acute MI. It is currently accepted that digitalis can be safely used during acute MI when indicated for control of supraventricular arrhythmias or CHF.[21] In the face of mild CHF one must consider the effects of any drug on the myocardial oxygen supply/demand ratio. If digitalis is used in a patient who starts out with a normal-sized heart, it will cause increased oxygen consumption by increasing contractility and possibly systemic vascular resistance without direct effects on left ventricular wall tension or heart rate. However, if cardiomegaly is present, digoxin may cause a reduction in left ventricular size, which reduces oxygen consumption.[22] In patients with moderate to severe CHF, digoxin does not acutely improve hemodynamic abnormalities.[23]

Case Study 2 Continued: Day 3

On the third day after the MI, the patient experienced the acute onset of shortness of breath. She became confused and disoriented but denied chest pain. Blood pressure was 80/40 mm Hg, pulse was 95 beats per minute, and respirations were 34/minute and severely labored.

Physical examination revealed rales over one half of the posterior thorax bilaterally and a grade 4/6 holosystolic murmur along the lower left sternal border radiating to the apex and right precordium. There was a palpable thrill along the lower left sternal border.

The patient was treated with morphine sulfate (10 mg IV in divided doses over 10 minutes) and Lasix (40 mg IV) and oxygen administered by face mask with an FI_{O_2} of 50%. An indwelling arterial catheter was inserted to monitor MAP and to facilitate serial arterial blood gas sampling. The initial arterial blood gas determination revealed a pH of 7.27, a PCO_2 of 48 mm Hg, a PO_2 of 44 mm Hg, and O_2 saturation of 75%.

An indwelling catheter was placed in the bladder and a flow-directed intrapulmonary catheter was inserted. Initial pressures were as follows: right atrial mean, 12 mm Hg; right ventricular pressure, 40/14 mm Hg; pulmonary artery; 40/20 mm Hg; and PAOP 18 mm Hg. The PAOP tracing did not reveal large C-V waves. Cardiac output by thermodilution was 2.8 L/minute with a CI of 1.9 L/minute/m². The $A - V_{O_2}$ difference was 3.3. Blood samples drawn simultaneously from the right atrium, pulmonary artery, and arterial line (Table 10–3) revealed a 4.2 vol% increase in oxygen content between the right atrium and pulmonary artery, suggesting a left-to-right shunt between these two sites.

During this time the MAP was 50–60 mm Hg, the urine output was less than 10 cc/hour, and the patient remained confused. Preparation was made for insertion of an intra-aortic balloon followed by emergency cardiac catheterization.

Discussion

Sudden, painless cardiovascular collapse associated with a new systolic murmur is an uncommon but ominous event following MI. The differential diagnosis is between papillary muscle rupture and interventricular septal rupture. The patient should be stabilized and the diagnosis sought as quickly as possible.

Papillary muscle rupture is found in approximately 1% of patients dying from an acute MI. It occurs more frequently with inferior than anterior MI because of the relatively poor collateral blood supply to the posterior papillary muscles.[24] The prognosis following papillary muscle rupture without surgical intervention is poor, with less than one half of patients alive after 24 hours. Rupture through the body of a papillary muscle almost always results in death, whereas rupture at the tip of a papillary muscle involves fewer chordae tendineae, causes less mitral regurgitation, and results in a greater chance of survival.[25]

Papillary muscle rupture occurs most commonly in the first week following an MI. Examination reveals signs of pulmonary edema and low cardiac output. A loud, harsh holosystolic murmur is usually heard at the apex and radiating toward the left sternal border and base.[26]

TABLE 10–3.—STEP-UP IN OYXGEN CONTENT

	RIGHT ATRIUM	PULMONARY ARTERY	ARTERIAL
Oxygen saturation	37%	58%	75%
Oxygen content (vol%)	7.2	11.4	14.7

Interventricular septal rupture is responsible for 1%–2% of deaths following an MI. It occurs most commonly in the first week and has an equal incidence in anterior and inferior wall MIs. Survival without surgery is dismal, with 50% dying in the first week. Like papillary muscle rupture, it manifests with the painless onset of forward and backward CHF. A loud, harsh holosystolic murmur is heard at the apex and lower left sternal border and not uncommonly radiates to the right precordium. A thrill is felt along the lower left sternal border in approximately 50% of patients.[26]

The differential diagnosis between papillary muscle rupture and interventricular septal rupture is best made by right heart catheterization. With papillary muscle rupture large C-V waves will be seen in the pulmonary artery occluded tracing. A step-up in oxygen content of 1 vol% or greater between the right atrium and right ventricle or pulmonary artery suggests a left-to-right shunt of blood (such as an interventricular septal rupture) between these sites.[27] A cross-sectional echocardiogram may also be helpful in differentiating these conditions. Discontinuity of the intraventricular septum suggests rupture there, while a flail leaflet suggests papillary muscle rupture.

In either condition, intra-aortic balloon counterpulsation is indicated. By reducing afterload, forward cardiac output should be increased. After stabilization, patients with interventricular septal rupture should be considered for early cardiac surgery to close the septal rupture.[28] Coronary artery revascularization can be done simultaneously. Early repair of a ruptured papillary muscle is also recommended.[29]

Case Study Continued

Insertion of an intra-aortic balloon resulted in an increase in the CI to 2.3 L/minute/m^2. The urine output remained 10–20 cc/hour while preparations were made for emergency cardiac catheterization.

The study revealed a posterior interventricular septal rupture and triple-vessel coronary artery disease. Because of the patient's tenuous hemodynamic status it was decided to proceed with emergency surgery. A Teflon patch was sewn over the interventricular septal rupture and three bypass grafts were placed. The postoperative course was uneventful and the patient left the hospital 14 days later.

REFERENCES

1. Scheidt S., Ascheim R., Killip T.: Shock after acute myocardial infarction: A clinical and hemodynamic profile. Am. J. Cardiol. 26:556–564, 1970.
2. Gutovitz A.L., Sobel B.E., Roberts R.: Progressive nature of myocardial injury in selected patients with cardiogenic shock. Am. J. Cardiol. 41:469–475, 1978.
3. Miller R.R., Olson H.G., Vismara L.A., et al.: Pump dysfunction after myocardial infarction: Importance of location, extent, and pattern of abnormal left ventricular segmental contraction. Am. J. Cardiol. 37:340–344, 1976.

4. Page D.L., Caulfield J.B., Kastor J.A., et al.: Myocardial changes associated with cardiogenic shock. *N. Engl. J. Med.* 285:134–137, 1971.
5. Wackers F.J., Lie K.I., Becker A.E., et al.: Coronary artery disease in patients dying from cardiogenic shock or congestive heart failure in the setting of acute myocardial infarction. *Br. Heart J.* 38:906–910, 1976.
6. Mason D.T., Amsterdam E.A., Miller R.R., et al.: Pathophysiology of myocardial infarction shock, in Eliot R.S., Wolf F.L., Forker A.D. (eds.): *Cardiac Emergencies.* Mt. Kisko, NY, Futura Publishing Co, Inc., 1977, pp. 11–39.
7. Cohn J.N.: Blood pressure measurement in shock. *JAMA* 199:118–122, 1976.
8. Weber K.T., Ratshin R.A., Janicki J.S., et al.: Left ventricular dysfunction following acute myocardial infarction: A clinicopathologic and hemodynamic profile of shock and failure. *Am. J. Med.* 54:697–705, 1973.
9. Scheinman M., Evans G.T., Weiss A., et al.: Relationship between pulmonary artery end-diastolic pressure and left ventricular filling pressure in patients in shock. *Circulation* 57:317–324, 1973.
10. Rackley C.E., Russell R.O. Jr., Mantle J.A., et al.: Right ventricular infarction and function. *Prog. Cardiol.* 101:215–218, 1981.
11. Gregoratos G., Gleeson E.: Initial therapy of acute myocardial infarction, in Karliner J.S., Gregoratos G. (eds.): *Coronary Care.* New York, Churchill Livingstone, Inc., 1981, pp. 127–166.
12. Danzig R.: Current status of oxygen therapy in acute myocardial infarction. *Cardiovasc. Med.* 4:1245–1248, 1979.
13. Kaplan K., Davison R., Parker M., et al.: Intravenous nitroglycerin for the treatment of angina at rest unresponsive to standard nitrate therapy. *Am. J. Cardiol.* 51:694–698, 1983.
14. Crexells C., Chatterjee K., Forrester J.S., et al.: Optimal level of filling pressure in the left side of the heart in acute myocardial infarction. *N. Engl. J. Med.* 289:1263–1266, 1973.
15. Goldberg L.I.: Dopamine: Clinical uses of an endogenous catecholamine. *N. Engl. J. Med.* 291:707–710, 1974.
16. Sonnenblick E.H., Frishman W.H., LeJemtel T.H.: Dobutamine: A new synthetic cardioactive sympathetic amine. *N. Engl. J. Med.* 300:17–22, 1979.
17. Mason D.T., Amsterdam E.A., Miller R.R.: Treatment of myocardial infarction shock, in Eliot R.S., Wolf G.L., Forker A.D. (eds.): *Cardiac Emergencies.* Mt. Kisko, NY, Futura Publishing Co, Inc., 1977, pp. 209–243.
18. McEnany M.T., Kay H.R., Buckley M.J.: Clinical experience with intra-aortic balloon pump support in 728 patients. *Circulation* 58(suppl. I):I124–I132, 1978.
19. Sclarovsky S., Zafrir N., Strasberg B.: Ventricular fibrillation complicating temporary ventricular pacing in acute myocardial infarction: Significance of right ventricular infarction. *Am. J. Cardiol.* 48:1160–1166, 1981.
20. Heikkila J.: Mitral incompetence complicating acute myocardial infarction. *Br. Heart J.* 29:162–169, 1967.
21. Rahimtoola S.H., Gunnar R.M.: Digitalis in acute myocardial infarction: Help or hazard? *Ann. Intern. Med.* 82:234–240, 1975.
22. Mason D.T.: Digitalis pharmacology and therapeutics: Recent advances. *Ann. Intern. Med.* 80:520–530, 1974.
23. Goldstein R.A., Passamani E.R., Roberts R.: A comparison of digoxin and dobutamine in patients with acute infarction and cardiac failure. *N. Engl. J. Med.* 303:846–850, 1980.
24. Sanders R.J., Neubeurger K.T., Rabin A.: Rupture of papillary muscles: Occurrence of rupture of the posterior muscle in posterior myocardial infarction. *Dis. Chest* 31:316–323, 1957.
25. Vlodaver A., Edwards J.E.: Rupture of ventricular septum or papillary muscle complicating myocardial infarction. *Circulation* 55:815–822, 1977.
26. Kaplan K., Talano J.V.: Systolic murmurs following myocardial infarction. *Pract. Cardiol.* 5:25–39, 1979.

27. Meister S.G., Helfant R.H.: Rapid bedside differentiation of ruptured interventricular septum from acute mitral insufficiency. *N. Engl. J. Med.* 287:1024–1025, 1972.
28. Montoya A., McKeever L., Scanlon P., et al.: Early repair of ventricular septal rupture after infarction. *Am. J. Cardiol.* 45:345–348, 1980.
29. Nishimura R.A., Schaff H.V., Shub C., et al.: Papillary muscle rupture complicating acute myocardial infarction: Analysis of 17 patients. *Am. J. Cardiol.* 51:373–377, 1983.

11 / Shock and Coagulopathy in Gram-Negative Bacteremia

RICHARD DAVISON, M.D.
DAVID GREEN, M.D.

BACTEREMIA due to gram-negative bacilli knows no medical specialty boundary in its steadily increasing frequency. It is presently the most commonly encountered serious infection in American hospitals. Some of the factors responsible for this increment are the increasing age and severity of illness in hospitalized patients, the widespread use of antibiotics, and the ever-growing population of immunocompromised individuals.

One fourth to one third of all patients with documented gram-negative bacteremia (GNB) die. If this overall mortality is scrutinized more carefully, it becomes obvious that the majority of deaths occur in the 40%–50% of patients with GNB who go into shock.[1, 2]

The hemodynamic and metabolic disturbances found in GNB complicated by shock have been extensively investigated.[3-5]

It is now generally accepted that this condition evolves in two distinct stages.[6] Initially there occurs a fall in peripheral vascular resistance that is accompanied by the anticipated high cardiac output state. Several mechanisms have been postulated to explain this early vasodilation, including the release of histamine,[7] β-endorphins,[8] and/or kinins[9]; as well as the intravascular activation of the complement system with the generation of anaphylatoxins.[10] In a later phase, a progressive decrease in effective blood volume is associated with worsening myocardial function. This results in a low output state with heightened sympathoadrenal and angiotensin activity, peripheral vasoconstriction, and generalized tissue hypoperfusion. This disturbance in physiology serves the purpose of redirecting a dwindling cardiac output to the more "essential" organs such as the heart and the brain. On the other hand, it is maladaptive because it causes parenchymal and endothelial cells to suffer an additional ischemic insult that can damage them irreversibly. Recovery in a patient with GNB and shock that is allowed to reach this stage is exceptional.

CASE STUDY

A 60-year-old diabetic woman was brought to the emergency room with a 12-hour history of shaking chills, weakness, and diarrhea. Vital signs on admission were as follows: pulse, 120 beats per minute; temperature, 103.6° F; blood pressure (BP) by cuff, 90/60 mm Hg, and respirations, 36/minute. The patient was alert but somnolent. The skin was warm and moist and the peripheral pulses weak but present. Lung fields were clear on auscultation and percussion. The cardiac examination was unremarkable. Pain was provoked on palpation of the left costovertebral angle, and there was abdominal distention with some diffuse tenderness and hypoactive bowel sounds. The complete blood cell count showed a normal hematocrit, a white blood cell count of $4,500/\text{mm}^{-3}$ with a marked shift to the left, and a platelet count of $210,000/\text{mm}^{-3}$. Blood chemistry studies revealed a blood sugar level of 480 mg/dl, a blood urea nitrogen (BUN) of 40 mg/dl, and normal electrolyte values except for a bicarbonate of 20 mEq/L. Arterial blood gas determination on room air disclosed a P_{O_2} of 56 mm Hg, a P_{CO_2} of 20 mm Hg, and pH of 7.40. Microscopic examination of the urine showed more than 100 WBCs per high power field, many in clumps, and 4+ bacteria. Serum ketones were faintly positive in an undiluted sample. Chest x-ray film showed clear lung fields and a normal cardiac silhouette. An electrocardiogram (ECG) demonstrated sinus tachycardia and nonspecific ST and T wave abnormalities. In the emergency room the patient was given 2 L of intravenous (IV) normal saline. Appropriate antibiotic therapy for urinary tract infection was initiated and a Foley catheter was inserted. Prior to transfer, 7,000 mg of IV hydrocortisone was given.

Discussion

The history, physical findings, and initial laboratory determinations are consistent with a urinary tract infection with associated GNB. As soon as baseline cultures are obtained, antibiotics should be started promptly and fluid administration initiated on the assumption that the patient's blood volume is deficient secondary to increased capillary permeability and vasodilation. The choice of fluids for this purpose—colloids versus crystalloids—is not easy.[11] It is generally accepted that smaller total amounts of colloid solutions are required to restore an effective blood volume. Critics point out that the risk of volume overload is greater, that colloids are expensive, and that, in conditions associated with an enhanced capillary permeability, the egress of colloids into the interstitial tissues (such as those of the lung) can be deleterious. Conversely, lowering of the plasma colloid osmotic pressure following the infusion of large amounts of crystalloid solutions has been incriminated in the development of "noncardiogenic" pulmonary edema.[12] More recently the use of a hypertonic albumin-containing fluid has been proposed as an alternative that minimizes interstitial edema during fluid resuscitation.[13] In fact, there are no currently available data to indicate that the agent used for fluid resuscitation has any influence on the eventual outcome.

Even more incompletely defined is the role, if any, that corticosteroids play in the treatment of GNB. As many proponents as opponents can be found, each voicing persuasive arguments that are almost invariably supported by scientifically unacceptable data. Although far from ideal, the only study available that merits some credence offers the following guidelines: (1) corticosteroids should be given in a single dose equivalent in potency to 30 mg/kg of methylprednisolone; (2) this dose may be repeated *once* after 4 hours; and (3) which particular steroid is used probably makes no difference.[14] In the case under study, an equipotent dose of hydrocortisone was given.

Case Study Continued

The patient was taken to the intensive care unit. Pulmonary and radial artery catheters were placed and the following hemodynamic values were obtained: cardiac output, 5.2 L/minute, mean right atrial pressure, 5 mm Hg; mean pulmonary artery pressure, 25 mm Hg; mean pulmonary artery occluded pressure (PAOP), 10 mm Hg; A−Vo₂ content difference, 4.0 vol%; and mean arterial pressure (MAP), 55 mm Hg. Urine output for the previous hour was 15 cc. Over the next 3 hours the patient received another 3 L of a crystalloid solution and the urine output averaged 25 cc/hour. At this point repeated measurement of hemodynamic parameters demonstrated a cardiac output of 4.8 L/minute, a mean right atrial pressure of 10 mm Hg, a mean pulmonary artery pressure of 32 mm Hg, a mean PAOP of 16 mm Hg, an A−Vo₂ content difference of 4.4 vol%, and a MAP of 60 mm Hg. Further volume expansion resulted in an increase in PAOP but failed to correct any of the abnormal parameters.

Discussion

Taken in isolation, the initial hemodynamic measurements, other than for a modestly depressed MAP, are not alarming. But when integrated with the rest of the clinical data, indications of early tissue hypoperfusion become evident. Seriously ill, febrile patients increase their oxygen delivery via a hyperdynamic circulation that is associated with a narrow arteriovenous oxygen content difference.[15] In this setting a "normal" A−Vo₂ content difference suggests that a deficient blood flow is being compensated for by an increased oxygen extraction. Consistent with this interpretation is the finding of a poor urinary output, since curtailment of renal blood flow occurs very early in the course of low perfusion states.

Diastolic volume, or preload, is one of the main determinants of myocardial function, the other two being afterload and the contractile state of the myocardium (see Chapter 1). In the clinical circumstance there is no practical method to obtain serial determinations of diastolic volume; therefore, this value is inferred from measurement of the filling pressures, that is, PAOP.

Human studies have shown that the normal resting left ventricle in the supine position has a filling pressure in the upper limits of normal (about 10 mm Hg). This pressure provides a diastolic volume that places the left ventricle close to its peak performance. Further elevation of the left ventricular end-diastolic pressure results in relatively minor increases in diastolic volume.[16] Unlike the normal heart, volume loading that raises PAOP well above normal values has been shown to improve the output of the ischemic left ventricle.[17] This is an expression of the disturbed diastolic pressure-volume relationship, or compliance of the diseased myocardium. Because of this fact, in any instance other than the normal state, an isolated PAOP measurement gives little information on the degree of diastolic left ventricular filling unless the value obtained is below normal. A poor correlation between PAOP and left ventricular diastolic volumes has been well demonstrated in seriously ill septic and cardiac patients.[18] It is only by assessing the cardiac output response to an induced modification in the filling pressures that a valid estimation can be made of the ventricular preload at that particular point in time. If, with the increased PAOP, the cardiac output improves, the range of filling pressures at which the change takes place will provide a rough approximation of the ventricular compliance and identify valid end points for future manipulations of the intravascular volume.

In the present case, the cardiac output was initially recorded as being within the upper limits of normal. In the context of an acutely ill individual that is septic and most likely has an elevated oxygen consumption, a "normal" cardiac output must be considered an inadequate cardiac response to the illness. Even after a sizable elevation in the filling pressures was induced the cardiac output failed to rise, indicating a depressed myocardial function.

Myocardial depression during sepsis has long been recognized and probably is not the result of a direct effect of the bacteria or their toxins on the myocardium, but rather is mediated by plasma factors.[19] Although the origin, character, and even existence of the "myocardial depressant factor(s)" remain quite controversial,[20] there is good evidence that irreversible myocardial dysfunction develops 4–6 hours following the induction of endotoxin shock in dogs.[21] Earlier studies that were unable to demonstrate myocardial failure in the isolated perfused heart had not exposed the preparation to blood from an animal in septic shock for a long enough time.[22, 23]

Certainly these findings coincide with the clinical observation of a time-dependent deterioration in cardiac output in the course of human GNB with shock. They also provide support for the concept that time is of the essence in the treatment of this condition. Once myocardial dysfunction develops, the addition of β-adrenergic agents such as dopamine is standard therapy, although evidence is lacking that their administration modifies prognosis.

There is little to suggest at this time that a relative or absolute deficiency in coronary blood flow plays a primary role in the causation of myocardial failure during GNB. Conversely, pulmonary hypertension is almost invariably associated with this syndrome and is an important contributing factor to the mortality.

Case Study Continued

An IV infusion of 5 μg/kg/minute of dopamine was initiated and hemodynamic parameters were remeasured as follows: cardiac output, 6.6 L/minute, mean right atrial pressure, 9 mm Hg; mean PAOP, 13 mm Hg; MAP, 65 mm Hg; and $A - Vo_2$ content difference, 3.6 vol%. The urine output increased to 60–80 cc/hour. These data suggest that the dopamine was exerting a positive inotropic effect as well as probably inducing renal vasodilation by direct dopaminergic stimulation. The reduction in systemic vascular resistance provides reassurance that, at the dose given, the α (vasoconstrictive) activity of this drug was not prominent. Oozing from the puncture site and emesis of coffee ground material were noted and led to assessment of clotting parameters. The following values were obtained: platelet count, 52,000/μl; activated partial thromboplastin time (APTT), 60 seconds (control, 35 seconds); prothrombin time (PT), 18 seconds (control, 11.2 seconds); fibrin degradation products (FDP) greater than 40. The relatively rapid onset of a hemorrhagic diathesis, accompanied by thrombocytopenia, prolongation of the APTT and PT, and an increase in FDP, is characteristic of disseminated intravascular coagulation (DIC).

Discussion

In 1968, Corrigan et al.[24] performed detailed coagulation analyses in 36 septic patients. They reported that various changes in the clotting mechanism were encountered irrespective of the infectious agent but apparently related to BP. The coagulation changes, regularly noted in patients with hypotension or shock, were interpreted as being secondary to DIC. Similar changes were not seen in patients with normal BP. Their conclusion that most patients with septicemia and low BP have DIC has been confirmed by many workers in the last 15 years.

The pathogenesis of the coagulopathy associated with septic shock requires the intravascular elaboration of thrombin. Thrombin is generated when either factor XII is activated or tissue factor is released. Endotoxin and bacterial coat lipopolysaccharides can activate factor XII.[25, 26] Activated factor XII converts prekallikrein to kallikrein, and kallikrein in turn further augments activation of factor XII. In patients with septic shock, the levels of factor XII, prekallikrein, and kallikrein inhibitors decrease.[27] Endotoxin stimulates monocytes to shed tissue factor[28] and granulocytes to release cytosolic procoagulant material.[29] In rabbits, depletion of granulocytes prevents the development of endotoxin-induced DIC.[30, 31]

When thrombin is generated, clotting factors V and VIII are consumed, and fibrinogen is converted to fibrin. The deposition of fibrin on endothelial cells leads to the release of plasminogen activator,[32] which converts plasminogen to plasmin.[33] Plasmin is a potent proteolytic enzyme which digests factors V, VIII, and fibrinogen. Cleavage of fibrinogen results in the formation of FDP, which impair platelet aggregation, inhibit the action of thrombin on fibrinogen, and interfere with fibrin polymerization.

Thrombin induces platelet activation, and the activated platelets become adherent to areas of the vessel wall damaged by endotoxin. Platelets may also become coated with antigen-antibody complexes; such complexes consist of endotoxin or various bacterial products and their respective antibodies. These coated platelets are readily ingested by macrophages, contributing to the development of thrombocytopenia. Bleeding occurs in patients with septicemia because of endothelial cell injury due to endotoxin and/or antigen-antibody complexes, the depletion of platelets and clotting factors, an increase in systemic fibrinolytic activity, and the anticoagulant effects of FDP.

In some patients with septic shock, thrombosis rather than hemorrhage predominates. Hypotension results in impaired hepatic perfusion; the liver normally removes activated clotting factors from the circulation.[34] Retention of these activated clotting intermediates predisposes to continuing coagulation. Protein C and antithrombin III are two naturally occurring inhibitors of coagulation; they are rapidly depleted during the course of DIC.[35, 36] In addition, the levels of the potent vasoconstrictor and platelet-aggregating agent, thromboxane A_2 (as reflected by measurements of thromboxane B_2), are markedly increased.[37] Intense vasoconstriction and partial occlusion of the microcirculation by platelet-fibrin thrombi lead to tissue hypoxia, with release of tissue procoagulants and proteases, further endothelial cell damage, and fragmentation of erythrocytes. Adenosine diphosphate escaping from red cells may contribute to the formation of platelet thrombi.[38] The resulting microinfarcts contribute to multiple organ dysfunction. The effects of DIC on hemostasis are summarized in Table 11–1.

The diagnosis of DIC is based on the clinical picture and a characteristic constellation of laboratory abnormalities. Oozing from venipuncture sites, extensive ecchymoses, and bleeding from the gastrointestinal or genitouri-

TABLE 11–1.—Effects of DIC
on Hemostasis

HEMORRHAGE
Endothelial cell injury (hypoxia, endotoxin)
Consumption of:
Platelets
Factors V, VIII, XIII
Fibrinogen
Anticoagulant effects of FDP
Depletion of antiplasmin
THROMBOSIS
Elaboration of thrombin:
Platelet aggregation
Fibrin formation
Deposition of platelets and fibrin on
injured vessel wall
Consumption of:
Protein C
Antithrombin III
Plasminogen

nary tract are typically observed. In the patient in whom thrombosis predominates, patchy areas of skin necrosis, gangrene of the tip of the nose, ears, or digits, and renal failure secondary to renal cortical necrosis will be observed. With either presentation, there will be thrombocytopenia and elevated FDP levels; the latter will cause the thrombin time to be prolonged. In patients with severe sepsis, such as the subject of our case presentation, there will be hypofibrinogenemia and depletion of factors V and VIII, with marked prolongation of the APTT and PT. Antithrombin III titers will be reduced, and fragmented erythrocytes will be seen on peripheral smear.

The differential diagnosis of DIC, shown in Table 11–2, includes thrombocytopenia due to antigen-antibody complexes, major hemorrhage (usually acute erosive gastritis or gastroenteritis), acute bone marrow suppression due to infection, drugs, or folate deficiency, and drug-induced immune thrombocytopenia (due to cardioactive agents, antibiotics, or heparin). In a study of patients with septicemia, Kelton et al.[39] found an excellent correlation between the severity of thrombocytopenia and the concentration of platelet-associated IgG, the latter probably representing immune complexes adherent to platelets. Kreger et al.[40] observed thrombocytopenia without evidence of DIC in 100 of 222 episodes of GNB, emphasizing the high frequency with which thrombocytopenia alone occurs in septicemia.

Prolongation of the APTT and PT may be due to vitamin K deficiency, a rather common occurrence in the poorly nourished patient receiving

TABLE 11–2.—HEMOSTATIC ABNORMALITIES IN ACUTELY
ILL PATIENTS WHICH MAY BE MISINTERPRETED
AS SIGNS OF DIC

ABNORMALITY	PROBABLE CAUSE
Thrombocytopenia	Platelet-associated antigen-antibody-complexes
	Secondary to major hemorrhage
	Bone marrow suppression
	Folate deficiency
	Drug-induced (for example: heparin)
Prolongation of APTT and PT	Vitamin K deficiency
	Blood collection thru heparin lock
Elevated FDP levels	Hematomas, pulmonary emboli
	Renal failure
All of the above plus hypofibrinogenemia	Liver disease

broad-spectrum antibiotics. Abnormalities of these clotting times may also be artifactual, due to the collection of blood from a heparin lock, since very small amounts of heparin (0.1U) are capable of considerably prolonging the APTT. Elevated FDP levels may be associated with the breakdown of thrombi in organizing hematomas or pulmonary emboli, or the accumulation of these degradation products in the patient with renal failure. Finally, liver disease may be associated with thrombocytopenia, prolongation of clotting times, hypofibrinogenemia, and elevated FDP levels. This coagulopathy may be distinguished from DIC by the clinical findings of jaundice, hepatosplenomegaly, and markedly abnormal liver function tests, and by coagulation abnormalities specific for DIC or liver disease. The former include a reduction in factor VIII coagulant activity, elevated fibrinopeptide A levels, and positive ethanol or protamine paracoagulation tests.[41] Liver disease is usually associated with enhanced plasma proteolytic activity as measured by euglobulin lysis tests and caseinolytic assays.

The management of DIC in the septic patient is directed toward the control of hemorrhage and the neutralization of thrombin. In the severely thrombocytopenic patient with persistent oozing of blood from the nose, gastrointestinal tract, or tracheostomy site, platelet transfusion should be given to maintain the platelet count above 20,000/μl. Platelets derived from a single blood donation ordinarily will increase platelet numbers by 5,000/μl; 10 units of platelets should provide a platelet count in the recipient of 50,000/μl. The platelet survival in these patients may be extremely abbreviated due to the presence of immune complexes, active bleeding, fever, etc., and daily transfusions may be required until the patient's condition has stabilized. Hypofibrinogenemia can be corrected by administering cryoprecipitate; each bag contains sufficient fibrinogen to increase fibrinogen levels by 5 mg/dl. A fibrinogen level greater than 50 mg/dl will generally provide adequate hemostasis. Clotting factors V and VIII may be supplemented by giving fresh frozen plasma; a dose of 15–20 ml/kg will raise factor levels by 25%, sufficient to prevent spontaneous bleeding.

A major concern is that thrombin generated by the underlying septic process will result in the continuing consumption of the transfused platelets and clotting factors, resulting in additional platelet-fibrin thrombi in the microvasculature and further organ dysfunction. Therefore, efforts to neutralize thrombin have been attempted, usually by administering heparin. Originally, full-dose heparin therapy (5,000–15,000 U as an initial bolus, followed by 10,000–30,000 U/24 hours) was recommended,[42] but when reports of disastrous hemorrhage with such therapy were published,[43] the pendulum swung toward avoidance of heparin except for specific indications such as purpura fulminans or venous thromboembolism.[41] On the other hand, there is a rationale for the use of minidose heparin in DIC.[36] As previously mentioned, antithrombin III is depleted in DIC, and small amounts of heparin are known to potentiate antithrombin III activity.[44] Potentiation of antithrombin III would serve to neutralize thrombin and limit the extent of the intravascular coagulation. Furthermore, heparin in doses of 5,000 U subcutaneously every 12 hours does not appear to increase the bleeding tendency. In patients with very low levels of antithrombin III, the levels of this inhibitor may be supplemented with plasma infusions. Thus, the principles of management in the patient with septic shock and DIC are (1) vigorous treatment of the sepsis and hypotension, as previously described, (2) infusion of platelets and clotting factors to control hemorrhage, and (3) use of minidose heparin to retard the ongoing intravascular coagulation.

Case Study Continued

The patient received several units of fresh frozen plasma, two single-donor platelet transfusions, and was started on subcutaneous heparin, 5,000 U every 12 hours. The abnormal clotting profile improved and bleeding from puncture site subsided. Tachypnea became progressively worse, and diffuse, fine rales were heard over both lung fields. A chest roentgenogram demonstrated bilateral infiltrates with an "alveolar" pattern. On an F_{IO_2} of 0.6, arterial blood gas values were as follows: P_{O_2}, 46 mm Hg; P_{CO_2}, 38 mm Hg; pH, 7.22; QSp/QT, 30%; and $A - V_{O_2}$ content difference, 4.2 vol%. Other pertinent findings on physical examination were a dulled sensorium, easily palpable peripheral pulses, cyanotic nail beds, and a cool, clammy skin. Endotracheal intubation was performed and abundant serous secretions were suctioned. With the addition of 15 cm H_2O of continuous positive airway pressure (CPAP), arterial blood Po_2 rose to 88 mm Hg and QSp/QT was measured at 20%. The significant reduction in intrapulmonary shunting and improvement in oxygenation with CPAP supports the diagnosis of adult respiratory distress syndrome (ARDS) (see chapter 12).

Discussion

Patients with GNB and associated shock and coagulopathy are at high risk for the development of ARDS and the closely related entity of noncardiogenic pulmonary edema.[45] Experimentally, the effects of GNB on the lung have been studied in the isolated perfused dog lung following the infusion of live gram-negative bacteria. There is a prompt rise in pulmonary vascular resistance, a marked decrease in surfactant activity, and a rapid onset of pulmonary venous hypoxia. Examination of the preparation with the electron microscope demonstrates that large numbers of capillaries have become obstructed by platelet thrombi and leukocyte plugs, and that extravasation of fluid has occurred around vessels and small airways.[46] Similar involvement of the human pulmonary microcirculation is probably responsible for the genesis of pulmonary hypertension in GNB. This is a common observation in septic patients; it is not secondary to elevated left ventricular filling pressures, hypoxemia, or acidosis and usually augurs a poor prognosis.[47]

To return to the clinical discussion, the finding of an $A - Vo_2$ content difference that remains narrow in the setting of a mounting metabolic acidosis is a most ominous sign. The most frequently invoked explanation is that the increasing vasoconstriction and diffuse damage to the microvasculature virtually limit blood flow to a "core perfusion." Thus, even though peripheral pulses may be easily palpable and the BP maintained at satisfactory levels, manifestations of severe tissue hypoperfusion persist. An alternate hypothesis emphasizes a cellular defect in oxygen uptake rather than a diminished capillary blood flow to explain the impaired oxygen extraction seen in severe GNB.[48]

Case Study Continued

Controlled ventilation became mandatory with the development of ventilatory failure. The metabolic acidosis worsened and was only temporarily alleviated by the administration of sodium bicarbonate. The rate of the dopamine infusion had to be increased into the α range to maintain arterial pressure. Eventually ventricular fibrillation supervened and was refractory to resuscitative efforts.

Discussion

It is an unfortunate fact that the majority of seriously ill patients with shock complicating GNB die, no matter how vigorously currently accepted therapy is administered. In the future, innovative approaches may prove that what has been traditionally accepted as irreversible shock may not truly be an irrevocable state. Along these lines, a significant reduction in the mortality of such high-risk patients has been recently reported after the early administration of endotoxin antiserum.[49]

REFERENCES

1. Young L.S., Martin W.J., Meyer R.D., et al.: Gram-negative rod bacteremia: Microbiologic, immunologic and therapeutic considerations. Ann. Intern. Med. 86:456–471, 1977.
2. Kreger B.E., Craven D.E., Carling P.C., et al.: Gram-negative bacteremia: III. Reassessment of etiology, epidemiology and ecology in 612 patients. Am. J. Med. 68:332–355, 1980.
3. Gunnar R.M., Loeb H.S., Winslow E.J., et al.: Hemodynamic measurements in bacteremia and septic shock in man. J. Infect. Dis. 128 (suppl.):295–298, 1973.
4. Siegel J.H., Cerra F.B., Coleman B., et al.: Physiological and metabolic correlations in human sepsis. Surgery 86:163–193, 1979.
5. Nishijima H., Weil M.H., Shubin H., et al.: Hemodynamic and metabolic studies on shock associated with gram-negative bacteremia. Medicine 52:287–294, 1973.
6. Hess M.L., Hastillo A., Greenfield L.J.: Spectrum of cardiovascular function during gram-negative sepsis. Prog. Cardiovasc. Dis. 23:279–298, 1981.
7. Hinshaw L.W., Vick M.M., Jordan M.M., et al.: Vascular changes associated with development of irreversible endotoxin shock. Am. J. Physiol. 202:103–110, 1962.
8. Faden A.I., Holaday J.W.: Experimental endotoxin shock: The pathophysiologic function of endorphins and treatment with opiate antagonists. J. Infect. Dis. 142:229–238, 1980.
9. O'Donnell T.F. Jr., Clowes G.H.A. Jr., Talamo R.C., et al.: Kinin activation in the blood of patients with sepsis. Surg. Gynecol. Obstet. 143:539–545, 1976.
10. Robinson J.A., Klodnycky M.L., Loeb H.S., et al.: Endotoxin, prekallikrein, complement and systemic vascular resistance. Am. J. Med. 59:61–67, 1975.
11. Shine K.I., Kuhn M., Young L.S., et al.: Aspects of the management of shock. Ann. Intern. Med. 93:723–734, 1980.
12. Stein L., Beraud J.J., Morissette M., et al.: Pulmonary edema during volume infusion. Circulation 52:483–489, 1975.
13. Jelenko C. III, Williams J.B., Wheeler M.L., et al.: Studies in shock and resuscitation: I: Use of a hypertonic, albumin-containing, fluid demand regimen (HALFD) in resuscitation. Crit. Care Med. 7:157–167, 1979.
14. Schumer W.: Steroids in the treatment of clinical septic shock. Ann. Surg. 184:333–341, 1976.
15. Harrison R.A., Davison R., Shapiro B.A., et al.: Reassessment of the assumed A−V oxygen content difference in the shunt calculation. Anesth. Analg. 54:198–202, 1975.
16. Parker J.O., Case R.B.: Normal left ventricular function. Circulation 60:4–12, 1979.
17. Crexels C., Chatterjee K., Dikshit K., et al.: Optimal level of ventricular filling pressure in the left side of the heart in acute myocardial infarction. N. Engl. J. Med. 289:1263–1266, 1973.
18. Calvin J.E., Driedger A.A., Sibbald W.J.: Does the pulmonary capillary wedge predict left ventricular preload in critically ill patients? Crit. Care Med. 9:437–443, 1981.
19. Raffa J., Trunkey D.D.: Myocardial depression in sepsis. J. Trauma 18:617–621, 1978.

20. Lefer A.M., Martin J.: Origin of myocardial depressant factor in shock. *Am. J. Physiol.* 218:1423–1427, 1970.
21. Hinshaw L.B., Archer L.T., Black M.R., et al.: Myocardial function in shock. *Am. J. Physiol.* 226:357–366, 1974.
22. Hinshaw L.B., Archer L.T., Greenfield L.J., et al.: Effect of endotoxin on myocardial performance. *J. Trauma* 12:1056–1062, 1973.
23. Hinshaw L.B., Greenfield L.J., Owen S.E., et al.: Cardiac response to circulating factors in endotoxin shock. *Am. J. Physiol.* 222:1047–1053, 1972.
24. Corrigan J.J., Ray W.L., May N.: Changes in the blood coagulation system associated with septicemia. *N. Engl. J. Med.* 279:851–856, 1968.
25. Yoshikawa T., Tanaka R., Guze L.B.: Infection and disseminated intravascular coagulation. *Medicine* 50:237–258, 1971.
26. Cronberg S., Skonsberg P., Nivenios–Larsson K.: Disseminated intravascular coagulation in septicemia caused by beta-hemolytic streptococci. *Thromb. Res.* 3:405–411, 1973.
27. Mason J.W., Kleeberg U., Dolan P., et al.: Plasma kallikrein and Hageman factor in gram-negative bacteremia. *Ann. Intern. Med.* 73:545–551, 1970.
28. Edwards R.L., Rickles F.R., Bobrove A.M.: Mononuclear cell tissue factor: Cell of origin and requirements for activation. *Blood* 54:359–370, 1979.
29. Niemetz J., Fani K.: Role of leukocytes in blood coagulation and the generalized Schwartzman reaction. *Nature* 232:247–248, 1971.
30. Thomas L., Good R.A.: Studies on the generalized Schwartzman reaction: I. General observations concerning the phenomenon. *J. Exp. Med.* 96:605–624, 1952.
31. Muller-Berghous G., Eckardt T.: The role of granulocytes in the activation of intravascular coagulation and the precipitation of soluble fibrin by endotoxin. *Blood* 45:631–641, 1975.
32. Bernik M.B., Kwaan H.C.: Plasminogen activator activity in cultures from human tissues: An immunological and histochemical study. *J. Clin. Invest.* 48:1740–1753, 1969.
33. Colman R.W.: Activation of plasminogen by human plasma kallikrein. *Biochem. Biophys. Res. Commun.* 35:272–279, 1969.
34. Wessler S.: Studies in intravascular coagulation: III. The pathogenesis of serum-induced venous thrombosis. *J. Clin. Invest.* 34:647–651, 1955.
35. Griffin J.H., Mosher D.F., Zimmerman T.S., et al.: Protein C, an antithrombotic protein, is reduced in hospitalized patients with intravascular coagulation. *Blood* 60:261–264, 1982.
36. Bick R.L.: Disseminated intravascular coagulation (DIC) and related syndromes, in Fareed J., Messmore H.L., Fenton J.W., Brinkhous K.M. (eds.): *Perspectives in Hemostasis.* New York, Pergamon Press, 1981, pp. 122–138.
37. Reines H.D., Cook J.A., Halushka P.V., et al.: Plasma thromboxane concentrations are raised in patients dying with septic shock. *Lancet* 2:174–175, 1982.
38. Born G.V.R.: Haemodynamic and biochemical interactions in intravascular platelet aggregation, in *Blood Cells and Vessel Walls: Functional Interactions.* Amsterdam, Excerpta Medica, 1980, pp. 61–77.
39. Kelton J.G., Neame P.B., Gouldie J., et al.: Elevated platelet-associated IgG in the thrombocytopenia of septicemia. *N. Engl. J. Med.* 300:760–764, 1979.
40. Kreger B.E., Craven D.E., McCabe W.R.: Gram-negative bacteremia: IV. Reevaluation of clinical features and treatment in 612 patients. *Am. J. Med.* 68:344–355, 1980.
41. Feinstein D.I.: Diagnosis and management of disseminated intravascular coagulation: The role of heparin therapy. *Blood* 60:284–287, 1982.
42. Wolf P.L.: Disseminated intravascular coagulation: Principles of diagnosis and management, in Schmer G., Strandjord P.E. (eds.): *Coagulation.* New York, Academic Press, 1973, pp. 17–44.
43. Green D., Seeler R.A., Allen N., et al.: The role of heparin in the management of consumption coagulopathy. *Med. Clin. North Am.* 56:193–200, 1972.
44. Rosenberg R.D.: Heparin, antithrombin and abnormal clotting. *Annu. Rev. Med.* 29:367–378, 1978.

45. Kaplan R.L., Sahn S.A., Petty T.L.: Incidence and outcome of the repiratory distress syndrome in gram-negative sepsis. *Arch. Intern. Med.* 139:867–869, 1979.
46. Harrison L.H., Hinshaw L.B., Coalson J.J., et al.: Effects of *E. coli* septic shock on pulmonary hemodynamics and capillary permeability. *J. Thorac. Cardiovasc. Surg.* 61:795–803, 1971.
47. Sibbald W.J., Patterson N.A.M., Holliday R.L., et al.: Pulmonary hypertension in sepsis: Measurement by the pulmonary arterial diastolic-pulmonary wedge pressure gradient and the influence of passive and active factors. *Chest* 73:583–591, 1978.
48. Wright C.J., Duff J.H., McLean A.P.H., et al.: Regional capillary blood flow and oxygen uptake in severe sepsis. *Surg. Gynecol. Obstet.* 132:637–644, 1971.
49. Ziegler E.J., McCutchan J.A., Fierer J., et al.: Treatment of gram-negative bacteremia and shock with human antiserum to a mutant *Escherichia coli. N. Engl. J. Med.* 307:1225–1230, 1982.

12 / Noncardiogenic Edema, Adult Respiratory Distress Syndrome, and PEEP Therapy

BARRY A. SHAPIRO, M.D.

SEVERE PHYSIOLOGIC STRESS potentially affects all organ systems, irrespective of the primary etiology or pathophysiology. The lungs are extremely vulnerable to such stress, which is why pulmonary dysfunction is so prevalent in critically ill patients. This chapter addresses two common lung sequelae of severe physiologic insult—noncardiogenic edema (NCE) and the adult respiratory distress syndrome (ARDS). The major supportive therapy for such pulmonary pathology is positive end–expiratory pressure (PEEP), which will be reviewed in that context.

PARENCHYMAL ANATOMY AND PHYSIOLOGY

Endothelial Permeability

The pulmonary endothelial cells are either joined together by adhesion at the luminal and medial surfaces or form gaps of about 4 nm between adjacent cells.[1] To explain the differential passage of substances of varying molecular weight across the endothelium, pores of small and large capacity are postulated to exist (Fig 12–1). The small pores are thought to be the gaps between cellular junctions whose diameters increase with increasing intravascular pressure[2, 3] and are postulated to be the site of diffusion of water and small water–soluble molecules. Molecules of larger size, such as plasma proteins, are believed to be transported through the pinocytotic vesicles, which are referred to as large pores.[4]

Acute increases in capillary hydrostatic pressure (cardiogenic edema) result in greater small pore movement of water into the interstitial space while large pore function is unaltered. This increase in interstitial water results in decreased interstitial oncotic pressure while vascular oncotic pressure remains unchanged. Thus, the oncotic gradient is increased, which tends to offset the increased hydrostatic pressure gradient and serves to limit fluid translocation from the vascular to the interstitial space.[5] Obviously, in lung pathology primarily involving increases in capillary endothelial permeability (NCE), this safety factor limiting interstitial water accumulation is lost.

Lung Interstitium and Lymphatics

The interstitial space of the lung is composed primarily of hyaluronic acid molecules constrained within a network of collagen fibers.[6] Interstitial fluid is contained in and around the interstices of the collagen web, forming a gel-like matrix that contains the alveoli (Fig 12–2). Gas exchange primarily occurs across the interstitial *tight space*—areas where capillary endothelium and alveolar epithelium come into close proximity. Most of the lung interstitium, however, exists as the *loose space* located in the alveolar septa adjacent to the tight space and surrounding the bronchioles, bronchial arteries, and veins. The loose space also contains lymphatic vessels, interstitial cells, smooth muscle, and nerve tissue[7] and has an extremely high compliance.

Normally, lung interstitial pressure is negative relative to atmospheric pressure and the compliance of the interstitial space is low (Fig 12–3). However, as the interstitial pressure approaches atmospheric pressure, the compliance increases dramatically, enabling large volumes of fluid to accumulate within the interstitial space without significant increases in interstitial pressures.[8] Interstitial water content can increase by at least 30% before significant increases in interstitial pressure occur.[8, 9]

The pulmonary lymphatic capillaries arise in the loose space as terminal sacs that become true lymphatic capillaries containing one-way valves. The lymphatic channels contain smooth muscle in their walls and eventually merge to become the larger collecting vessels that have an active peristaltic capability regulated by the autonomic nervous system.[10] Normal lung lymph flow is 5–6 ml/hour/100 gm of lung tissue[9]; however, lymph flow has been demonstrated to increase by 20-fold.[5, 7, 9] This capability of increasing lymph flow in conjunction with the dynamic nature of the interstitial space compliance allows for increases of up to 300% in capillary hydrostatic pressures without physiologically significant increases in interstitial pressure.[5]

Lung Epithelium

Ninety percent of the alveolar surface is covered by type 1 alveolar cells, which play the major integumentary role in the maintenance of the air-

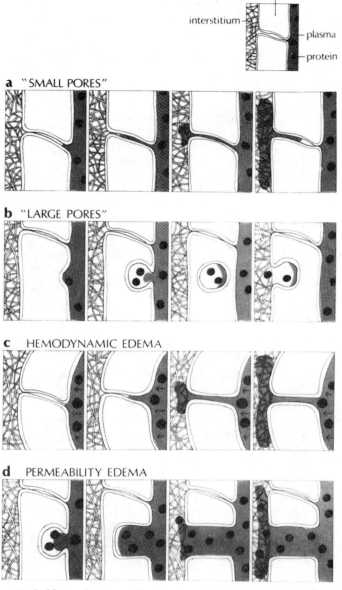

Fig 12–1.—*Probable mechanisms of pulmonary endothelial permeability. a, cytoplasmic junctions are either open or apposed at luminal and interstitial surfaces and are referred to as the "small pores." These junctions allow water and small water-soluble molecules to pass from lumen to interstitium. The controlling mechanisms are unknown, although intraluminal pressure is believed*

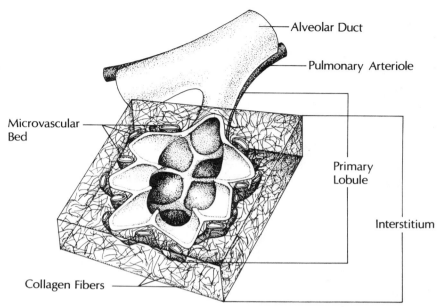

Fig 12–2.—*A schematic representation of a primary lobule arising from an alveolar duct. The single pulmonary arteriole gives rise to a complex network of capillaries referred to as the microvascular bed. The alveoli are in closely packed clusters and are shaped as tetrahedrons, an extremely stable geometric configuration. The interstitium is composed primarily of hyaluronic acid molecules and water constrained within a threadlike network of collagen fibers. This gel-like matrix is an important support for the microvascular bed and is responsible for both supporting and shaping the alveoli. In addition, the interstitium is believed to place limitations on alveolar distensibility.*

---

to play a role. Note that protein molecules cannot traverse these small pores and that transendothelial water conductance is independent of this mechanism. b, pinocytosis forms vesicles at the luminal surface that encase both fluid and protein molecules. These vesicles traverse the cytoplasm and extrude their contents into the interstitium. The pinocytotic vesicles are referred to as the "large pores." The endothelial cell mechanisms responsible for the pinocytosis are unknown. c, increased transmural pressure gradients result in continuously open junctions, resulting in an increased flow of water to the interstitium. Transendothelial water conductance and rate of protein transfer are unchanged. The resulting hemodynamic edema is identified in the research animal by an increased lymph flow with an unchanged protein content. d, endothelial cell injury may cause deficiencies in the transendothelial pinocytotic process, functionally resulting in transcytoplasmic fenestrations. The transendothelial water conductance and rate of protein transfer are increased. The resulting permeability edema is identified in the research animal by an increase in lymph flow and an increase in the protein content of lymph. (From Shapiro B.A., Cane R.D.: Metabolic malfunction of lung: Noncardiogenic edema and adult respiratory distress syndrome. Ann. Surg. 13:271–298, 1981. Used by permission.)

177

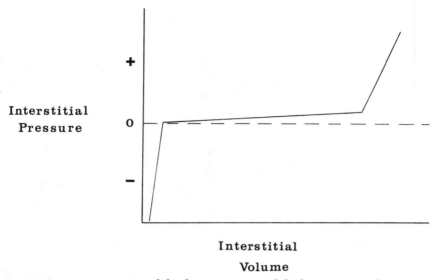

Interstitial
Volume

Fig 12–3.—Representation of the dynamic nature of the lung interstitial space compliance. Interstitial pressure is expressed relative to atmospheric pressure (760 mmHg-0).

blood barrier.[11] The cytoplasmic junctions between alveolar cells are extremely tight under normal conditions and are impermeable to water.[12] Alveolar type 2 cells (granular pneumocytes) constitute approximately 80% of alveolar epithelial cells[11] and produce the pulmonary surfactant and fluid which completely covers the alveolar epithelium.[13, 14] However, only 40%–50% of the type 2 cell enzymatic activity can be accounted for by the production, storage, and secretion of the surfactant complex and the fluid lining.[15] It is highly probable that other functions exist that are not related to the formation of the surfactant system or the alveolar fluid lining.

Damage to alveolar epithelium has profound effects on lung function. Type 1 cells are extremely vulnerable to injury and limited in reparative capabilities.[16] At least three pathophysiologic phenomena accompany type 1 cell damage: (1) alveolar edema secondary to loss of the watertight barrier[12, 17, 18]; (2) atelectasis resulting from the loss of geometric alveolar stability secondary to alveolar fluid[6, 7]; and (3) decreased lung compliance due to atelectasis and loss of the type 1 cell stretchability.[11, 19]

Type 2 cells are far less susceptible to injury and have remarkable reparative capabilities.[16, 20–22] Severe injury to these cells may result in irreversible damage.[15, 22] Damage results in two predictable and clinically identifiable conditions: severely decreased lung compliance, and alveolar atelectasis secondary to surfactant malfunction.

PULMONARY EDEMA

Pulmonary edema may be broadly defined as excessive vascular fluid egress with abnormal accumulation in the interstitial and air spaces of the lung. Such accumulation of extravascular water affects pulmonary function and gas exchange to varying degrees, depending on both the site of accumulation (interstitial versus alveolar) and the quantity of fluid involved.

Cardiogenic Edema

Pulmonary edema is most readily recognized when fluid collects in the corners of the tetrahedron-shaped alveoli, causing geometric instability and rapid collapse.[7] Theoretically, *rapid* movement of fluid into the tight space results in sudden high pressures that may lead to destruction of the epithelium as an effective barrier to fluid passing into the alveolar space. Although this is speculative, it is a probable mechanism by which acute left ventricular failure (cardiogenic edema) results in alveolar fluid accumulation. The common clinical symptoms of dyspnea, rales, and severe hypoxemia are primarily attributable to the alveolar fluid accumulation.

Noncardiogenic Edema

In the absence of direct epithelial damage by toxic inhalants, the alveolar epithelium appears to remain an effective water barrier as long as *rapid* fluid movement is avoided. Most noncardiogenic causes of pulmonary edema involve less rapid water movement than left ventricular failure and therefore primarily involve interstitial accumulation of water without accumulation of alveolar fluid. Thus, the clinical symptoms are those of increased interstitial pressure impinging on bronchioles and blood vessels, resulting in increased airway and vascular resistances leading to abnormal distribution of perfusion and ventilation.[9]

The most common genesis of pulmonary NCE in critically ill patients is believed to result from both increased permeability of the endothelium to proteins[23-26] and increased water conductance across the endothelial cells. Such abnormal endothelial cell function is identified in the animal model by increased pulmonary lymph flow with a concomitant increase in protein content.[7, 24, 26] Even though reliable laboratory models for the study of permeability NCE are available,[7, 26] etiologies in man are not clearly delineated. However, correlations between laboratory investigations and clinical observations allow the following generalizations to be made with a reasonable degree of confidence.

1. Certain blood-borne toxins such as bacterial endotoxins[27] and drugs[28-30] result in significant alteration of endothelial permeability. A

high incidence of permeability edema is known to occur following sepsis in man.

2. Microemboli produce endothelial humoral and cytoplasmic changes that affect permeability.[23-25, 31, 32] This is believed to be the primary mechanism of development of NCE following disseminated intravascular coagulopathy (DIC) and fat emboli.[33-35]

3. Most investigators agree that the initial parenchymal damage from inhaled toxins is endothelial, which helps explain the NCE that often occurs in man after exposure to inhaled toxins.[7, 23, 24, 26]

ADULT RESPIRATORY DISTRESS SYNDROME

Since the introduction of the term "adult respiratory distress syndrome" in 1967, *epithelial* cell involvement has been a consistent feature in the syndrome's morphological description.[36-40] This epithelial cell involvement includes both type 1 cell sloughing and type 2 cell dysfunction.[41] The latter involves abnormal surfactant production resulting in reduced lung compliance and collapse of numerous gravity-dependent alveoli.[42, 43] Gravity-dependent alveolar collapse leads to an increase in unventilated but perfused areas of lung (zero V/Q), which will result in an arterial hypoxemia that is relatively refractory to increases in the inspired oxygen concentration.[44] The combination of refractory hypoxemia, severely decreased lung compliance, and diffuse involvement on chest x-ray studies has become the clinical hallmark of ARDS.[39, 45-48] Despite other uses of the acronym ARDS, the literature consistently indicates that it should be used to refer only to a severe and diffuse parenchymal abnormality involving epithelial as well as endothelial cell dysfunction.

ACUTE LUNG INJURY

Acute lung injury (ALI) may be characterized as a spectrum of abnormal parenchymal cell function, starting with predominately endothelial cell malfunction, resulting in NCE, and progressing to both epithelial and endothelial cell malfunction, resulting in ARDS. Table 12–1 summarizes this concept.

The diagnosis of ALI requires maintaining a high index of suspicion in those patients having a compatible history. There appears to be general agreement that patients with multiple trauma[48], sepsis[27], and DIC[33] are at high risk. Combinations of other physiologic insults (e.g., alveolar hyperoxia, aspiration, fat embolism, hypotension, interstitial pneumonia, multiple transfusions, operative procedures lasting over 5 hours, poor nutritional status) have been suggested as predisposing factors.[49]

The more severe form of ALI—ARDS—is readily identified by (1) a

TABLE 12–1.—CLINICAL SPECTRUM OF ACUTE LUNG INJURY (ALI)*†

| | ENDOTHELIAL CELL DYSFUNCTION | | EPITHELIAL CELL DYSFUNCTION |
	INCREASED PERMEABILITY		DIMINISHED SURFACTANT FUNCTION
Spectrum of ALI	Mild ────────→	Moderate ────────→	Severe
Clinical diagnosis	NCE		ARDS
Degree of hypoxemia	Moderate		Severe
Response to F_{IO_2}	Responsive		Refractory
Lung compliance	Moderate decrease		Severe decrease

*NCE, noncardiogenic edema; ARDS, adult respiratory distress syndrome.
†From Shapiro et al.[50] Reproduced by permission.

patible clinical history and physical findings, (2) refractory hypoxemia (arterial PO_2 <60 mm Hg at an F_{IO_2} of 0.5 or higher), (3) a markedly diminished pulmonary compliance, and (4) a chest radiograph showing diffuse bilateral parenchymal infiltrates.[50, 51] The less severe or earlier form of this pathology—NCE—is more difficult to diagnose. The following features are reasonably reliable: (1) a compatible clinical history, (2) an F_{IO_2} of 0.35 or higher required to maintain the arterial PO_2 above 60 mm Hg, (3) absence of chronic lung disease and cardiogenic edema, and (4) chest x-ray findings compatible with NCE and without pneumonic infiltrate or atelectasis.[50, 51]

MANAGEMENT OF ALI

The initial factor leading to ALI is increased pulmonary endothelial permeability. There are presently no scientifically documented means of directly enhancing the ability of these cells to recover from the insult.[24] Therefore, therapy directed toward the underlying etiology (e.g., antibiotics in sepsis) must be emphasized, along with supportive pulmonary therapy to ensure an optimal milieu for patient survival as well as reversal of the pulmonary pathology. Essential goals of supportive therapy include (1) maintaining adequate vascular volume and perfusion, (2) ensuring tissue oxygenation by maintaining adequate hemoglobin concentration and an arterial PO_2 of at least 55–60 mm Hg, and (3) limiting inspired oxygen concentrations to less than 50%.

Fluid Balance

Relative hypervolemia results in elevation of capillary hydrostatic pressures and increased pulmonary extravascular water (EVW), a phenomenon that occurs to a greater extent and at lower hydrostatic pressures in the presence of NCE.[24, 52] Since there are no data suggesting that in the presence of NCE the increased EVW resulting from transient fluid overload is removed from the lung when euvolemia is reinstated, meticulous care must be taken to *avoid* relative hypervolemia.

Although it has been demonstrated that vigorous volume depletion with diuretics may limit accumulation of EVW,[53] there is little evidence to suggest that severe volume depletion enhances mobilization of preexisting EVW. Since severe volume depletion may decrease cardiac output and perfusion, common sense dictates that maintaining a hypovolemic state in these patients is not desirable. It appears that careful titration of vascular volume and vascular space requirements to maintain euvolemia will provide adequate perfusion without excessive pulmonary microvascular pressures.

The administration of intravenous (IV) colloid solutions has been proposed as a therapy for NCE based on the oversimplified rationale that increasing plasma oncotic pressures will prevent accumulation of interstitial lung water or possibly enhance removal of water from the pulmonary interstitium.[54] Since oncotic gradients are minimal in normal lung and nearly ablated in NCE, there can be no scientific validity to the assumption that colloid administration will remove EVW in this disease entity. Present knowledge of lung parenchymal function leads to the conclusion that colloid administration should lead to increased net filtration of water and protein into the interstitium, and therefore is inherently deleterious to the lung with NCE. Administration of albumin to burn patients has been shown to increase lung water.[55] The clinical decision to administer colloid to a patient with NCE must be based on specific indications that override the potential harm to the lungs.

Alveolar Oxygen Tension and ALI

ALI results when small mammals breathe 100% oxygen for several days, the parenchymal hyperoxia affecting endothelial cells to a greater degree than epithelial cells.[14, 56–58] The last parenchymal cell type to demonstrate dysfunction secondary to hyperoxia in primates is the alveolar type 2 cell.[59, 60] However, endothelial cell and type 1 cell damage appears to place metabolic stress on type 2 cells which may leave them more susceptible to hyperoxic damage.[61, 62] Correlation of high F_{IO_2}, duration of exposure to high oxygen concentrations, and degree of lung fibrosis has been demonstrated in models of ALI,[52, 63–65] which may partly explain why alveolar hyperoxia with NCE appears to promote progression to ARDS.

Augmentation of the inspired oxygen concentration up to 40% should be effective for maintaining adequate arterial oxygenation in mild forms of NCE. There are ample indirect data to support the clinical warning that oxygen concentrations in excess of 50% threaten to impose hyperoxic damage on the already metabolically stressed pulmonary endothelial cells and may lead to more severe pathology, i.e., ARDS.[52, 63, 64, 66–71]

When the diagnosis of NCE is made, it is a reasonable clinical goal to limit the $F_{I_{O_2}}$ to 0.40 or less. In most instances the proper application of PEEP therapy enables this goal to be attained.

PEEP THERAPY

For purposes of this discussion, PEEP shall refer to the existence of an airway pressure above ambient at the end of exhalation, independent of inspiratory dynamics.[51, 72] Continuous positive airway pressure (CPAP) shall refer to PEEP in conjunction with spontaneous ventilation through a device that provides inspiratory gas flow when minor airway pressures below the PEEP level are generated. Continuous positive pressure ventilation (CPPV) shall refer to control or assist/control ventilation with PEEP.

Pulmonary Effects of PEEP

Three mechanisms have been postulated to explain the improvement in pulmonary function and gas exchange following PEEP therapy: (1) alteration of small airway closure in gravity-dependent lung areas; (2) decreased lung EVW, and (3) increased functional residual capacity (FRC).

Although it has been demonstrated that the lung volume at which small airway closure occurs often rises above FRC in anesthetized man,[73, 74] the effect of PEEP on arterial oxygenation as related to the FRC–closing volume relationship is not well documented and is often conflicting.[75, 76] Although future studies may substantiate a beneficial relationship between PEEP and lung volumes at which airway closure occurs, the present data are inconclusive.

The direct effects of PEEP on extravascular lung water are difficult to evaluate because of the complex factors governing lung water distribution. However, there is sufficient evidence to support the statement that extravascular lung water is derived from both juxta-alveolar and extra-alveolar vessels and that the fluid flux varies with the degree of alveolar inflation, pulmonary artery pressure, and pleural pressures.[10–12] The overwhelming balance of evidence suggests that PEEP results in either a significant increase or no change in interstitial water.[77, 78]

Increased FRC

It is well documented that PEEP increases FRC, which appears to be the main mechanism by which pulmonary function and gas exchange are improved. However, to what extent the FRC improvement is accomplished by increases in alveolar volume or by alveolar recruitment is controversial.

Daly and associates[79] utilized incidence light photomicrography to study normal rat alveolar characteristics at various levels of PEEP. They demonstrated that (1) alveolar diameters increased linearly with 0–10 cm H_2O; (2) end-expiratory diameters increased to a greater degree than end-inspiratory diameters; (3) beyond 10 cm H_2O PEEP, the increase in alveolar diameters progressively diminished and reached a plateau at approximately 15 cm H_2O PEEP; and (4) beyond 15 cm H_2O PEEP, alveolar pressure increased without measurable increase in alveolar diameters. These data suggest that there is an upper limit to the distensibility of normal alveoli and that within those limits, PEEP can increase FRC simply by increasing alveolar size.

"Alveolar recruitment" is a term commonly used to refer to an increase in FRC secondary to inflation of previously collapsed alveoli. Indirect evidence that PEEP may recruit alveoli was first presented in 1969 by McIntyre and associates,[80] who demonstrated that both arterial oxygenation and pulmonary compliance were rapidly improved when PEEP was applied to lung models with decreased surfactant activity. Recent studies[81] reaffirm this phenomenon occurring within minutes of the application of PEEP therapy.

Cardiac Effects of PEEP

Reduction of cardiac output coincident with PEEP therapy is due to a combination of mechanisms, of which reduction in right heart venous return is undoubtedly the primary and most frequently encountered.[82, 83] When PEEP therapy produces clinically significant reductions in cardiac output despite reasonable intravascular volume augmentation, an element of ventricular dysfunction most likely exists. Currently available information suggests this is most often related to increased right heart afterload with right ventricular dilation and leftward interventricular septal deviation resulting in decreased left ventricular output.[84, 85] Biventricular dysfunction has also been implicated.[86] Inotropic support is rarely necessary at PEEP levels less than 20 cm H_2O.[86] In each patient there appears to be a PEEP level at which reduction of cardiac output is of greater detriment to tissue oxygenation than the effects of improved arterial oxygen content are beneficial. Fortunately, these detrimental PEEP levels are usually above those that significantly improve arterial oxygen content when the patient is not hypovolemic.

THERAPEUTIC PEEP LEVELS

To determine the most desirable levels of PEEP, numerous clinical studies have been undertaken in patients with acute respiratory failure and clinical signs compatible with ALI.[88–92] These studies utilized an end point of achieving an arterial P_{O_2} above 60 mm/Hg with an $F_{I_{O_2}}$ below 0.5 without detriment to the cardiac output. This end point is clinically valid in ALI because (1) the most readily monitored effect of PEEP in acute lung injury is the improvement in arterial oxygen tension; (2) assuming adequate hemoglobin content and maintenance of adequate cardiac output, an arterial P_{O_2} of 60 mm Hg (90% oxyhemoglobin) is adequate for oxygen delivery to tissues; and (3) there are data to suggest that adequate arterial oxygenation at an $F_{I_{O_2}}$ below 0.5 may avoid cellular hyperoxic conditions that alter or depress pulmonary parenchymal metabolic function.

Table 12–2 summarizes data from six studies utilizing the above-described clinical end point for determining appropriate levels of PEEP therapy. The data demonstrate that only 5% of patients with ALI required PEEP levels above 30 cm H_2O, and 80% required 20 cm H_2O or less. The required PEEP correlates with severity of lung injury, while correlations between these therapeutic PEEP levels and factors such as mortality, required fluid therapy, and incidence of pneumothorax are not well established.

PULMONARY COMPLIANCE AND PEEP

Pulmonary compliance may be conveniently estimated in conjunction with control mode positive pressure ventilation by dividing the exhaled tidal volume by the pressure change from baseline to end-inspiratory pla-

TABLE 12–2.—Therapeutic PEEP in Man

STUDY	NO. OF PTS.	PROBABLE PATHOLOGY*	INSP. MODE	PEEP RANGE (MEAN)
Gallagher and Civetta[87]	315	Mixed	IMV	6–45 (15.3)
Downs et al.[88]	12	NCE-ARDS	IMV	6–20 (13.2)
Falke[89]	7	NCE-ARDS	CMV	5–15
Kirby et al.[90]	28	ARDS	IMV	15–44 (25)
Suter et al.[91]	15	NCE-ARDS	CMV	0–15
Venus et al.[92]	15	NCE-ARDS	SPONT	10–25

*NCE, noncardiogenic edema; ARDS, adult respiratory distress syndrome.

teau—a measurement referred to as effective static compliance (ESC). Some investigators noted that optimal PEEP levels and best pulmonary compliance often coincide and have suggested that ESC may be a useful clinical guide to determine optimal PEEP.

Although changes in *lung* compliance may correlate with the optimal PEEP level, the utilization of the ESC measurement (a reflection of both lung and chest cage compliance) is not always reliable. Although chest wall compliance may remain relatively constant when comatose or paralyzed patients are being controlled on positive pressure ventilation, it is subject to much variation when the patient breathes spontaneously on an intermittent mandatory ventilation (IMV) device, is on assist/control mode, or "fights" the ventilator for any reason.

SPONTANEOUS VENTILATION AND PEEP

Zarins and associates[93] studied, in six normal primates, the effects on cardiac function of 20 cm H_2O PEEP in conjunction with both IMV and controlled mechanical ventilation (CMV). They found that all the animals manifested similar decreases in cardiac output irrespective of the presence of spontaneous ventilation. Considering that PEEP levels of 20 cm H_2O in normal lungs results in significant reduction of cardiac output without improvement in V/Q relationships,[94, 95] a logical explanation for Zarin's findings is that "excessive" PEEP decreases cardiac output without physiologic benefit, regardless of the mode of ventilation.

Downs et al[96] compared CMV at a rate of 12/minute without PEEP to IMV (2/minute) with 0, 5, and 10 cm H_2O of PEEP and found that spontaneous ventilation associated with the IMV mode resulted in less positive intrapleural pressures. Venus and associates[97] reported similar findings in dogs following acid aspiration supported with 10 cm H_2O of PEEP in conjunction with both IMV and CMV. In addition, they found significantly less depression of cardiac output when spontaneous ventilation was present. Shah and associates[98] reported similar findings in nine patients convalescing from multiple trauma.

The available data strongly support the thesis that spontaneous ventilation in conjunction with PEEP therapy enhances the pulmonary effects (increased transpulmonary pressures) while reducing detrimental alterations in cardiovascular function secondary to a rise in intrapleural pressures.

EARLY APPLICATION OF PEEP THERAPY

There is prospective evidence to suggest significant benefit from early application of low levels of PEEP when the inspired oxygen concentration is kept below 40% in surgical and trauma patients at risk for developing ARDS.[99, 100] In addition, McAslan and Cowley[101] reported on 1,676 major trauma patients who had routinely received 5 cm H_2O of PEEP on admission to the trauma center. The PEEP was increased as necessary to maintain an arterial P_{O_2} of 60 mm Hg at less than 0.4 $F_{I_{O_2}}$. PEEP of 10 cm H_2O was commonly required, while more than 15 cm H_2O was seldom necessary. This patient group was retrospectively compared with a similar group of major trauma victims in whom PEEP therapy had not been used until significant respiratory failure was clinically evident. The "early PEEP" group showed significantly diminished pulmonary morbidity.

It appears that serious consideration for applying early PEEP therapy should be given to patients at risk for ALI who require over 35% inspired oxygen to maintain an arterial P_{O_2} of 60 mm Hg or greater. Technical improvements in CPAP masks now make clinically practical the early application of low-level PEEP therapy to the unintubated patient at risk for developing ALI.

SUMMARY OF PEEP THERAPY IN ALI

INDICATIONS.—The principal clinical indication for PEEP therapy is the diagnosis of ALI. Initiation of PEEP therapy should be seriously considered as soon as the diagnosis is clinically evident.

GOALS.—The primary goal of PEEP therapy in ALI is to accomplish adequate arterial oxygen content (adequate hemoglobin content plus an arterial P_{O_2} greater than 60 mm Hg) without significant reduction in cardiac output at an $F_{I_{O_2}}$ below 0.5. This should provide adequate tissue oxygenation while avoiding potentially detrimental alveolar oxygen concentrations. Our experience is that an $F_{I_{O_2}}$ of 0.4 is an attainable and practical goal in most circumstances.

THERAPEUTIC LEVELS.—Utilizing the concept of ALI representing a spectrum of pulmonary damage from the less severe or earlier form (NCE) to the more severe form (ARDS): NCE usually shows significant improvement in gas exchange with 5–15 cm H_2O of PEEP, with most patients responding optimally by 10 cm H_2O PEEP; while ARDS is usually improved with 10–30 cm H_2O of PEEP, and most of these patients manifest an optimal response between 10 and 20 cm H_2O of PEEP.

METHODOLOGY.—PEEP should be increased or decreased in increments of 3–5 cm H_2O and effects should be evaluated within 20 minutes. We prefer increments of 5 cm H_2O, since this is reliably attainable and rarely excessive. The patient should be allowed to breathe spontaneously to whatever degree is compatible with cardiovascular and clinical stability.

Spontaneous breathing appears to be an advantage in PEEP therapy but by no means a necessity. Although PEEP is most consistently and reliably administered via endotracheal or tracheostomy tube, mask CPAP up to 15 cm H_2O PEEP is technically feasible and may prove beneficial in many unintubated patients.

MONITORING.—Essential monitoring includes vital signs, continuous ECG, serial arterial blood gas measurement, and appropriate nurse/respiratory therapist availability. Appropriate monitoring of the respiratory equipment, inspired gas concentration, and system flow is essential since technical malfunction is not uncommon.

A pulmonary artery flotation catheter is warranted when more than 20 cm H_2O of PEEP is required or there is uncertainty concerning the diagnosis of ALI, the cardiovascular status, or the intravascular fluid volume. The clinically useful information available by means of a pulmonary artery catheter in relation to PEEP therapy includes measurement of arteriovenous oxygen content difference and cardiac output measurements to aid the assessment of perfusion and oxygen extraction; intrapulmonary shunt calculations to aid assessment of the pulmonary effects of PEEP; and pulmonary artery occlusion pressures to aid in the assessment of intravascular fluid administration.

CARDIOVASCULAR SUPPORT.—Correction of hypovolemia should ideally be achieved prior to initiation of PEEP therapy; however, intravascular volume augmentation is frequently required during or following application of PEEP therapy. Reasonable IV fluid administration in conjunction with PEEP levels up to 20 cm H_2O usually compensates for reductions in cardiac output secondary to reduction in venous return. PEEP therapy seldom requires inotropic support at levels below 20 cm H_2O.

CONTRAINDICATIONS.—There are no absolute contraindications to the use of PEEP therapy in ALI. There do not appear to be data substantiating the concept that clinically appropriate levels of PEEP should be withheld for fear of producing barotrauma. While patients requiring PEEP therapy for severe ALI (ARDS) have an increased incidence of barotrauma, this appears to be related to the severity of the parenchymal disease rather than the level of applied airway pressure therapy.

CASE STUDY 1

A 59-year-old man was involved in a head-on motor vehicle accident at 10:00 P.M. The paramedics reported unfastening his seat belt and shoulder strap before removing him from the vehicle. They splinted his right leg, placed an 18-gauge IV catheter in the right forearm, and administered normal saline prior to bringing him to the emergency room.

He arrived in the emergency room at 10:30 P.M. awake but disoriented. His skin was cool and clammy to the touch; blood pressure (BP) was 60 mm Hg systolic, pulse was 130 beats per minute and regular, and respiratory rate was 30/minute and nonlabored. A 6-cm diameter echymosis without laceration was noted above the right eyebrow. Pupils were equal and reactive, fundi were normal. The neck was supple. Clear breath sounds were present bilaterally. Heart tones were without murmurs or extra sounds. The abdomen was distended and tense without bowel sounds. The right thigh was swollen, discolored, and painful; the skin was intact. He could move his foot and toes on command. Neurologic status was grossly intact.

Two 16-gauge peripheral IV catheters were placed and a central catheter was placed via the right subclavian vein. Peritoneal tap returned blood that did not clot. Blood was obtained for typing, crossmatching, and other laboratory tests. The operating room staff was notified.

An electrocardiogram (ECG) revealed sinus tachycardia. Right thigh x-ray revealed a displaced femoral fracture. Hemoglobin was 11 gm/dl and WBC count was $8,500/cc^{-3}$. The patient had been placed on a 40% Venturi-type mask; arterial blood gas analysis revealed a pH of 7.41, a PCO_2 of 32 mm Hg, and a PO_2 of 95 mm Hg.

Over the next hour the patient received 4 units of whole blood, 1 L of hetastarch, and 2 L of crystalloid solution. On transfer to the operating room the patient was alert and oriented, with a BP of 100/50 mm Hg, a pulse of 110 beats per minute, a respiratory rate of 30/minute, and a CVP of 8 cm H_2O.

In the operating room an inhalation anesthetic with muscle relaxant was administered without event. The induction was without any suspicion of aspiration. The BP remained over 100 mm Hg systolic, pulse 100–110 beats per minute and CVP 7–11 cm H_2O. A right radial arterial catheter was placed. The spleen was removed and liver lacerations were repaired. An open reduction of the right femur was accomplished. A nasogastric tube and a nasotracheal tube were placed at the end of the operation.

The patient arrived in the surgical intensive care unit at 3:00 A.M. and was placed on a volume-limited ventilator. Fluids administered since admission were 6 units of whole blood, 10 units of packed RBCs, 3 L of hetastarch, and 7 L of crystalloid fluid, with an estimated blood loss in the operating room of 4,500 ml and a urine output of 700 ml. Assessment of cardiopulmonary function and arterial blood gases revealed the following: BP, 120/60 mm Hg; pulse, 100 beats per minute; respirations, 10/minute; mechanical tidal volume, 1,200 ml; pH, 7.42; PCO_2, 36 mm Hg; PO_2, 120 mm Hg; FI_{O_2}, 0.50; CVP, 10 cm H_2O; temperature, 35° C; hemoglobin, 12 gm/dl; and normal serum electrolyte levels.

Discussion

The patient tolerated the surgery well and appeared to be no longer bleeding. There are a number of factors to consider in the immediate postoperative care that are important in decreasing the incidence of complications. The main factors are (1) maintaining adequate perfusion without fluid overload, (2) maintaining urine output above 50 ml/hour to reduce the chances of acute tubular necrosis (ATN), and (3) maintaining adequate arterial oxygenation without exposing the lungs to unnecessary hyperoxia. Additional factors are pain management and ventilator discontinuance.

The most reasonable clinical course is to assume that the patient is in adequate fluid balance since the hemodynamic and perfusion status are acceptable. Some overall plan for fluid administration is essential and must be based on the principle that urine and nasogastric fluid losses should be replaced with appropriate electrolyte solutions plus a minimal amount of free water. If the hemodynamic status should deteriorate, fluid challenges of 50–100 ml should be administered to reestablish an adequate vascular volume/vascular space relationship (see chapter 1). Of course, frequent evaluation for further bleeding is essential.

A reasonable urine output should be maintained to diminish the incidence of ATN. Although controversial, a urine output above 50 ml/hour is a reasonable goal. Following assurance of adequate intravascular volume and, if needed, renal perfusion, dopaminergic stimulation or intermittent diuretic therapy can be employed singly or in combination.

Certainly an FI_{O_2} above 0.5 is undesirable and one of 0.4 or less is preferred, since some pulmonary parenchymal insult must be assumed, as the patient's Pa_{O_2} is only 120 mm Hg on 50% oxygen. Appropriate levels of PEEP (5–10 cm/H_2O) should accomplish this goal with only small increments of additional vascular volume required to maintain cardiac output.

The patient should be warmed slowly by covering him with warm blankets. Shivering increases oxygen consumption and carbon dioxide production and should be avoided. The muscle relaxant (Pancuronium) should be redistributed and excreted over the next several hours. Spontaneous ventilation should be evaluated as muscle strength returns. It is essential to remember that the patient will have pain as he emerges from the hypothermia and general anesthesia. Pain will raise catecholamine levels and create arteriolar and venous constriction. When narcotics are administered for pain relief, this catecholamine level will diminish and hypotension may result. The best way to avoid this circumstance is to administer adequate analgesia from the beginning and avoid the pain and anxiety that leads to stress reactions. Morphine sulfate, 1–4 mg IV, may be administered each hour and as necessary to establish and maintain an adequate analgesic level without significantly depressing respiratory drive. Conventional analgesic administration of larger doses of narcotics given intramuscularly results in widely fluctuating serum drug concentrations, poor pain control, and greater potential for adverse side effects.

Case Study Continued

At 7:00 A.M. the patient was awake and oriented. He had received 2 mg of morphine sulfate IV on six occasions and complained only of mild right thigh pain. His urine output was 150 ml since returning from the operating room, and he had received 350 ml of 5% dextrose in 0.45% saline. His rectal temperature was 37.2° C. PEEP, 5 cm H_2O, was added to the ventilator regimen and enabled a decrease in $F_{I_{O_2}}$ to 0.4.

Spontaneous ventilatory efforts began at 5:00 A.M. and the IMV rate was gradually decreased to 4/minute. At this time the vital signs and blood gases were as follows: BP, 140/75 mm Hg; pulse, 90 beats per minute; respiratory rate (V)—4/minute, (S)—20/minute, TV(V)—1,200 ml, (S)—300 ml, MV—12.8 L, VC—1.4 L; pH, 7.44; P_{CO_2}, 34 mm Hg; P_{O_2}, 100 mm Hg; $F_{I_{O_2}}$, 0.40; and CVP, 9 cm/H_2O.

The patient was taken off the ventilator and placed on a CPAP system at 5 cm H_2O of PEEP with an $F_{I_{O_2}}$ of 0.4. His vital signs changed only in that the heart rate increased to 95 beats per minute. Arterial blood gas analysis after 20 minutes revealed a pH of 7.41, a P_{CO_2} of 38 mm Hg, and a P_{O_2} of 95 mm Hg.

Between 7:00 A.M. and 3 P.M. the patient received 1 L of D5W/0.45 saline plus 40 mEq of potassium chloride. Urine output was 650 ml and nasogastric drainage 200 ml. Morphine sulfate, 4 mg IV, had been given each hour. A 2 μg/kg/minute infusion of dopamine was running and two 10-mg doses of furosemide had been given to maintain urine output. Six hours later assessment of the patient revealed a BP of 110/70 mm Hg, a pulse of 95 beats per minute, respiratory rate of 22/minute, TV of 400 ml, MV of 8.8 L, pH of 7.43, P_{CO_2} of 38 mm Hg, P_{O_2} of 55 mm Hg, $F_{I_{O_2}}$ of 0.4 and CVP of 9 cm H_2O.

Heart tones were clear and no murmurs were heard. Bilateral breath sounds were present with scattered rhonchi; no rales or wheezing were noted. A chest x-ray film revealed an appropriately placed endotracheal tube and no infiltrates or atelectasis.

Discussion

The patient was developing progressive hypoxemia which did not appear due to obvious hypervolemia, cardiogenic edema, pneumonia, atelectasis, or retained secretions. The most probable cause is NCE. If the P_{O_2} dropped further, it would be advisable to increase PEEP rather than increase $F_{I_{O_2}}$, as a low Pa_{O_2} on 40% oxygen implies a significant amount of lung with either very low V/Q ratios or zero V/Q ratios.

Case Study Continued

At 3:30 P.M. the vital signs were unchanged but the arterial P_{O_2} was 52 mm Hg. CPAP was increased to 10 cm H_2O without a change in vital signs or respiratory pattern. Arterial blood gas values were as follows: pH, 7.43; P_{CO_2}, 38 mm Hg; and P_{O_2}, 87 mm Hg on 40% inspired oxygen.

The remaining course was uneventful. The $F_{I_{O_2}}$ was decreased to 0.35 and the CPAP to 5 cm H_2O by the second postoperative day. The patient was extubated and placed on a 35% air entrainment mask, with the following arterial blood gas values: pH, 7.41; P_{CO_2}, 39 mm Hg; and P_{O_2}, 82 mm Hg.

Careful titration of supportive therapy (fluids, diuretics, oxygen, PEEP, airway care) provided an optimal milieu for avoiding cardiac, pulmonary, and renal complications and ensuring a satisfactory outcome.

CASE STUDY 2

A 62-year-old woman with a 40-year history of malabsorption syndrome (nontropical sprue) experienced a 30-pound weight loss secondary to emotional stress and noncompliance with her glutin-free diet. After thorough investigation to rule out other causes for the weight loss, she was placed on a strict diet but did not gain weight over 1 month. It was decided to place her on parenteral nutrition, in response to which she gained over 10 pounds in 14 days. On the 15th day she became febrile to 103° F, complained of chills and dizziness, and suffered mild hypotension. Empirical therapy for assumed gram-negative sepsis (subsequently confirmed by blood culture) consisted of an aminoglycoside and cephalosporin. Her fever defervesced the next day, but she was noted to bruise easily and had two episodes of hemoptysis. Coagulation studies confirmed a mild DIC. That evening she complained of dyspnea and an arterial blood gas analysis revealed a pH of 7.53, a Pco_2 of 32 mm

Hg, and a Po_2 of 48 mm Hg (Fi_{O_2} of 0.2). She was placed on 50% oxygen and transferred to the medical intensive care unit.

On admission to the intensive care unit she was awake, anxious, and alert, sitting up in bed and complaining of severe shortness of breath. She was markedly cachectic. BP was 90/50 mm Hg, pulse was 120 beats per minute, and respiratory rate was 28/minute and labored, with a tidal volume of 250 ml and a vital capacity of 1.4 L. She was using accessory muscles to breath. Bilateral breath sounds were heard with no wheezes, rales, or rhonchi. Air entry was better at the apices than the bases. Attempts at coughing produced neither sputum nor relief. Heart tones were clear without murmers or extra sounds. On 50% inspired oxygen the pH was 7.51, Pco_2 was 32 mm Hg, and the Po_2 was 42 mm Hg. Hemoglobin was 9.1 gm/dl; WBC count, 12,500/mm^{-3} (down from 21,000 2 days earlier); and electrolytes, normal.

Discussion

This patient's cachexia, in addition to the recent sepsis and DIC, placed her at risk for ALI. Her refractory hypoxemia suggested significant areas of lung with zero V/Q ratios and intrapulmonary right-to-left shunting which, in the absence of pneumonia and/or atelectasis, made the most probable pulmonary diagnosis ARDS.

Since the sepsis was being adequately treated, the next most important factor is to ensure adequate perfusion and oxygenation while relieving the work of breathing and hopefully decreasing the Fi_{O_2} to at least 0.4. Since it can be predicted that at least 15 cm H_2O of PEEP will be required to achieve these aims, an endotracheal tube is indicated. This will also allow safe tracheal suction and positive pressure ventilation if the work of breathing is not sufficiently relieved by CPAP.

This patient's cardiovascular reserves are questionable because of her age and long-standing cachexia. A pulmonary artery catheter would be the safest and surest means of monitoring the cardiopulmonary response to her pathology and therapy. Additionally, an arterial line would facilitate blood gas monitoring and provide continuous BP monitoring.

Packed RBC infusion will improve the oxygen-carrying capacity of the blood. However, it is advisable to transfuse after the pulmonary artery line is established so that careful hemodynamic monitoring can be accomplished during the transfusions.

Case Study Continued

The entire situation was carefully explained to the patient and the need for her cooperation was stressed. A right radial arterial catheter was placed. Because of her inability to lie flat and because of the mild coagulopathy, a pulmonary artery catheter was placed via the right basilic vein by a cutdown procedure. After placement of the pulmonary artery catheter a no. 8 nasotracheal tube was placed after adequate topical anesthesia had been established. The patient was placed on a CPAP system at 5 cm H_2O with an FI_{O_2} of 0.70. After allowing 15 minutes for the patient to stabilize, assessment revealed the following: BP, 90/60 mm Hg; pulse, 120 beats per minute; respirations, 30/minute; tidal volume, 250 ml; MV, 7.5 L/minute; pH, 7.51; PCO_2 32 mm Hg; PO_2, 41 mm Hg; FI_{O_2}, 0.7; PV_{O_2}, 32 mm Hg; PAOP, 14 mm Hg; cardiac output,

7.0 L/minute; $DA - V_{O_2}$, 2.2 vol%; QSp/QT, 43%; and hemoglobin, 9.2 gm/dl.

The CPAP was increased to 10 cm H_2O with essentially no changes occurring after 15 minutes. The CPAP was then increased to 15 cm H_2O, and 20 minutes later the patient indicated her breathing was easier. Approximately 500 ml of crystalloid solution had been administered since the intubation. At this time the patient's vital signs, hemodynamic parameters, and blood gas values were as follows: BP, 90/60 mm Hg; pulse, 110 beats per minute; respirations, 25/minute; tidal volume, 250 ml; MV, 6.25 L/minute; pH, 7.49; PCO_2, 35 mm Hg; PO_2, 65 mm Hg; FI_{O_2}, 0.7; PV_{O_2}, 32 mm Hg; PAOP, 13 mm Hg; cardiac output 5.5 L/minute; $DA - V_{O_2}$, 3.2 vol%; QSp/QT, 32%; and hemoglobin, 9.2 gm/dl.

Discussion

The patient's pulmonary status had significantly improved. That she was not using accessory muscles to breathe indicated it was much easier to breathe. The respiratory rate decreased and the arterial oxygenation markedly improved. The decrease in cardiac output was probably secondary to the improved arterial oxygenation, which was reflected in the markedly diminished intrapulmonary shunt. There can be no argument that PEEP was beneficial to this point; the critical question is whether or not it should then be increased further.

Two of the three clinical goals of PEEP therapy in ARDS have been met, namely, perfusion has been adequately maintained and the arterial PO_2 increased to above 60 mm Hg. However, the third goal, to decrease the FI_{O_2} to 0.4 or less, has not yet been met. One option is to wait and see if the arterial P_{O_2} continues to improve, which will allow the $F_{I_{O_2}}$ to be decreased and at the same time one could transfuse with RBCs. However, this would ignore the overwhelming evidence that hyperoxic alveolar gas is detrimental to the lung parenchyma in this disease process. The other option is to increase the CPAP to 20 cm H_2O. Although many physicians are anxious about this level of PEEP therapy, there are little data to suggest that this level is deleterious in patients with severe disease.

Case Study Continued

The CPAP was increased to 20 cm H_2O and 20 minutes later reassessment revealed considerable improvement in oxygenation with no major hemodynamic changes. The arterial blood gas analysis and shunt study revealed an arterial pH of 7.43, a Pa_{CO_2} of 42 mm Hg; a Pa_{O_2} of 128 mm Hg ($F_{I_{O_2}}$ = .07); Pv_{O_2} of 37 mm Hg; and a QSp/QT of 24%.

RBC transfusion was started and the $F_{I_{O_2}}$ decreased to 0.5, which resulted in an arterial P_{O_2} of 72 mm Hg. The patient remained comfortable. Four units of packed RBCs were administered over the next 2 hours. Reassessment revealed the following values: BP, 100/70 mm Hg; pulse, 100 beats per minute, respirations, 20/minute; tidal volume, 220 ml; MV, 4.4 L/minute; pH, 7.43; P_{CO_2}, 42 mm Hg; P_{O_2}, 84 mm Hg; $F_{I_{O_2}}$, 0.5; Pv_{O_2}, 37 mm Hg; PAOP, 16 mm Hg; cardiac output, 5.1 L/minute; $D_A - v_{O_2}$, 3.8 vol%; QSp/QT, 22%; and hemoglobin, 11.3 gm/dl.

No rales were heard, and a repeated chest x-ray film showed increased lung volume with no infiltrate or atelectasis. No S_3 or S_4 was noted. The $F_{I_{O_2}}$ was reduced to 0.4 and the Pa_{O_2} was 64 mm Hg, with no significant change in any other clinical parameters.

The patient remained comfortable and stable for the next 18 hours, at which time her cardiovascular function remained unchanged and her Pa_{O_2} was 80 mm Hg ($F_{I_{O_2}}$ = 0.4) and QSp/QT was 18%.

The CPAP was reduced to 15 cm H_2O which resulted in an acceptable Pa_{O_2} of 68 mm Hg ($F_{I_{O_2}}$ = 0.4) and QSp/QT of 23%.

Four hours later the arterial P_{O_2} had risen to 79 mm Hg and the $F_{I_{O_2}}$ was reduced to 0.35. The pulmonary artery catheter was removed. The next morning, on 15 cm H_2O CPAP, the patient had a BP of 100/60 mm Hg, pulse of 90 beats per minute, was breathing with a tidal volume of 275 ml, and had an arterial pH of 7.42, a Pa_{CO_2} of 38 mm Hg, and a Pa_{O_2} of 82 mm Hg ($F_{I_{O_2}}$ = 0.35).

The CPAP was reduced to 10 cm H_2O and oxygenation remained satisfactory. The patient continued to improve and the next day the CPAP was decreased to 5 cm H_2O and the patient extubated 3 hours later. She was discharged from the intensive care unit the following day receiving 2 L of oxygen via a nasal cannula. Arterial blood gas values at that time were pH, 7.41; P_{CO_2}, 38 mm Hg; and P_{O_2}, 72 mm Hg.

REFERENCES

1. Scheeberger E.E.: Ultrastructural basis for alveolar-capillary permeability to protein. *Ciba Found. Symp.* 38:3, 1976.
2. Karnovsky M.J.: The ultrastructural basis of transcapillary exchange. *J. Gen. Physiol.* 52:645, 1967.
3. Fishman A.P., Petra G.G.: Permeability of pulmonary vascular endothelium. *Ciba Found. Symp.* 38:29, 1976.

4. Bruns R.R., Palade G.E.: Studies on blood capillaries: II. Transport of ferritin molecules across the wall of muscle capillaries. *J. Cell Biol.* 3:277–282, 1968.
5. Civetta J.M.: A new look at the Starling equation. *Crit. Care Med.* 7:84–91, 1979.
6. Zweifach B.W., Silberberg A.: The interstitial lymphatic flow system, in Guyton A.C., Young D.B. (eds.): *International Review of Physiology, Cardiovascular Physiology III.* Baltimore, University Park Press, 1979, pp. 215–260.
7. Staub N.C.: Pulmonary edema. *Physiol. Rev.* 54:678, 1974.
8. Guyton A.C., Granger H.J., Taylor A.E.: Interstitial fluid pressure. *Physiol. Rev.* 51:527, 1971.
9. Iliff L.D., Green R.E., Hughes J.M.B.: Effect of interstitial edema on distribution of ventilation and perfusion in isolated lungs. *J. Appl. Physiol.* 33:462, 1972.
10. Klika E.: The ultrastructure of pulmonary lymphatic vessels and capillaries. *Acta Univ. Carol.* [*Med.*] 21:23, 1975.
11. Weibel E.R., Gehr P., Haies D., et al.: The cell population of the normal lung, in Bouhuys A. (ed.): *Lung Cells in Disease.* Amsterdam, Elsevier/North-Holland, Inc., 1976.
12. Staehlin L.A.: Structure and function of intracellular junctions. *Int. Rev. Cytol.* 39:191, 1974.
13. Kikkawa Y., Yoneda K., Smith F., et al.: The type II epithelial cells of the lung: II. Chemical composition and phospholipid synthesis. *Lab. Invest.* 32:295,1975.
14. Mason R.J.: Phospholipid synthesis in primary culture of type II alveolar cells, abstracted. *Am. Rev. Respir. Dis.* 115(part 2):352,1977.
15. Fishman A.P.: Non-respiratory function of lung. *Chest* 72:84, 1977.
16. Bachoven M., Weibel E.R.: Basic pattern of tissue repair in human lungs following unspecific injury. *Chest* 65:145, 1974.
17. Kuhn C.: The cells of the lung and their organelles, in Crystal R.D. (ed.): *The Biochemical Basis of Pulmonary Function.* New York, Marcel Dekker, 1976, pp. 3–48.
18. Naimark A.: Clinical implications of research in lung disease, in Bouhuys A. (ed.): *Lung Cells in Disease.* Amsterdam, Elsevier/North-Holland, Inc., 1976, pp. 315–328.
19. Rosenbaum R.M., Picciano P.: The type 1 alveolar lining cells of the mammalian lung. *Am. J. Pathol.* 90:123, 1978.
20. Adamson I.Y.R., Bowden D.H.: The type 2 cell as a progenitor of alveolar regeneration: A cytodynamic study in mice after exposure to oxygen. *Lab. Invest.* 30:35, 1974.
21. Evans M.J., Cabral L.J., Stephens R.J., et al.: Transformation of alveolar type 2 cells to type 1 cells following exposure to NO_2. *Exp. Mol. Pathol.* 22:142, 1975.
22. Lamy M., Fallat R.J., Koeniger E., et al.: Pathologic features and mechanisms of hypoxemia in adult respiratory distress syndrome. *Am. Rev. Respir. Dis.* 114:267, 1976.
23. Fishman A.P.: Pulmonary edema: The water exchange function of the lung. *Circulation* 46:390, 1972.
24. Robin E.D., et al.: Medical progress: Pulmonary edema. Parts 1 & 2. *N. Engl. J. Med.* 288:239, 1973.
25. Hurley J.V.: Current views on the mechanics of pulmonary edema. *J. Pathol.* 125:59, 1978.
26. Staub N.C.: Pulmonary edema due to increased microvascular permeability to fluid and protein. *Circ. Res.* 43:143, 1978.
27. Bessa S.D., Dalmasso A.P., Goodale R.L. Jr.: Studies on the mechanism of endotoxin-induced increase of alveolocapillary permeability. *Proc. Soc. Exp. Biol. Med.* 147:701, 1974.
28. Addington W.W., Cugell D.W., Bazeley E.S., et al.: The pulmonary edema of heroin toxicity: An example of stiff lung syndrome. *Chest* 62:199, 1972.
29. Karliner J.S., Steinberg A.D., Williams M.H.: Lung function after pulmonary edema associated with heroin overdosage. *Arch. Intern. Med.* 124:350, 1969.
30. Burton W., Vender J., Shapiro B.A.: Adult respiratory distress syndrome following Placidyl abuse. *Crit. Care Med.* 8:48, 1980.
31. Malik A.B., VanderZee H.: Mechanisms of pulmonary edema induced by microembolization in dogs. *Circ. Res.* 42:72, 1978.

32. Malik A.B., VanderZee H.: Lung vascular permeability following progressive pulmonary embolization. *J. Appl. Physiol.* 45(4):590, 1978.
33. Bone R.C., Francis P.B., Pierce A.K.: Intravascular coagulation associated with the adult respiratory distress syndrome. *Am. J. Med.* 61:585, 1976.
34. Deykin D.: Emerging concepts of platelet function. *N. Engl. J. Med.* 290:144, 1974.
35. Josephson S., Swedenborg J., Dahlgren S.E.: Delayed lung lesion in dogs after thombin-induced disseminated intravascular coagulation. *Acta Chir. Scand.* 140:431, 1974.
36. Bachoven M., Weibel E.R.: Alterations of gas exchange apparatus in adult respiratory insufficiency associated with septicemia. *Am. Rev. Respir. Dis.* 116:589, 1977.
37. Bergofsky E.H.: The acute respiratory insufficiency syndrome following nonthoracic trauma: The lung in shock. *Am. J. Cardiol.* 26:619, 1970.
38. Blaisdell F.W.: Pathophysiology of the respiratory distress syndrome. *Arch. Surg.* 108:44, 1974.
39. Blaisdell F.W., Schlobohm R.M.: The respiratory distress syndrome: A review. *Surgery* 74:251, 1973.
40. Nash G., Foley F.D., Langlinais P.C.: Pulmonary interstitial edema and hyaline membranes in adult burn patients: Electron microscopic observations. *Hum. Pathol.* 5:149, 1974.
41. Katzenstein A.A., Bloor C.M., Leibow A.A.: Diffuse alveolar damage: The role of oxygen, shock, and related factors. A review. *Am. J. Pathol.* 85:210, 1976.
42. Clements J.A., Brown E.S., Johnson R.P., et al.: Pulmonary surface tension and the mucous lining of the lungs: Some theoretical considerations. *J. Appl. Physiol.* 12:262, 1958.
43. Collier C., Hackney J.D., Rounds D.E., et al.: Alterations of surfactant in oxygen poisoning. *Dis. Chest* 48:233, 1965.
44. James O.: Respiratory failure after injury: A review and plea for accuracy. *Heart Lung* 6:303, 1977.
45. Dowd J., Jenkins I.C.: The lung in shock: A Review. *Can. Anaesth. Soc. J.* 19:309, 1972.
46. Petty T.L., Ashbaugh D.G.: The adult respiratory distress syndrome: Clinical features, factors influencing prognosis and principles of management. *Chest* 60:233, 1971.
47. Rosen A.J.: Shock lung: Fact or fancy? *Surg. Clin. North Am.* 55:613, 1975.
48. Webb W.R.: Pulmonary complications of non-thoracic trauma: Summary of the national research council conference. *J. Trauma* 9:700, 1969.
49. Pepe P.E., Potkin R.T., Reus D.H., et al.: Clinical predictors of the adult respiratory distress syndrome. *Am J. Surg.* 144:124, 1982.
50. Shapiro B.A., Cane R.D., Harrison R.A.: Positive end-expiratory pressure in acute lung injury. *Chest* 83:358, 1983.
51. Shapiro B.A., Cane R.D., Harrison R.A.: Positive end-expiratory pressure therapy in adults with special reference to acute lung injury: A review of the literature and suggested clinical correlations. *Crit. Care Med.* 12:127–141, 1984.
52. Rinaldo J.E., Rogers R.M.: Adult respiratory disease syndrome: Changing concepts of lung injury and repair. *N. Engl. J. Med.* 306:900, 1982.
53. Robin E.D., Carey I.C., Grenvik A., et al.: Capillary leak syndrome with pulmonary edema. *Arch. Intern. Med.* 130:66, 1972.
54. DaLuz P., Shubin H., Weil M.H.: Pulmonary edema related to changes in colloid osmotic pressure and pulmonary artery wedge pressure in patients after acute myocardial infarction. *Circulation* 51:350, 1975.
55. Goodwin G.W., Dorethy J., Lam V., et al.: Randomized trial of efficacy of crystalloid and colloid resuscitation on hemodynamic response and lung water following thermal injury. *Ann. Surg.* 197, 1983.
56. Kistler G.S., Caldwell P.R.B., Weibel E.R.: Development of fine structural damage to alveolar and capillary lining cells in oxygen-poisoned rat lungs. *J. Cell Biol.* 32:605, 1967.
57. Block E.R.: Recovery from hyperoxic depression of pulmonary 5-hydroxytryptamine clearance: Effect of inspired Po_2 tension. *Lung* 155:131, 1978.
58. Block E.R., Cannon J.K.: Effect of oxygen exposure on lung clearance of amines. *Lung* 155:287, 1978.

59. Evans M.J., Dekker N.P., Cabral-Anderson L.J., et al.: Quantitation of damage to the alveolar epithelium by means of type 2 cell proliferation. *Am. Rev. Respir. Dis.* 118:787, 1978.
60. Frank L., Massaro D.: The lung and oxygen toxicity. *Arch. Intern. Med.* 139:347, 1979.
61. Frank L., Bucher J.R., Roberts R.J.: Oxygen toxicity in neonatal and adult animals of various species. *J. Appl. Physiol.* 45:699, 1978.
62. Hyers T.H.: Pathogenesis of adult respiratory distress syndrome: Current concepts. *Semin. Respir. Med.* 11:104, 1981.
63. Witschi H.R., Haschek W.M., Klein-Szanto A.J., et al.: Potentiation of diffuse lung damage by oxygen: Determining variables. *Am. Rev. Respir. Dis.* 123:98, 1981.
64. Hackney J.D., Evans M.J., Spier C.E., et al.: Effect of high concentrations of oxygen on reparative regeneration of damaged alveolar epithelium in mice. *Exp. Mol. Pathol.* 34:338, 1981.
65. Matalon S., Egan E.A.: Effects of 100% O_2 breathing on permeability of alveolar epithelium to solute. *J. Appl. Physiol.* 50(4):859, 1981.
66. McCord J.M., Fridovich I.: The biology and pathology of oxygen radicals. *Ann. Intern. Med.* 89:122, 1978.
67. Winter P., et al.: The toxicity of oxygen. *Anesthesiology* 37:210, 1972.
68. Suttorp N., Simon L.M.: Lung cell oxidant injury: Enhancement of polymorphonuclear leukocyte-mediated cytotoxicity in lung cells exposed in sustained in vitro hyperoxia. *J. Clin. Invest.* 70:342, 1982.
69. Shasby D.M., Van Benthuysen K.M., Tate R.M., et al.: Granulocytes mediate acute edematous lung injury in rabbits and isolated rabbit lungs perfused with phorbol myristate acetate: Role of oxygen radicals. *Am. Rev. Respir. Dis.* 125:443, 1982.
70. Johnson K.H., Fantone J.C., Kaplan J., et al.: In vivo damage of rat lungs by oxygen metabolites. *J. Clin. Invest.* 67:983, 1981.
71. Tate R.M., Van Benthuysen K.M., Shasby D.M., et al.: Oxygen radical-mediated permeability edema and vasoconstriction in isolated perfused rabbit lungs. *Am. Rev. Respir. Dis.* 126:802, 1982.
72. Kacmarek R.M., Dimas S., Reynold J., et al.: Technical aspects of positive and expiratory pressure: Parts I–III. *Respir. Care* 27:1478, 1982.
73. Weenig C.S., Pietak S., Hickey R.F., et al.: Relationship of preoperative closing volume to FRC and alveolar-arterial oxygen difference during anesthesia with controlled ventilation. *Anesthesiology* 41:3–7, 1974.
74. Hedenstierna G., Santesson J., Norlander O.: Airway closure and distribution of inspired gas in the extremely obese, breathing spontaneously and during anesthesia with intermittent positive pressure ventilation. *Acta Anaesthesiol. Scand.* 20:334–342, 1976.
75. McCarthy G.S., Hedenstierna G.: Arterial oxygenation during artificial ventilation: The effect of airway closure and its prevention by positive end expiratory pressure. *Acta Anaesthesiol. Scand.* 22:563–569, 1978.
76. Wyche M.D., Teichner R.L., Kallos T., et al.: Effects of continuous positive-pressure breathing on functional residual capacity and arterial oxygenation during intra-abdominal operations. *Anesthesiology* 38:68–74, 1973.
77. Demling R.H., Staub N.C., Edmonds L.H.: Effect of end expiratory airway pressure on accumulation of extra-vascular lung water. *J. Appl. Physiol.* 38:907–912, 1975.
78. Caldini P., Leith J.D., Brennan M.J.: Effect of continuous positive pressure ventilation (CPPV) on edema formation in dog lung. *J. Appl. Physiol.* 39:672–679, 1975.
79. Daly B.D.T., Edmonds C.H., Norman J.C.: In vivo alveolar morphometrics with positive end expiratory pressure. *Surg. Forum* 24:217–219, 1973.
80. McIntyre R.W., Laws A.K., Ramachandran P.R.: Positive expiratory pressure plateau: Improved gas exchange during mechanical ventilation. *Can. Anaesth. Soc. J.* 16:477–486, 1969.
81. Rose D.M., Downs J.B., Heenan T.J.: Temporal responses of functional residual capacity and oxygen tension to changes in positive end-expiratory pressure. *Crit. Care Med.* 9:79–82, 1981.
82. Qvist J., Pontoppidan H., Wilson R.S.: Hemodynamic responses to mechanical ventilation with PEEP. *Anesthesiology* 42:45–55, 1975.

83. Perschau R.A., Pepine C.J., Nichols W.N., et al.: Instantaneous blood flow responses to positive end-expiratory pressure with spontaneous ventilation. *Circulation* 59:1312–1318, 1979.
84. Haynes J.B., Carson S.D., Whitney W.P., et al.: Positive end-expiratory pressure shifts left ventricular diastolic pressure area curves. *J. Appl. Physiol.* 48:670–676, 1980.
85. Jardin F., Farcot J., Boisante L., et al.: Influence of positive end-expiratory pressure left ventricular performance. *N. Engl. J. Med.* 304:387–392, 1981.
86. Liebman P.R., Patten M.T., Manny J., et al.: The mechanism of depressed cardiac output on positive end expiratory pressure (PEEP). *Surgery* 83:594–598, 1978.
87. Gallagher T.J., Civetta J.M.: Goal-directed therapy of acute respiratory failure. *Anesth. Analg.* 59:831–834, 1980.
88. Downs J.B., Klein E.F., Modell J.H., et al.: The effect of incremental PEEP on Pa_{O_2} in patients with respiratory failure. *Anesth. Analg. Curr. Res.* 52:210–215, 1974.
89. Falke K.J.: Do changes in lung compliance allow the determination of "optimal PEEP"? *Anaesthesist* 29:165–168, 1980.
90. Kirby R.R., Downs J.B., Civetta J.M., et al.: High level positive end-expiratory pressure (PEEP) in acute respiratory insufficiency. *Chest* 67:156–163, 1975.
91. Suter P.M., Fairley H.M., Isenberg M.D.: Optimum end-expiratory airway pressure in patients with acute pulmonary failure. *N. Engl. J. Med.* 292:284–289, 1975.
92. Venus B., Jacobs H.K., Lim L.: Treatment of the adult respiratory distress syndrome with continuous positive airway pressure. *Chest* 76:257–261, 1979.
93. Zarins C.K., Bayne C.G., Rice C.L., et al.: Does spontaneous ventilation with IMV protect from PEEP induced cardiac output depression? *J. Surg. Res.* 22:299–304, 1977.
94. Dueck R., Wagner P.D., West J.B.: Effects of positive end-expiratory pressure on gas exchange in dogs with normal and edematous lungs. *Anesthesiology* 47:359–366, 1977.
95. Hammon J.W., Wolfe W.G., Moran J.F., et al.: The effect of positive end expiratory pressure on regional ventilation and perfusion in the normal and injured primate lung. *J. Thorac. Cardiovasc. Surg.* 72:680–689, 1976.
96. Downs J.B., Douglas M.E., Sanfelippo P.M., et al.: Ventilatory pattern, intrapleural pressure and cardiac output. *Anesth. Analg. Curr. Res.* 56:88–94, 1977.
97. Venus B., Jacobs K.H., Mathru M.: Hemodynamic responses to different modes of mechanical ventilation in dogs with normal and acid aspirated lungs. *Crit. Care Med.* 8:620–627, 1980.
98. Shah D.M., Newell J.C., Dutton R.E., et al.: Continuous positive airway pressure versus positive end-expiratory pressure in respiratory distress syndrome. *J. Thorac. Cardiovasc. Surg.* 74:557–562, 1977.
99. Schmidt G.B., O'Neill W.W., Kotb E., et al.: Continuous positive airway pressure in the prophylaxis of the adult respiratory distress syndrome. *Surg. Gynecol. Obstet.* 143:613–618, 1976.
100. Weigelt J.A., Mitchell R.A., Snyder W.H. III: Early positive end-expiratory pressure in the adult respiratory distress syndrome. *Arch. Surg.* 114:497–501, 1979.
101. McAslan, T.C., Cowley R.A.: The preventive use of PEEP in major trauma. *Am. Surgeon* 45:159–167, 1979.

13 / Management of Infection in the Compromised Host

JOHN P. PHAIR, M.D.

INFECTION is a major cause of morbidity and mortality in patients with defects in the immune or inflammatory system.[1] Compromised ability to produce antibody, deficiencies in the lymphocyte-macrophage system of cell-mediated resistance, defects in the complement cascade, or an inadequate number or dysfunction of polymorphonuclear leukocytes (PMNLs) can lead to invasion by a wide variety of microorganisms. Such defects in host defense against infection can be the result of congenital deficiencies, acquired disease, or therapy. Management of infection in the compromised host requires aggressive attempts to establish an etiology and prompt, effective, therapeutic intervention.

PATHOGENESIS OF INFECTION AND PRINCIPLES OF MANAGEMENT IN THE COMPROMISED HOST

There are several principles relevant to a rational approach to the management of infection in compromised patients. First, specific infectious agents are associated with specific defects in host defenses (Table 13–1). The absence of antibody is associated with infection due to the pyogenic encapsulated microorganisms such as *pneumoniae, Neiserria meningitidis,* and *Hemophilus influenzae.*[2] The capsule of these organisms represents a virulence factor which enables the bacteria to resist phagocytosis in the absence of opsonins (antibody and/complement). Examples include dysgammaglobulinemia, multiple myeloma, and chronic lymphocyte leukemia. A deficiency in cell mediated immunity is associated with infection due to intracellular pathogens.[3] The classic association is tuberculosis or cryptococcal meningitis with Hodgkin's disease.

The central and complex role of the complement system in the inflammatory response has been recently reviewed.[4] The complement system is composed of 14 proteins, or complement components, which circulate as inactive precursors in serum, and several biologically active and inactive

TABLE 13–1.—SOME HOST DEFECTS, DISEASE STATES, AND MICROORGANISMS

DEFECT	DISEASE	MICROORGANISMS
Absent or low antibody concentration	Multiple myeloma Chronic lymphocytic leukemia X-linked hypogammaglobulinemia Common variable hypogammaglobulinemia	S. pneumoniae H. influenzae N. meningitidis
Complement deficiency		
C3	Congenital absence	S. aureus
C5–9	Congenital absence	N. gonorrhoeae
Deficient or defective polymorphonuclear leukocytes	Cirrhosis (chemotactic factor inactivator) Chronic granulomatous disease (killing) Neutropenia (absence) Diabetes (chemotaxis) Corticosteroid therapy (adherence)	Aerobic gram-negative bacilli S. aureus Fungi Aerobic gram-negative bacilli
Deficient cell-mediated immunity	Hodgkin's disease Corticosteroid therapy Acquired immunodeficiency syndrome Sarcoidosis Protein-calorie malnutrition Postoperative state	Fungi Mycobacterium Herpes virus Simplex Zoster Cytomegalovirus

factors which are released following activation of the sequence. A major aspect of defense against infection provided by this humoral system is facilitation of phagocytosis of microorganisms. Opsonization or coating of bacteria aids the ingestion of the organisms by phagocytic cells and occurs after fixation of the first protein in the complement sequence, C1q, by antibody. The interaction of C1q with antibody follows the combination of antibody with antigen, in this case the surface of the invading microorganisms. The fixation of C1 activates the classical complement pathway and results in deposition of the third component of the cascade, C3, on the cell wall of the microorganisms. Phagocytic cells have receptors for C3 which facilitate attachment of the cell to the microorganism, thus initiating the process of engulfment. Some bacteria and fungi react directly with C3, bypassing the requirement for specific antibody. Activation of the terminal components of complement (C5 through C9) by this mechanism requires components of the alternative or properdin pathway. In addition to facilitating phagocytosis, byproducts of activated C3 and C5 attract PMNLs to areas of inflammation. Finally, the terminal components of this cascade, when activated and deposited on bacterial surfaces, are able to lyse susceptible organisms. Congenital absence of C1q results in multiple infections, as does a deficiency of C3. Kindreds which lack C2 have a high incidence of collagen vascular disease, and individuals who lack terminal complement components have recurrent meningococcemia and gonococcemia.

A defect in function or inadequate numbers of PMNLs results in an increased susceptibility to infection due to staphylococci, including both S. *aureus* and S. *epidermidis*, aerobic gram-negative bacilli, and fungi.[5] Such infections are common in the prototypic example of PMNL dysfunction, chronic granulomatous disease, a congenital defect in cellular oxidative metabolism that results in a failure of intracellular killing of catalase-negative microorganisms.[6] However, the most common infectious problem associated with PMNL abnormalities is sepsis occurring in neutropenic patients.

The second principle requiring emphasis is the need for early, accurate diagnosis to facilitate the management of infection in compromised patients. There is solid evidence that in this group of patients, early appropriate therapy results in an improved prognosis. The survival of bacteremic patients who receive two effective bactericidal antibiotics approaches 70%. If the organisms are susceptible to only one agent or if no effective antibiotic is given, survival decreases.[5] Similarly, survival of patients developing invasive pulmonary aspergillosis is totally dependent on early diagnosis and initiation of antifungal chemotherapy.[7]

A third point which must be borne in mind is that institution of therapy in specific situations must often be empirical. Waiting for results of culture and susceptibility testing before initiating antibiotics in febrile neutropenic patients results in an unacceptable mortality.[5] In patients with defects in cell-mediated immunity, prompt therapy is also necessary, but there is not the same urgency as in the neutropenic individual.

Finally, following initiation of therapy, close observation of the patient must continue. The response to therapy, the search for superinfection, and need for alternative treatment must be reevaluated daily. Superinfection represents a major problem due to persistence of the underlying host defect and the alteration in normal flora resulting from the use of antibiotics. In addition, "new" infections can arise during the initial treatment regimen. Examples include development of *Pneumocystis carinii* pneumonia, disseminated herpes zoster, or tuberculosis. Presumably these infections represent reactivation of previously dormant organisms, a common sequela of corticosteroid or other immunosuppressive therapy, the stress of infection, or the basic disease state.

CASE STUDY 1

A 45-year-old man presented with fatigue and 5-pound weight loss over several weeks. He had noted minimal bleeding when brushing his teeth and some increase in bruising. Physical examination revealed pale mucous membranes and conjunctivae; there was no lymphadenopathy, splenomegaly, or hepatomegaly. A complete blood cell count was remarkable for a hemoglobin value of 8 gm/dl and a total white blood cell (WBC) count of 1,500/mm^{-3}. The differential WBC count revealed 30% segmented neutrophils and blast forms; a paucity of platelets was noted on smear. The patient was admitted to the hospital, and bone marrow aspiration and biopsy confirmed the diagnosis of acute nonlymphocytic leukemia. Combination induction therapy consisting of Adriamycin, cyclophosphamide, 6-thioguanine, and cytosine arabinoside was begun. There was a progressive fall in the total WBC count over the next 8 days. On the tenth day of hospitalization, the total WBC count was 100/mm^3 and no segmented neutrophils were seen. The platelet count was 7,000/mm^3 and bleeding at sites of intravenous (IV)

lines was apparent. Platelet transfusions were administered. During the hospitalization, the patient gargled twice a day with Mycostatin, which was administered to prevent oropharyngeal fungal infection. On the 12th day, the patient's temperature rose to 103.7° F; no localizing symptoms were noted. Physical examination revealed no source of the fever. A chest radiograph was unchanged from admission; no infiltrates were noted. Blood and urine were obtained for culture. The patient was unable to produce sputum. Ticarcillin and amikacin were initiated as empirical antibiotic therapy.

Discussion

The appropriate decision was made to begin antibiotic therapy with a β-lactam antibiotic and an aminoglycoside. Fever in a profoundly neutropenic patient, even in the absence of localizing signs or symptoms, must be treated as infection, even if blood products have been recently administered. The choice of antibiotics should be dictated by the flora isolated in the unit where the patient is hospitalized. Oncology services should be monitored to determine the etiology of recent bacterial infections. Some units routinely obtain specimens of stool and skin and from the anterior nares and pharynx for culture to determine the microorganisms colonizing patients. The organisms most frequently cited as causing bacteremia in neutropenic patients include *Pseudomonas aeruginosa*, *Klebsiella pneumoniae*, *Escherichia coli*, and *Staphyloccus aureus*.[5]

Various combinations of antibiotics have been used in empirical therapy of the febrile neutropenic patient. In the past several years, it has become clear that an aminoglycoside alone does not provide adequate therapy. However, a combination of an aminoglycoside with a β-lactam antibiotic improves patient survival.[5] The currently available aminoglycosides are, in order of introduction of clinical practice, gentamicin, tobramycin, and amikacin. Gentamicin, which has been in clinical use since 1969, is familiar to physicians and has a wide spectrum of activity against the majority of aerobic gram-negative bacilli, including *P. aeruginosa* and staphylococci. The disadvantages of gentamicin include development of significant resistance, especially among *Pseudomonas sp.*, in specific centers.[8] In addition, ototoxicity and nephrotoxicity occur with prolonged use of this agent or when the dose administered is too high for a given patient's renal status. Tobramycin, the second broad-spectrum aminoglycoside introduced into practice, is approximately twice as effective as gentamicin against *P. aeruginosa* on a weight-for-weight basis but is less effective in the treatment of *Serratia narcescens* infection. Resistance to this agent in certain centers is also high. Well-controlled studies have demonstrated less nephrotoxicity in patients receiving tobramycin than in patients receiving gentamicin. Amikacin, the most recently available aminoglycoside, has the widest spectrum of activity against aerobic gram-negative bacilli. In addition, the pharmacokinetics of this agent differ from those of gentamicin and tobramycin, and there is an increase in the therapeutic to toxic ratio. Thus, serum concentrations achieved with amikacin are usually well above the minimal concentrations required to inhibit growth of aerobic gram-negative bacilli yet are below toxic levels. There are no well-designed studies comparing the nephrotoxicity of amikacin and tobramycin. It is generally thought that amikacin is intermediate in toxicity between gentamicin and tobramycin.[9]

The majority of published studies of treatment of febrile neutropenic patients have combined an aminoglycoside with a third-generation penicillin, such as carbenicillin or ticarcillin. One multicenter study compared carbenicillin/gentamicin with cephalothin/gentamicin and cephalothin/carbenicillin regimens.[10] Overall, there was little difference between these three regimens; *Pseudomonas* infections responded better to the first combination and *Klebsiella* to the second. Interestingly, bacteremia due to *S. aureus* was treated effectively by the combination of carbenicillin and gentamicin.[10] There are no definitive studies comparing the use of the newly available wider spectrum cephalosporins (cefotaxime, moxalactam, cephaperazone) plus aminoglycosides with either the third- or fourth-generation penicillins (piperacillin/mezlocillin/azoloccin) plus aminoglycosides in treatment of febrile neutropenic patients. Also, there is no information that would support the use of the newer β-lactam antibiotics alone in treatment of these patients. Our current practice is to treat febrile neutropenic patients with a broad-spectrum penicillin with activity against *P. aeruginosa* (carbenicillin, ticarcillin, mezlocillin or piperacillin) and an aminoglycoside (Table 13–2).

It should be kept in mind that in the absence of segmented neutrophils, the signs and symptoms that serve to identify the site of infection are often muted.[11] A perirectal abscess or urinary tract infection may be asymptomatic and manifest with none of the classic physical findings. The patient with pneumonia has cough and dyspnea, but sputum production is usually scanty and the sputum rarely contains inflammatory cells. The chest film, which demonstrates fluid exudation into alveoli, reveals infiltrates even in the absence of segmented neutrophils.

After initiating empirical antibiotic therapy, the physician must continue

TABLE 13–2.—ANTIBIOTICS USEFUL IN NEUTROPENIC PATIENTS

AGENTS	SPECTRUM	ADVERSE EFFECTS
β-Lactam antibiotics		
Penicillins		
Carbenicillin	P. aeruginosa	Allergy
Ticarcillin	Enterobacteria	Hypokalemia
Mezlocillin	Streptococci	Inhibition of platelet aggregation
Piperacillin		
Cephalosporins		
First generation (cephalothin)	S. aureus	Allergy
	Enterobacteriaceae	
Second generation (cefamandole)	Streptococci	Inhibition of platelet aggregation
Third generation	Enterobacteriaceae	Prolonged prothrombin time
Moxalactam	Some P. aeruginosa	Superinfection
Cefotaxime	Streptococci	
Cephaperazone		
Sulfonamides		
Trimethoprim-sulfamethoxazole	Enterobacteriaceae	Allergy
	Streptococci	Superinfection
	P. carinii	Marrow suppression
Aminoglycosides		
Gentamicin	Enterobacteriaceae	Nephrotoxicity
Tobramycin	S. aureus	Ototoxicity
Amikacin	P. aeruginosa	
Other		
Vancomycin	S. aureus	Phlebitis
	S. epidermidis	Nephrotoxicity
	Enterococcus	Allergy
	J. K. corynebacteria	
Amphotericin	Candida sp.	Acute fever, chills, nausea, phlebitis,
	Aspergillus sp.	chronic nephrotoxicity, anemia
	Phycomyces	
	Cryptococci	

to reevaluate the clinical situation. If appropriate agents are chosen, the patient usually stabilizes. Ultimately, however, the prognosis depends on the response of the bone marrow. Thus, patients who rapidly develop leukocytosis do better than those whose granulocyte count remains below 500/mm^3.[12]

Case Study Continued: Day 6 of Antibiotic Therapy

The patient, following initiation of antibiotic therapy, remained febrile; his temperature rose daily to 101° F or higher. Blood samples obtained for culture at the onset of fever and during antibiotic treatment were sterile. The number of segmented neutrophils remained under 100/mm^3. Candida stomatopharyngitis, which had been noted 3 days earlier, progressed in spite of continued Mycostatin gargles. The patient complained of difficulty swallowing and sticking of food at the level of the midsternum. A barium swallow confirmed the diagnosis of esophagitis.

A test dose of amphotericin B, 1 mg suspended in 125 ml of 5% dextrose in water, was infused over 2 hours. There was no reaction, and following premedication with acetylsalicylic acid and compazine, 15 mg of the antifungal agent was administered in 250 ml of dextrose and water over 4 hours. The following day 30 mg of amphotericin B was given, followed on day 8 by 50 mg, which was then continued on a daily basis. Serum creatinine and potassium levels were measured every third day to monitor renal toxicity and renal potassium wasting, known complications of amphotericin B therapy. A complete blood cell count was also frequently done, as ane-

mia due to ineffective erythropoiesis also commonly occurs with amphotericin therapy.

After 10 days of antifungal treatment and a total of 17 days of antibiotic therapy, the patient noted less discomfort on swallowing and the pharyngeal exudate had markedly decreased. The number of peripheral segmented neutrophils had increased to 500/mm^3. On the 20th day of antibiotic therapy, the count had risen to 1,100/mm^3. The patient's temperature continued to rise daily to 101° F in association with the infusion of amphotericin. All antibiotics were discontinued and he became afebrile. A repeated bone marrow aspiration demonstrated a complete remission.

Discussion

When a patient remains neutropenic and febrile after 5–7 days of antibiotic therapy, a second critical decision faces the physician. In the patient whose case was presented here, there was good evidence of probable invasive fungal infection, an extremely common infection in neutropenic patients. Involvement of the gastrointestinal tract and later dissemination are the usual course of this infection if unrecognized.[5] Diarrhea, renal insufficiency, and indurated erythematous skin lesions have been associated with disseminated *Candida tropicalis* infection.[13] This organism is more invasive than *C. albicans*, which more commonly colonizes mucous membranes of neutropenic patients. Daily fundoscopic examination should be carried out to look for evidence of *Candida* endophthalmitis, another sign of disseminated infection.

Amphotericin B is the treatment of choice for fungal infection in the neutropenic patient. However, it does produce acute toxic effects, including nausea, vomiting, rigors, and fever. With rapid infusion, ventricular arrhythmias have been reported. Prolonged therapy results in renal insufficiency and ineffective erythropoiesis.[14]

When blood cultures are positive and the bacterial isolate is susceptible to the antibiotics being administered, granulocyte transfusions have been reported to benefit patients with continued evidence of infection.[15] To be useful, the granulocyte transfusions should be given daily. The ultimate prognosis again is dependent on reversal of the marrow aplasia. With negative blood cultures, granulocyte transfusions are reported to be of less benefit.

Reevaluating the patient must include repeated blood cultures and a renewed search for a focus of infection. Careful examination of the rectum, pharynx, sinus, and sites of IV lines, removal of any catheters that have been in place for 3 or more days, culture of catheter tips, and culture of blood drawn through long-line (i.e., Hickman) catheters should be carried out. A long-line catheter should be removed if cultures are positive. Organisms recently implicated as causes of sepsis in this situation include S. epidermidis[16] and Corynebacterium CDC-JK,[17] which in the past were dismissed as contaminants. In some centers, isolation of these organisms is frequent enough to justify the empirical addition of vancomycin to the antibiotic combination already in use. These bacteria are generally resistant to β-lactam antibiotics.

Currently, the safest approach to unexplained fever in the neutropenic patient is to continue the antibiotics rather than discontinue therapy and reevaluate the patient.[18] A more recent study provided evidence to support the addition of amphotericin B to the antibiotic regimen to treat probable fungal infections.[19] If the fever responds, therapy should be continued until the segmented neutrophil count returns to at least 1,000/mm^3.

Alternatively, the patient may develop evidence of a focus of infection such as pneumonia. Some findings can suggest an etiology. For example, colonization of the nose with Aspergillus sp. has preceded development of pulmonary infection due to this organism.[20] Empirical initiation of amphotericin B with the development of signs of pulmonary infection in a patient with positive nasal cultures has been recommended. It is also important to keep in mind that Aspergillus infection of the lung may be associated with pleuritic pain and hemoptysis and may mimic pulmonary infarction.[7]

Commonly, however, pneumonia appears without providing clues to the etiology. Cultures of sputum and blood are often not helpful and aggressive attempts to define the etiology are required. Bronchoscopy with brushing and transbronchial biopsy under coverage of platelet transfusions should be carried out before the patient is extremely hypoxemic. The range of potential etiologies is extremely broad. Total empirical therapy requires the use of many agents with a great potential for toxicity. Thus, an aggressive, diagnostic approach represents the most conservative management.

CASE STUDY 2

A 25-year-old man with hemophilia A was admitted to the neurosurgical service following an episode of head trauma. He presented with obtundation and seizures. Computerized axial tomography revealed a subdural hematoma. During his hospitalization he was begun on carbamazepine, which controlled his convulsions. Ten days after discharge he returned to the emergency room with a severe sore throat and a fever of 102.5° F measured orally. Examination revealed a patient in moderate distress due to difficulty in swallowing. Severe stomatopharyngitis with whitish plaques in the pharynx, on the tongue, and on the buccal mucosa was present. The remainder of the examination was noncontributory; specifically, the lung fields were clear. Laboratory studies revealed a total WBC of 4,300/mm^3 with less than 10% segmented neutrophils. A chest radiograph showed no changes from the film obtained 2 weeks before; there were no infiltrates. The patient was admitted to the hospital. IV ticarcillin and amikacin and Mycostatin mouth gargles were begun. Carbamazepine was discontinued and phenobarbital substituted as anticonvulsant therapy. Within 96 hours, the patient's peripheral smear revealed metamyelocytes and band forms indicating a return of the bone marrow to normal function. The highest daily temperature recorded

was 100° F orally and the patient felt somewhat improved. It was decided to continue antibiotics until the patient's neutrophil count was 1,000/mm^3 or greater. On the seventh hospital day the WBC count and differential were normal; however, the patient's temperature rose to 102° F, and cough and dyspnea had developed. Arterial blood gas analysis revealed a pH of 7.45, a P_{CO_2} of 20 mm Hg, and a P_{O_2} of 50 mm Hg on room air. A chest film revealed bilateral nodular densities. Bronchoscopic brushings were positive for *P. carinii*. Ticarcillin and amikacin were discontinued and IV trimethoprim-sulfamethoxazole was initiated. Over the ensuing 3 weeks there was gradual improvement and the patient was discharged. Following recovery, it was determined that the patient was anergic when skin-tested with *Candida*, histoplasmin, mumps, *Tricophyton* antigens, and purified protein derivative. His absolute lymphocyte count was 1,488/mm^{-3} and the T helper/T suppressor lymphocyte ratio was 0.59 (normal range, 1.0–2.5).

Discussion

This patient illustrates the necessity for aggressive diagnostic efforts in infected patients who are immunocompromised even after initiating empirical broad-spectrum antibiotic therapy. This individual, who received 90,000 units/year of factor VIII for hemophilia, also had acquired immunodeficiency syndrome (AIDS). This form of immune defect has been reported in previously healthy homosexually active males, patients with hemophilia A, IV drug abusers, and Haitian emigrants. The cause is unknown.[21] The patient's rehospitalization was initially due to infection (stomatopharyngitis) secondary to neutropenia which was the result of the anticonvulsant therapy. With recovery of the bone marrow and appropriate antibiotic treatment, his temperature responded. However, during the hospitalization he developed infection with *Pneumocystis carinii*. The fact that this patient had hemophilia A in conjunction with the changes seen on a chest radiograph alerted his physicians to the possibility of an opportunistic infection. The appropriate test, bronchoscopy, was immediately carried out. Trimethoprim-sulfamethoxazole was instituted and resulted in recovery.

The pathogenesis of AIDS lies in an altered cell-mediated immune regulation.[21] Infections due to facultative intracellular pathogens and malignant disease, primarily Kaposi's sarcoma, have been reported in these patients. Common sites of infection include the lungs, meninges, and gastrointestinal tract. In addition to *P. carinii*, common pathogens include *Nocardia*, cytomegalovirus, herpes simplex, mycobacteria (especially of the *avian-intracellulare* group), and fungi, particularly *Candida* sp. and *Cryptococcus neoformans*. This pattern of infection is similar to that seen in patients with Hodgkin's disease, lymphoma, or patients receiving corticosteroids.[31] It should be noted that pneumonia due to *Legionella pneumophila* and related organisms also occurs with increased frequency in patients receiving corticosteroids or with defective cell-mediated immunity. It is of interest that *L. pneumophila* is killed intracellularly by activated mononuclear phagocytes (macrophages and histiocytes), not by segmented neutrophils.[22]

It is not uncommon to be faced with a septic patient with multiple causes of increased susceptibility to infection who has pneumonia.[23] In such circumstances, although the chest radiograph can be suggestive, a definitive diagnosis can only be made following identification of a specific pathogen in bronchial washings, brushings, or tissue. It is especially useful to demonstrate tissue invasion histologically. The bronchoscopist in collaboration with the infectious disease consultant should decide which cultures are most appropriate for a specific patient. The number of specimens should be dictated by the differential diagnosis. If available, the shielded brush is essential to prevent contamination by the aerobic and anaerobic flora of the oropharynx. The shielded brush, which is disposable, can be clipped with sterile wire cutters and placed in appropriate media for culture. This technique usually provides a large specimen for staining and inoculation of appropriate cultures. Quantitative cultures can help interpretation when there is a high suspicion that flora usually resident in the oropharynx may be the cause of pulmonary infection. Topical anesthesia should be administered via inhalation, not through the bronchoscope, to avoid contamination of the area to be sampled. Appropriate smears and cultures should be secured by alerting the diagnostic microbiology laboratory that the procedure is imminent. Table 13–3 outlines the appropriate handling of specimens obtained by bronchoscopic brushing. If definitive results are not immediately available, empirical therapy with IV trimethoprim-sulfamethoxazole and erythromycin should be started. Once the pathogen has been identified, therapy can be altered in 24 hours.

Very hypoxemic patients who do not respond to oxygen therapy require open lung biopsy because of the drop in Po_2 which occurs during bronchoscopy and the associated risk of cardiac arrhythmias.[24, 25] An empirical

TABLE 13–3.—MICROBIOLOGY PROCESSING OF BRONCHOSCOPY SPECIMENS OBTAINED FROM IMMUNOCOMPROMISED HOSTS

MICROORGANISM	SPECIMEN	PROCEDURE	HANDLING
Anaerobic bacteria	1 brush in triple-lumen sheathed catheter	Anaerobic culture	Place brush in anaerobic pre-reduced broth with glass beads; vortex & culture on anaerobic media
Pneumocystis, yeasts	1 brush in triple-lumen sheathed catheter	Toluidine blue O, PAS silver methenamine stain	Place brush in 0.5 ml of sterile saline, vortex; use cell suspension for smears
Legionella	1 brush in triple-lumen sheathed catheter	Legionella culture and fluorescent stain	Place brush in 1.0 ml of sterile H_2O, vortex; use cell suspension for smears, culture
Routine aerobic bacteria & fungi	1 brush in triple-lumen sheathed catheter	Routine aerobic and fungal culture & gram stain	Place brush in 1.0 ml of sterile saline, vortex; use cell suspension for culture & smears
Virus	1 brush in triple-lumen sheathed catheter	Virus culture	Place brush in viral media, transport *promptly* to virology lab for tissue culture inoculation; if laboratory is closed, store in transport medium at 70° C
	1 brush nondisposable	Fluorescent stains for virus identification	Make 6 smears of brushed bronchial cells at bedside for fluorescent stains; air dry and bring to virology lab with culture specimen
Mycobacteria	1 brush or < 5 ml of bronchial washings	Mycobacterial smear and culture	Place brush in 1.0 ml of tween albumin broth, vortex; use cell suspension for smear & culture; *or*, process bronchial washings according to standard lab protocol

trial of antimicrobial therapy results in delay, often with further worsening of the clinical situation, greater operative risk, and more confusion. Furthermore, the use of empirical therapy alone without a diagnosis can be hazardous. For example, trimethoprim-sulfamethoxazole has many adverse effects,[26] amphotericin B is nephrotoxic,[14] and erythromycin, isoniazid, and rifampin are hepatotoxic. Finally, in complicated cases, other entities can mimic pulmonary infection. Pulmonary pathology resembling infection can be due to earlier radiation, bleomycin therapy, hemorrhage, embolus, or progression of neoplastic disease.[27] Intelligent management of these critically ill patients requires knowledge of the cause of immunosuppression, careful evaluation of therapy to date and of the clinical situation, and appropriate use of invasive techniques.

REFERENCES

1. Allen J.C.: *Infection and Compromised Host*. Baltimore, Williams & Wilkins Co., 1976.
2. Hermans P.E., Diaz-Buxo J.P., Stobo J.D.: Idiopathic late-onset immunoglobulin deficiency: Clinical observations in 50 patients. *Am. J. Med.* 61:221, 1976.
3. Sharma S., Remington J.S.: The role of cell-mediated immunity in resistance to infection in the immunocompromised host, in Verhoef J., Peterson P.K., Quie P.K. (eds.): *Infection in the Immunocompromised Host: Pathogenesis, Prevention and Therapy*. Amsterdam, Elsevier/North Holland Biomedical Press, 1980, pp. 59-76.
4. Frank M.M.: The complement system in host defense and inflammation. *Rev. Infect. Dis.* 1:483, 1979.
5. Schmimpff S.C.: Therapy of infection in patients with granulocytopenia. *Med. Clin. North Am.* 61:1101, 1977.
6. Mills E.L., Quie P.C.: Congenital disorders of the function of polymorphonuclear neutrophils. *Rev. Infect. Dis.* 3:505, 1980.
7. Herbert P.A., Bayer A.S.: Fungal pneumonia: Invasive pulmonary aspergillosis. *Chest* 80:220, 1981.
8. Kauffman C.A., Ramundo N.C., Williams S.G., et al.: Surveillance of gentamicin-resistant gram-negative bacilli in a general hospital. *Antimicrob. Agents Chemother.* 13:918, 1978.
9. Smith C.R., Lietman P.S.: Comparative clinical trials of aminoglycoside, in Whelton A., Neu H.C. (eds.): *The Aminoglycosides: Microbiology, Clinical Use and Toxicology*. New York, Marcel Dekker, Inc., 1982, pp. 497–510.
10. The E.O.R.T.C. International Antimicrobial Therapy Project Group: Three antibiotic regimens in the treatment of infection in febrile granulocytopenic patients with cancer. *J. Infect. Dis.* 137:14, 1978.
11. Sickles E.A., Greene W.H., Wiernik P.H.: Clinical presentation of infection in granulocytopenic patients. *Arch. Intern. Med.* 135:715, 1975.
12. Bodey G.P., Buckley M., Sathe Y.S., et al.: Quantitative relationships between circulating leukocytes and infection in patients with acute leukemia. *Ann. Intern. Med.* 64:328, 1966.
13. Winegard J.R., Merz W.G., Saral R.: *Candida tropicalis:* A major pathogen in immunocompromised patients. *Ann. Intern. Med.* 91:539, 1979.
14. Bennett J.E.: Chemotherapy of systemic mycoses. *N. Engl. J. Med.* 290:30, 1974.
15. Schiffer C.A.: Principles of granulocyte transfusion therapy. *Med. Clin. North Am.* 61:1119, 1977.
16. Wade J.C., Schimpff S.C., Newman K.A., et al.: *Staphylococcus epidermidis:* An increasing cause of infection in patients with granulocytopenia. *Ann. Intern. Med.* 97:503, 1982.
17. Lipsky B.A., Goldberger A.C., Tompkins L.S., et al.: Infections caused by nondiphtheria corynebacterium. *Rev. Infect. Dis.* 4:1220, 1982.

18. Pizzo P.A., Robichaud K.J., Gill F.A., et al.: Duration of empiric antibiotic therapy in granulocytopenic patients with cancer. *Am. J. Med.* 67:194, 1979.
19. Pizzo P.A., Robichaud K.J., Gill F.A., et al.: Empiric antibiotic and antifungal therapy for cancer patients with prolonged fever and granulocytopenia. *Am. J. Med.* 72:101, 1982.
20. Aisner J., Murello J., Schimpff S.C., et al.: Invasive aspergillosis in acute leukemia: Correlation with nose cultures and antibiotic use. *Ann. Intern. Med.* 90:4, 1979.
21. Fauci A.: The syndrome of Kaposi's sarcoma and opportunistic infection: An epidemiologically restricted disorder of immunoregulation. *Ann. Intern. Med.* 96:777, 1982.
22. Horwitz M.A., Silverstein S.C.: Intracellular multiplication of Legionnaire's disease bacteria *(Legionella pneumophila)* in human monocytes is reversibly inhibited by erythromycin and rifampin. *J. Clin. Invest.* 71:15, 1983.
23. Phair J.P., Reising K.S., Metzger E.: Bacteremic infection and malnutrition in patients with solid tumors: Investigation of host defense mechanism. *Cancer* 45:2702, 1980.
24. Dubrausky C., Awe R.J., Jenkins D.E.: The effect of bronchofiberscopic examination on oxygenation status. *Chest* 2:137, 1975.
25. Katz A.S., Michelson E.L., Stawicki J.: Cardiac arrhythmias: Frequency during fiberoptic bronchoscopy and correlation with hypoxemia. *Arch. Intern. Med.* 141:603, 1981.
26. Lawson D.H., Pauce B.J.: Adverse reactions to trimethoprim-sulfamethoxazole. *Rev. Infect. Dis.* 4:429, 1982.
27. Penning J.E.: Dilemma: Pneumonia in the immunocompromised patient. *J. Respir. Dis.* 3:25, 1982.

14 / Upper Gastrointestinal Tract Bleeding and Liver Failure

Donald M. Sinclair, M.D.

Bleeding from the upper gastrointestinal (GI) tract may be the primary reason for admission to an intensive care unit for some patients and frequently complicates the course of critically ill patients with non-GI tract pathology. There are three common causes of massive upper GI tract bleeding that account for 90%–95% of cases in which a definitive lesion can be identified. These are described below.

1. Peptic ulceration.—Peptic ulcer is probably the most common cause of upper GI tract bleeding. The majority of these ulcers are situated in the duodenum. Twenty to thirty percent of patients with peptic ulcer have had at least one prior episode of significant GI bleeding. When a patient with known peptic ulcer has GI hemorrhage, the ulcer is the most probable site of bleeding.

2. Erosive gastritis.—Gastritis may be associated with recent heavy alcohol ingestion or a history of ingestion of salicylates or other drugs. Similarly, gastric erosions and ulcerations may occur in "stressful" situations and are not infrequently found in patients with intracranial disease, burns, or recent trauma.

3. Variceal bleeding associated with portal hypertension.—Variceal hemorrhage usually occurs in conjunction with alcoholic cirrhosis but may occur in other forms of cirrhosis associated with portal hypertension, especially postnecrotic cirrhosis. Portal vein thrombosis may also lead to variceal hemorrhage in the absence of cirrhosis. Bleeding from varices tends to be abrupt and often massive. Minor bleeding from esophageal varices may occur for days before it is discovered. Upper GI tract bleeding in a patient with cirrhosis suggests a variceal source, but because patients with cirrhosis have a higher incidence of peptic ulceration, bleeding from the latter must be excluded. Furthermore, in the alcoholic patient with cirrhosis who has continued to drink prior to the onset of bleeding, bleeding from gastritis is not uncommon.

Differentiation of the cause of GI tract bleeding depends on a meticulous history and physical examination in conjunction with specific radiologic and endoscopic investigations.

As cardiopulmonary instability may result from blood loss of more than 1,000 ml, diagnostic steps may have to be taken concurrently with resuscitation or even temporarily delayed until the patient's condition has been stabilized.

Complete evaluation of the patient presenting with GI tract bleeding is extremely important, since a variety of systemic diseases may be associated with hemorrhage. A bleeding diathesis must always be ruled out. Investigation of hepatic function should be included, as cirrhosis of the liver is frequently associated with bleeding esophageal varices, gastric erosions, or peptic ulceration.

Less common causes of GI tract bleeding include esophagitis, esophageal carcinoma, peptic ulceration of the esophagus, lacerations of the mucosa of the distal end of the esophagus associated with severe vomiting, carcinoma of the stomach, mesenteric venous or arterial occlusion by embolism or thrombosis, aortic aneurysms, and primary blood dyscrasias, including leukemia, thrombocytopenic states, disseminated intravascular, coagulation, and the hemophilias.

Diagnosis

First, establish that the massive blood loss is indeed upper abdominal in origin. The majority of patients present with hematemesis, vomiting fresh blood. Rarely, the blood may have been swallowed from the nasopharynx and then returned as hematemesis. In other patients the blood may remain hidden from view in the GI tract or may be present rectally (hematochezia). In the occult presentation of a GI tract bleed, other causes of internal bleeding, such as a leaking abdominal aneurysm, colonic bleeding, and so forth, need to be excluded.

A history of peptic ulcer, or chronic epigastric pain, alerts one to the likelihood of an erosive bleed. A history of hepatitis, cirrhosis, jaundice, or chronic alcoholism may suggest varices, and confirmatory signs of portal hypertension (collateral vascular anastamoses via caput medusa or hemorrhoids, splenomegaly) and the effects of hypersplenism (e.g., anemia, thrombocytopenia, leukopenia) must be sought. A history of the recent ingestion of large quantities of alcohol or erosive drugs (commonly aspirin or indomethacin) may suggest erosive gastritis.

Examination, apart from looking for the signs of portal hypertension just mentioned, should include a search for the signs of liver failure: jaundice, ascites, spider nevi, and neurologic abnormalities. Abdominal palpation and thoracic percussion for liver size and consistency, splenomegaly, and epigastric tenderness or guarding are important.

Endoscopy is the primary diagnostic step in a patient with upper GI tract bleeding. If massive active bleeding is occurring endoscopy may be worthless; in any case, it must not interfere with resuscitative measures. Eiseman and Norton[1] point out that the introduction of routine endoscopy has led to more definitive diagnoses being made and most particularly to a fall in the incidence of diagnosis of esophageal varices in cirrhotics. These patients are most often found to have gastric erosions. Massive active bleeding may obscure the endoscopist's view, but in most cases a diagnosis can be established. Cautery may even be applied to the bleeding point via the endoscope if the bleeding is localized.

Radiologic examination includes contrast studies of the lumen of the GI tract and angiography.

Contrast studies such as a barium swallow may identify esophageal varices. Peptic ulceration may be shown by introduction of barium into the stomach; however, blood clots in the gastric lumen or ulcer bed will frequently negate any positive findings. Barium studies are best performed 12 hours after the bleeding has been controlled.

If bleeding persists, and gastroesophagoscopy and barium studies have not revealed the site of bleeding, the patient should be considered for emergency selective angiography. Angiography may demonstrate the site of active bleeding[2] and, if variceal hemorrhage is suspected, may confirm the presence of varices as well as portal hypertension. Occasionally one may be able to observe the leaking of contrast material from esophageal vessels. Angiography is also valuable in providing information on the patency of the portal, splenic, and left renal veins should surgical decompression of the portal system be contemplated.

Selective visceral angiography is indicated before barium examination when the history, physical examination, and endoscopy provide no clue to the source of bleeding.

If bleeding continues and gastric aspiration fails to reveal fresh bleeding into the stomach, blood loss may be occurring from a lesion beyond the pylorus. Selective celiac axis and mesenteric artery angiography may be useful to localize the cryptogenic bleeding site. However, extravasation of contrast material into the intestinal lumen can be shown only when bleeding is active and at a rate estimated to be greater than 0.5 ml/minute. Arteriography is helpful to reveal the site of bleeding; however, the cause of bleeding often cannot be determined unless an aneurysm, varix, or vascular malformation is present.

Additional laboratory investigations are sometimes helpful and should include determination of the hematocrit, hemoglobin, white blood cell count with differential, platelet count, prothrombin time, and coagulation studies. Although the initial studies are valuable and essential, repeated measurement and evaluation of the laboratory data are important as the clinical course of the bleeding evolves.

MANAGEMENT

Peptic Ulceration

Initial treatment following acute resuscitation involves placement of a nasogastric tube and gastric lavage with iced saline or milk. If bleeding persists despite gastric lavage, angiography is indicated, not only for diagnostic purposes but to enable specific therapy.

When a diagnosis of peptic ulcer has been made, either medical or surgical treatment is advised. A history of previous bleeding or failed medical treatment are relative indications for surgical management. Arterial embolization, freezing of the gastric mucosa, laser surgery, and intragastric, intra-arterial, or intraperitoneal vasoconstrictors may all be considered in patients with peptic ulcer.[3] Arterial embolization is associated with embolization to the lungs, which may produce strange new shadows on chest x-ray films.[4] Finally, the possibility of surgical intervention must be considered.

Erosive Gastritis

Cold lavage is the primary therapeutic step for patients with gastric erosions. If bleeding continues to be worrisome, angiography and vasopressin administration are indicated. As the erosion is seldom limited to a particular area of the stomach, partial surgical resection is unlikely to be useful. The use of cimetidine or other H_2-receptor antagonists prophylactically (e.g., in patients at a high risk of stress ulceration such as those with shock, burns, following major surgery, with major sepsis, following erosive drug ingestion, on steroids) or in all hyperacidic states should also be borne in mind. In the prevention of stress ulcers the dose is 300 mg intravenously (IV) qid. In hyperacidic states this therapy should be continued for 6 weeks orally. Cimetidine may interfere with the metabolism of other drugs, especially in the elderly and the acutely ill, and it does reduce liver blood flow. Use of intragastric antacids is a more old-fashioned but satisfactory mode of treatment. A combination of antacids and H_2-receptor blocker may give more protection than either therapy alone. Propranolol is also effective,[5] especially in cirrhotics.

Variceal Bleeding

If bleeding is active at the time of diagnosis it should be stopped if possible by direct pressure applied to the bleeding area by a Sengstaken-Blakemore tube. The triple-lumen tube is comprised of a relatively large-bore gastric tube with two inflatable balloons. The more distal balloon is round and should be situated in the stomach. The proximal balloon is sausage-shaped and should lie in the esophagus. With the gastric balloon inflated with 100–150 cc of air, traction is applied to pull it back into the gastroesophageal junction. It is taped into this position and the esophageal balloon is inflated to 33 mm Hg pressure to tamponade the bleeding vessel. Tamponade should be maintained for 48 hours (Fig 14–1).

Selective angiography of the left gastric and superior mesenteric arteries should be undertaken to enable infusion of a vasoconstrictor when balloon tamponade fails to control the bleeding. Vasopressin administered by continuous arterial infusion is effective in stopping the bleeding. The IV administration of a vasoconstrictor, particularly in a shocked patient, is to be condemned. The catheter is positioned in the desired artery under radio-

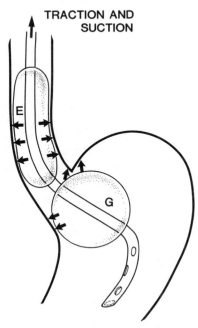

TRACTION AND SUCTION

E

G

Fig 14–1.—*Diagram showing placement of Sengstaken-Blakemore tube.* E = *esophageal balloon,* G = *gastric balloon pulled into gastroesophageal junction.*

logic control and an infusion of 0.1–0.4 units of vasopressin per minute is given by continuous infusion pump and continued for 2–3 days, with slow decrements in rate over this time.

COMPLICATIONS OF GI TRACT BLEEDING

Several complications may develop in patients with massive upper GI tract bleeding. Hypovolemic shock is common. These patients frequently require large volumes of blood and fluids for resuscitation, and hence may show the adverse effects of massive blood transfusion. Underlying liver disease is common in patients who present with major upper GI tract bleeding. The presence of large quantities of blood in the GI tract results in an acute increase in metabolic load on the liver and may precipitate hepatocellular failure in the patient with preexisting compromised liver function.

Hepatic Blood Flow

The liver has an abundant blood supply, receiving more than a fourth of the resting cardiac output, 1 L via the portal system and 400 cc via the hepatic artery per minute. The resistance in the liver to this large blood flow is low, with normally only an 8 mm Hg pressure difference between the portal vein (8 mm) and the hepatic vein (0 mm). Significant loss of sinusoid capacity must occur before there is a measurable rise in resistance to flow which manifests as a rise in portal vein pressure (portal hypertension). Once the portal vein pressure does start to rise there will be an associated marked increase in hepatic lymph production.

Liver Function

The functions of the liver can be conveniently considered in two categories: metabolic and conversion functions.

METABOLIC FUNCTIONS.—The liver is the central metabolic organ, playing an integral role in protein, carbohydrate, and lipid metabolism. Especially important is its role in protein metabolism. It is the largest protein exporter in the body, manufacturing most of the plasma proteins and many of the blood clotting factors. Normal production of albumin is 12 gm/day. This output may be increased to 100 gm/day when albumin losses are severe, as in patients with severe burns or the nephrotic syndrome. The catabolic aspects of protein metabolism involve deamination and transamination. Oxidative deamination of amino acids forms ketoacids and ammonia. Transamination results in the transference of amino groups into ketoacids, which are then able to enter the intermediary pathways of carbohydrate and lipid metabolism. In liver disease, decreased utilization of this process results in decreased amino acid incorporation into the citric acid cycle and aminoacidemia and aminoaciduria.

Ammonia is converted into urea in the liver for excretion in the urine. The detoxification of ammonia involves incorporation of ornithine, citrulline, arginine, and aspartic acid into the urea cycle and is catalyzed by many liver cell enzymes. Hepatocellular damage may result in decreased urea synthesis and elevation of the serum ammonia concentration. If portal hypertension accompanies hepatocellular failure, venous anastomoses between the portal vein and systemic venous channels allow ammonia to escape hepatic detoxification, leading to elevated systemic blood ammonia levels. Excessive nitrogenous material in the intestine (from bleeding or dietary protein) results in excessive amounts of ammonia being formed by bacterial deamination of amino acids. The liver is thought to manufacture certain specific substances essential for cerebral metabolic function.

The ability of the liver to increase the production of albumin ninefold is an example of the liver's large reserve capacity. If one adds to this the amazing regenerative capacity of the liver, it is obvious that by the time the liver exhibits "low output," the vast majority of the hepatocytes must be compromised.

CONVERSION FUNCTION.—The liver metabolizes endogenous and exogenous compounds (e.g., drugs), either converting them into more water-soluble forms which are readily excreted in the urine, making them more active (e.g., cortisone to cortisol), inactivating substances (e.g., estrogens), or, unfortunately, producing toxic metabolites (e.g., conversion of acetaminophen). The best-known hepatic conversion is that of fat-soluble bilirubin (indirect bilirubin), formed from the breakdown of heme molecules derived from the destruction of effete erythrocytes, into more water-soluble (direct) bilirubin. The conversion in this case entails the formation of the glucuronide salt of bilirubin. This is an example of a phase II conversion. Phase II conversion denotes a synthesizing process which creates a new, more water-soluble compound. In contrast, phase I conversions denote degradations, most often by oxidation, but also by desulfuration, dehalogenation, and so forth. Phase I conversions take place in the hepatocytes and involve enzyme systems such as the P-450 system which inactivate many compounds (e.g., barbiturates).

Many of the signs of liver failure are primarily due to disruption of these functions and the consequent changes in serum concentrations of various endogenous and exogenous compounds.

Acute Liver Failure and Encephalopathy

Acute liver failure will develop if more than 60% of hepatocytes are damaged, resulting in inability of the liver to perform its metabolic functions adequately. Failure may manifest as abnormal carbohydrate metabolism (a tendency to hypoglycemia or hyperglycemia), abnormal lipid metabolism (a fall in total serum cholesterol), and, most importantly, abnormal protein metabolism. Decreased protein production may lead to a low serum albumin level with a resultant lowering of plasma colloid osmotic pressure. Decreased production of clotting factors may lead to deranged blood clotting mechanisms. Urea synthesis may be depressed, resulting in a rising blood ammonia level and a low blood urea nitrogen (BUN) level. Elevation of ammonia levels will be augmented because ammonia absorbed from the gut may bypass the liver through collaterals and because hypokalemic metabolic alkalosis is common in patients with liver failure, which shifts the balance between ammonia and ammonium in the direction of ammonia. Ammonia (unionized) enters the brain readily and is also more easily reabsorbed from the urine than ammonium (ionized) (Fig 14–2).[6]

Decreased metabolism of hormones such as estrogens may lead to development of gynecomastia in males and spider nevi. Decreased conjugation of bilirubin may lead to jaundice, while decreased drug metabolism (e.g., of benzodiazepines) may lead to excessive drug effects. A history of the recent use of benzodiazepines is common in association with hepatic coma.

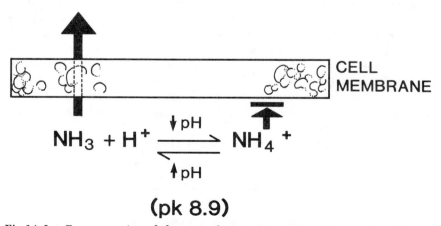

$$NH_3 + H^+ \underset{\uparrow pH}{\overset{\downarrow pH}{\rightleftarrows}} NH_4^+$$

(pk 8.9)

Fig 14–2.—*Representation of change in degree of ionization of ammonia with increases or decreases in pH. Note: NH$_3$ (ammonia) diffuses across cell membrane whereas NH$_4^+$ (ammonium ion) cannot diffuse across cell membrane.*

Acute liver failure therefore will manifest with jaundice, raised serum ammonia concentration and the effects thereof, with the signs of hepatic malfunction (fetor hepaticus, spider nevi, erythematous palms) and with ascites (decreased colloid osmotic pressure, increased portal pressure, increased aldosterone activity with water and sodium retention). These defects will be reflected in the function of other organs such as the brain and kidneys.

Hepatic Encephalopathy

The actual metabolic insult of hepatic encephalopathy is not known, but ammonia accumulation probably plays a role by depressing brain metabolism, leading to a lack of available energy for essential functions. Other protein and amino acid imbalances play important roles yet to be wholly defined. Ammonia levels probably reflect a general trend. While the severity of the encephalopathy usually parallels the rise of ammonia, there are many exceptions in which coma may ensue while the ammonia level is still low. Accumulation of intermediate chain fatty acids may also be important. False neurotransmitters may be manufactured and disrupt synaptic actions.

Whatever the metabolic basis, hepatic encephalopathy may start as a slight mood change, often associated with a flapping tremor (asterixis) and progressing to lethargy and coma. The altered states of consciousness of liver failure must be distinguished from other causes of impaired consciousness. It is possible to find signs of liver failure in patients with other pathologies either unrelated (e.g., cerebrovascular accident, CNS pathology, tumor) or semi-unrelated (e.g., chronic subdural hematoma in an alcoholic who had fallen during a drinking bout and who may or may not have had an associated clotting deficit). These treatable causes of disturbed consciousness must be ruled out. Patients with disturbed liver function are liable to develop hypoglycemia, which may aggravate hepatic coma. A typical EEG pattern of symmetric high-voltage waves, three to five per second, is seen in hepatic coma.

Hepatic coma may be staged for severity (Table 14–1).

TABLE 14–1.—STAGING OF HEPATIC COMA

STAGE	NEUROLOGIC CONDITION
I	Changed emotional state: euphoria or depression
II	Lethargy, confusion
III	Sleeping but rousable; incoherent when awakened
IV	Coma, not rousable

Hepatorenal Failure

Liver failure may be associated with renal failure. This probably occurs via a direct renal mechanism rather than secondary to abnormal aldosterone action. This primary renal mechanism is again due to direct interference with renal cellular metabolism by some of the accumulated products resulting from failure of hepatic metabolic processes. This failure is usually mild; however, more severe failure may be precipitated by the heavy-handed administration of diuretics and by the use of nephrotoxic antibiotics. The kidney, already weakened by toxins from the liver failure, is more sensitive to other nephrotoxins. The rapid loss of fluid and salt by overenthusiastic diuretic therapy or abdominal paracentesis in patients with ascites may further lead to severe fluid and electrolyte changes. GI tract bleeding may also adversely alter fluid, electrolyte, and hemodynamic parameters. A concentrated urine with a low sodium concentration is usually seen. However, if there is associated renal tubular damage, a high urinary sodium concentration may result due to impaired sodium reabsorption. Hepatorenal failure has a very poor prognosis, but the renal failure will reverse if liver function improves.

Treatment of Acute Liver Failure

1. Look for and treat any precipitating cause:
   a. An increased protein load in the form of either a sudden change in diet (e.g., an alcoholic "helped" by taking him off alcohol and put onto nourishing high-protein foods) or GI tract bleeding, which may flood the liver's urea-forming capacity.
   b. Intercurrent infection to which these patients are especially prone (poor nutrition, poor social circumstances, and compromised immune system) may tip the balance, possibly by increased protein catabolism.
   c. Sudden changes in hepatic function in an already borderline patient such as those with hepatitis or any other liver disease may lead to dramatic deterioration.
   d. Changes in renal function may lead to ammonia retention.
   e. A sudden increase in pH may lead to a sudden rise in serum ammonia concentration.
2. Decrease the protein load by stopping and later limiting dietary protein intake.
3. Empty the bowel of blood (enemas).
4. Sterilize the bowel (neomycin, 0.5 gm q6h orally).
5. Give lactulose by mouth or by enema. It is metabolized by colonic

    bacteria to acids and so lowers the bowel pH thereby decreasing ammonia absorption.

6. Watch fluids, electrolytes, and acid-base status very closely and restrict salt and fluid intake when necessary to limit ascites. Cautious diuretic therapy may be undertaken to reduce ascites.

7. Review all drugs that the patient is receiving and consider possible altered metabolism of them with consequent accumulation.

8. Where there is any sign of neurologic malfunction (e.g., Wernicke's encephalopathy) give thiamine parenterally.

9. Abdominal paracentesis is indicated if ascites is embarrassing respiration. Beware of tapping too much too fast, as this may precipitate hemodynamic instability.

10. Give vitamin K, 20 mg/day intramuscularly for 3 days, if prothrombin (PT) time is prolonged.

11. Monitor progress of liver failure with the use of liver function tests.

Liver Function Tests

    A large number of biochemical tests have been designated "liver function tests." Most in fact do not measure liver function directly but measure compounds, usually enzymes, that have leaked out of damaged or dead hepatocytes. Some of the tests measure change "that is more in keeping with ancient alchemy than with present day biochemistry and physiology."[7] For a more comprehensive discussion of liver function tests see work by Podolsky and Issenbacher[6] and Calibes and Schenker.[8]

    Four tests have proved useful in predicting the outcome in hepatic failure: blood glucose, blood ammonia, serum bilirubin, and serum albumin level determination. All these parameters reflect actual metabolic function of the liver and should be measured serially during the disease. To these four basic simple tests, we may add PT time[8] in monitoring hepatic metabolism.

    The serum enzymes (i.e., the enzymes lost from the damaged hepatocytes) are helpful in following the course of acute hepatic disease. When enzyme levels are high the disease is active and cells are severely compromised or dying. As the enzyme levels taper off the disease is entering a more quiescent phase and fewer hepatocytes are at risk. As the liver is "burnt out" and the disease reaches a terminal stage, the enzyme levels may fall while the disease progresses. These enzyme studies say nothing about hepatic function as such. The transaminases are the most frequently followed. Alkaline phosphatase may also be useful but is not of use in children, pregnant women, and patients with coexisting bone disease (Table 14–2).

TABLE 14-2.—LIVER FUNCTION TESTS

TEST	NORMAL VALUE	HEPATOCELLULAR INJURY*	OBSTRUCTION
HEPATOCYTE DAMAGE			
Enzyme leak from damaged hepatocytes			
Transaminases:			
SGOT/AST	< 40 Karmen units	200–3,000 units	200 units
SGPT/ALT	< 40 Karmen units		
Alkaline phosphatase	25–85 IU 1.5–4.5 Bodzansky units 4–13 King-Armstrong units	1–2X normal	2–10X normal (alkaline phosphatase concentration in microvilli of bile canaliculi)
LDH isoenzymes may also be used			
SYNTHETIC FUNCTION			
Serum albumin	3.5–5 gm/dl	3 gm/dl; this means severe loss of function	Normal
Prothrombin time	10–12 sec	> 16 sec after 48 hr vitamin K therapy means severe loss of function	Normal after vitamin K for 48 hr
CONVERSION AND EXCRETORY FUNCTION OF LIVER			
Bilirubin (total)	≤ 1 mg	2–10 mg	10–30 mg
BSP—not used any more			

*For example, viral hepatitis.

TABLE 14–3.—PROGNOSTIC
SCORE FOR LIVER FAILURE

Empirical scoring, 1 point each for:
Bilirubin, 2 mg/dl
Serum albumin < 3 gm/dl
Prothrombin time > 16 sec
Encephalopathy
History of varices

An empirical scoring system for predicting outcome in surgical patients with liver disease using serum levels of bilirubin, albumin and PT time combined with the presence or history of encephalopathy and of varices has been shown to correlate with hospital mortality in surgical patients (Table 14–3).[9]

CASE STUDY

A 46-year-old man was brought to the emergency room in the middle of the night after having vomited a large amount of blood. He was unkempt, smelled strongly of alcohol, was restless but sluggish, and was incoherently responsive to questioning. His clothing and body were filthy and covered with blood and vomitus. The ambulance drivers had collected him from a bar, where he had been drinking. No further history was available.

The patient had a blood pressure (BP) of 90/70 mm Hg, a pulse rate of 110 beats per minute, and relatively cold extremities. His respiratory rate was 32/minute. A peripheral 14-bore IV line was established and then an internal jugular Cordis cannula was introduced for central venous pressure (CVP) monitoring and to permit placing a pulmonary artery catheter later if such were required. Blood was sent to the blood bank for crossmatching and to the laboratory for serum electrolyte determination, CBC count, and coagulation profile. Arterial blood gas analysis revealed a pH of 7.30, a P_{CO_2} of 28 mm Hg, and a P_{O_2} of 65 mm Hg. A rapid infusion of 1½ L of Ringer's lactate brought the blood pressure up to 100/70 mm Hg; the pulse stayed at 110 beats per minute. The CVP had risen from −2 to 0, which suggested that only partial restoration of circulating blood volume had been achieved. The patient was given 4 L of oxygen by nasal cannula. Examination of the cardiovascular and respiratory system revealed no gross abnormalities. The patient had an enlarged nodular liver, splenomegaly, and ascites. Spider nevi were noted on the anterior chest wall. There were dilated veins on the anterior abdominal wall. The hemoglobin concentration was 10.4 gm/dl. Two units of whole blood were given.

Discussion

There is a natural inclination to give such a patient the widest possible berth, but beware. He is a mine of medical dangers and needs close examination, observation, and care. Immediate examination must establish his cardiovascular, CNS, and respiratory status. An alcoholic vomiting up blood is a nightmare and will keep you busy. Obviously your main attention must be on the bleeding, but do not forget the possibility, even the likelihood, of concomitant disease. Heavy alcohol use is frequently associated with other drug abuse and heavy cigarette consumption. Liver failure, infections, hypothermia, malnutrition, alcoholic myocarditis, and chronic obstructive pulmonary disease are all possibilities, quite apart from coronary artery disease and other diseases of the patient's age group. While pursuing the main problem, nurture a healthy awareness and suspicion for these other pitfalls.

In patients with hematemesis, try to establish how much blood has been vomited. All further blood loss in the hospital must be collected and measured. Do not forget that blood may be accumulating in the gut without being obvious on external assessment. If, for example, the patient's waist measurement was 40 inches, his abdominal volume would then be 20 L or more. Loss of 30% of the blood volume into the GI tract (i.e., 1.5–2 L) would increase his waist measurement only to 41½ inches. A reliable rule of thumb is 1 inch per liter. It is easy to miss hidden blood loss of considerable volume unless you search for it diligently. Clinical signs of blood loss are most important. The classic signs of hypovolemic shock are a cold, clammy skin, a fast pulse, and low BP. Alcohol ingestion may interfere with this presentation, leaving the patient more vasodilated and bradycardiac than might be expected.

At least one reliable large-bore IV line should be placed at a very early stage. Two IV routes are preferable, and if bleeding is vigorous, even more may be necessary.

An internal jugular or a subclavian line can be lifesaving. The internal jugular route may further be used for CVP, pulmonary artery pressure, and cardiac output monitoring. An excellent handbook by Rosen et al.[10] gives alternative approaches to all large vessels. The largest possible cannula should be used. To give 1 L of saline via an 18-gauge needle requires 6½ minutes under pressure but only 2½ minutes via a 12-gauge cannula.[11]

The central line must be connected to a manometer or pressure transducer for monitoring CVP, thereby enabling assessment of response to transfusion. If there is any history or clinical indication of preexisting heart disease, a pulmonary artery catheter should be placed to obtain pulmonary artery occluded pressures (PAOP), and thus to monitor both left and right atrial filling pressures. If the patient is severely ill, an arterial line and urine catheter should also be placed.

When the line is established, blood should be drawn and dispatched for blood bank crossmatching; measurement of hemoglobin, hematocrit, and serum electrolytes; clotting profile; and possible toxicologic investigation.

Fluid Therapy

Volume replacement must be begun as quickly as possible. Certainly do not wait for blood. Fluid replacement is begun with lactated Ringer's solution, a balanced salt solution that very satisfactorily compensates for volume loss.[12] Because the Ringer's solution is not confined to the intravascular compartment but moves into the interstitial compartment as well, about three times the volume of blood lost must be given.

As one starts with a very uncertain idea of the amount of blood lost, the best approach is to spend less time worrying about amount lost and more time in assessing *response* to volume given. Ringer's lactate, 1–1½ L, may be given rapidly and the effect on BP, pulse rate, CVP, PAOP, and urine production assessed.

If the parameters have returned to normal values, you have replaced a probable 500-cc blood loss adequately. If there is still not a sufficient response, further volume may be given. A certain amount of hemodilution is acceptable, even advantageous. An end hematocrit of 0.3–0.35 should be aimed for.[13] This gives a good balance between adequate oxygen-carrying capacity and viscosity. Experimental work by Takashi and Safar[14] showed that dogs could be bled to hematocrits of less than 0.2 and survive. This has frequently been borne out in clinical practice. So do not be afraid of hemodilution while awaiting blood.

Whole blood or packed cells are added to the regimen as they become available to achieve the desired hematocrit. This approach will result in a fall in colloid osmotic pressure due to hemodilution. Preexisting hypoalbuminemia in patients with liver disease will lead to even lower colloid osmotic pressure. Inclusion of osmotically active substances (albumen, starch) in the fluid therapy regimen may be considered to achieve normal levels.[15, 16] However, this practice is controversial, especially in the shocked patient, in whom administered colloid will simply leak out of the intravascular space.[18] Controlled trials have been unable to demonstrate physiologically significant differences in patients resuscitated with colloid or crystalloid fluids.[18–20]

IV fluids should be *warmed*. A drunken patient who has suffered exposure may already by hypothermic. Large amounts of room temperature fluid will further lower temperature. Rapid administration of cold banked blood may lead to hyperkalemia that can be dangerous, although warming will not wholly reverse this problem.[21, 22]

Case Study Continued

During administration of the second unit of blood the patient vomited another 800 cc of bright red blood and his BP dropped to 70/50 mm Hg, the CVP fell to below zero, and the heart rate rose to 140 beats per minute. Yet another IV line was established and an arterial line and urine catheter were placed. The mild metabolic acidemia shown on blood gas analysis was not corrected. The patient was now slightly more obtunded and was intubated to protect his airway and placed on a T piece with 40% oxygen. A portable chest x-ray film revealed no specific ab-

normalities and confirmed that the endotracheal tube was well positioned. A large-bore nasogastric tube was passed and a further 400 cc of blood and clot was aspirated. An additional 2 units of blood were given, the blood pressure was stabilized, right atrial filling pressure was +2 mm Hg, urine production was acceptable, and hemoglobin was 13 gm/dl.

Discussion

Further evaluation of the patient confirmed the earlier impression of liver disease, and in addition to the signs previously noted, palmar erythema and mild clubbing of the fingernail beds were observed. Blood was drawn for liver function tests.

Endoscopy was now performed using a fiberoptic esophagoscope in an attempt to identify the bleeding site. The gastric mucosa was found to be extremely hyperemic and a few areas of shallow erosion were seen, but there was no sign of bleeding from these sites. Rather, large lower esophageal varices were found with erosion and oozing.

Case Study Continued

Two hours later a further episode of bleeding occurred and 1,700 ml of blood was aspirated from the nasogastric tube. A Sengstaken-Blakemore tube was passed. The lower cuff was inflated and the tube pulled back to wedge the lower cuff in the cardioesophageal junction. The upper cuff was then inflated to a pressure of 30 mm Hg. The tube was aspirated intermittently. The patient required sedation for the passage of the tube and was given 2 mg of morphine sulfate IV.

The patient received an additional 3 units of whole blood and 1 L of Ringer's lactate to restore adequate cardiovascular junction. Following resuscitation his BP was 110/60 mm Hg, heart rate was 90 beats per minute, and the CVP was 4 cm H_2O. He was still obtunded but rousable and rated 3.5 on the coma scale. Respiratory rate was 18/minute

with good air entry bilaterally. No adventitious sounds were heard on auscultation of the chest.

An enema was given to clear the bowel of blood and the patient was started on a regimen of neomycin, 0.5 mg q6h, lactulose, and antacids administered via the gastric port of the Sengstaken-Blakemore tube. In view of the history of alcoholism and signs of liver disease he was given thiamine, 100 mg IV, and vitamin K, 15 mg IV.

Repeated laboratory measurements revealed the following values: serum Na, 145 mEq/L; serum K, 4.6 mEq/L; serum Cl, 100 mEq/L; BUN, 23 mg/dl; glucose, 250 mg/dl; serum albumin, 3.2 gm/dl; bilirubin, 2.8 mg/dl; and ammonia, 110 mg/dl. PT time was 16 seconds (control, 12 seconds), hemoglobin concentration was 11.0 gm/dl, and white blood cell count was 9,800/mm³. Arterial blood gas analysis with an F_{IO_2} of 0.4 revealed a pH of 7.33, P_{CO_2} of 32 mm Hg, and P_{O_2} of 152 mm Hg. The F_{IO_2} was reduced to 0.3. 0.5N saline with 5% dextrose was infused at 75 ml/hour with orders for a 250-ml bolus of 0.9N saline to be given if the CVP fell below 4 cm H_2O. Urine output was well maintained and the urine showed no evidence of free hemoglobin. No further episodes of bleeding occurred and the patient's level of consciousness steadily improved. Thirty-six hours later the patient was alert; serum ammonia levels were now 83 mg/dl. The Sengstaken-Blakemore tube was removed and the patient extubated. He was referred to the surgical service for further workup and surgery for portal hypertension.

Discussion

To achieve passage of the bulky Sengstaken-Blakemore tube, this restless patient required some sedation. Sedation of an alcoholic is a tricky business. Morphine and paraldehyde both may precipitate coma in a patient with hepatic failure. Morphine has the advantage that its action can be reversed with a specific antagonist, naloxone. If morphine is used it is wisest to give the drug in small increments, 0.5–1.0 mg IV, and to titrate the dose against response. Long-acting short chain barbiturates are mostly excreted by the kidney and may be used, but alcohol potentiates their action, and so dosage should be very cautious in a patient who may have been drinking prior to admission. Chlordiazepoxide and diazepam have a tendency to accumulate and may precipate delirium or coma in these patients. Lorazepam is better excreted in liver failure and is probably the most suitable sedative in patients with liver failure.[23] It may be given in incremental doses of 1 mg IV up to a dose of 5 mg.

This patient required 7 units of blood during his initial resuscitation and management, which raises the possibility of problems arising related to large blood transfusions. Disadvantages of blood transfusion include: (1) transmission of disease (e.g., hepatitis); (2) pyrogenic reactions due to polysaccharides derived from bacterial metabolism contaminating blood containers or anticoagulants; (3) incompatibility and hemolytic reactions due to infusion of mismatched blood; (4) allergic reactions, which may manifest as rashes, urticaria, bronchospasm, edema, etc.; (5) possible development of coagulation disturbances due to low concentrations of platelets and blood clotting factors in stored blood; and (6) citrate toxicity leading to hypocalcemia and acidemia. Citrate derived from the acid-citrate-dextrose anticoagulant in stored blood is usually rapidly metabolized by the liver but may accumulate in the presence of liver disease, severe shock, or hypothermia. Ionized calcium levels may fall in the presence of rapidly infused citrate-phosphate-dextrose or acid-citrate-dextrose anticoagulated blood. This calcium lack may depress myocardial function. The free citrate itself may also have a depressant effect on myocardial function.[24, 25] Calcium should be given in cases where ionized calcium levels are shown to be low or where depressed myocardial function is suspected. Most texts caution against its use in these circumstances, but I give 5 cc of 10% $CaCl_2$ slowly through a separate IV line for every 2 units of blood transfused. The use of calcium for clotting defects in massive transfusions was shown to be unnecessary by Loranto and Howland.[26] Fresh frozen plasma, or better still, fresh blood, 1 unit for every 10 units of blood, should also be given during massive transfusion. This ensures adequate clotting factors for hemostasis. Although controversy exists over such a policy, one does not have the luxury during massive hemorrhage to indulge in the niceties of debate.

A play-safe game plan of giving calcium with every second unit and a fresh unit of blood every tenth unit assures minimal chances of myocardial depression and adequate hemostatic mechanisms.

Other problems that may arise with the infusion of large amounts of blood include:

7. Potassium intoxication. The serum concentration of potassium in stored blood rises with time and may reach levels as high as 30 mEq/L.

8. Accumulation of microaggregates derived from cellular debris, small fibrin clots, leukocyte, and platelet aggregates, leading to pulmonary damage and the development of clinical problems such as the adult respiratory distress syndrome. Because particulate matter accumulates in stored blood, blood filters are necessary with all blood transfusions. With a routine filter particles of 170 μ or larger are filtered out. However, up to 100,000 aggregates per milliliter may still be left in blood after such filtration.[27]

Combinations of screen and depth filters that filter out particles to 20 μ are effective and do not prevent rapid transfusion if pressure bags are used. Swank remains the standard filter against which all others are judged.

9. 2,3-Diphosphoglycerate concentrations are low in stored blood, which may have an adverse effect on delivery of oxygen to the tissues.

10. Acidemia may result, as the pH of stored blood ranges from 7.1 to 6.6. Serum lactic acid concentration is on the order of 20 mg/dl in freshly stored blood but with time may rise above 100 mg/dl. It is controversial whether routine administration of bicarbonate is necessary during transfusions of large amounts of blood. Massive transfusion coupled with metabolic acidosis due to poor circulation may cause severe acidosis. Routine administration of sodium bicarbonate, about 10 mEq per unit, has been shown to increase survival.[28] Pursual of such a routine combined with good hemodynamics means that when the crisis is over, one may well be confronted with an extremely alkalotic patient due to an excess of bicarbonate from exogenous administration and the metabolism of lactate and citrate. Banked blood may already be low in 2,3-DPG and thus may have a shift to the left of the oxygen dissociation curve which will be worsened with a

pH rise. It is seldom necessary to give bicarbonate for correction of the blood transfusion alone, provided transfusion is begun early and is vigorous enough. Blood gas analysis should guide bicarbonate therapy. This can as satisfactorily be measured on central venous as well as arterial blood.[29]

11. Other factors of particular importance in patients with liver diseases, such as ammonia intoxication or hypothermia, may develop, as stored blood has high ammonia concentrations (80–700 mg/dl) and is cold. Ideally, relatively fresh blood should be employed for transfusions in patients with hepatic disease, and all blood and fluids should be warmed when large volumes are being infused rapidly.

Table 14–4 summarizes recommendations for large-volume blood transfusions.

When hemorrhage is copious one can become more and more involved in pumping volume in an attempt to keep the patient "afloat." Remember that it is essential to be constantly monitoring the effects of your efforts. The BP, CVP or wedge pressure, peripheral temperature, and urine production are guides to the adequacy of volume. Hematocrit, clotting profile, and arterial blood gas values are guides to the adequacy of the fluids used to achieve volume replacement. Also bear in mind the possibility of other complications of blood transfusion, especially reactions to the transfusion. Special care must be exercised to avoid mismatching in the hustle of a massive bleed. Reactions must be treated immediately.[30]

Several additional problems could have arisen during the management of a patient with massive upper GI tract bleeding. These include: (1) Al-

TABLE 14–4.—MASSIVE BLOOD TRANSFUSION

With every unit of blood given:
   Check group, compatibility, state of blood, etc.
   Warm blood.
   Filter blood.
   Watch for reaction to blood.
   Assess physiologic response.
With every second unit of blood given:
   Give 5 cc of 10% $CaCl_2$ slowly IV.
   (Via a second IV—clotting!)
With every fifth unit, or as per manufacturer's instructions:
   Change filter in blood line.
   Also whenever resistance to infusion rises (check IV too!).
    use microfilter for large transfusions.
With every tenth unit of blood given:
   Give 1 unit of fresh frozen plasma.
   Give 1 unit of fresh blood, if available.
   Assess acid-base status and correct if necessary.
   Assess volume in versus volume out.
   Review overall plan: hemostasis, blood supply, more help,
    etc.

cohol withdrawal, which can prove very stormy and even fatal. Hyperpyrexia, hypoglycemia, and convulsions may occur from this cause alone. (2) Further bleeding may have necessitated an emergency portacaval shunt with the associated problems of anesthesia for the patient with liver failure.[31, 32] Postanesthetic jaundice may have developed and may require further assessment.[33] (3) Frank hepatic failure with coma and hepatorenal failure with its associated very guarded prognosis could have led to a less satisfactory outcome.[34]

REFERENCES

1. Eiseman B., Norton L.: *Massive Upper Intestinal Haemorrhage in Recent Advances in Intensive Therapy.* Edinburgh, Churchill Livingstone, Inc. 1977.
2. Eisenberg H., Laufer I., Skillman J.: Arteriographic diagnosis and management of suspected chronic diverticular haemorrhage. *Gastroenterology* 64:1091–1100, 1973.
3. Oh T.E.: *Acute Upper Gastrointestinal Bleeding: Intensive Care Manual.* Sydney, Butterworth, 1981, pp. 81–82.
4. Leitman B.S., McCauley D.I., Firooznia H.: Multiple metallic pulmonary densities after therapeutic embolization. *JAMA* 248:2155–2156, 1982.
5. Lebrec D., Poynard T., Hilton P., et al.: Propranolol for prevention of recurrent gastrointestinal bleeding in patients with cirrhosis. *N. Engl. J. Med.* 305:1371–1374, 1981.
6. Podolsky D.K., Issenbacher, K.J.: Derangements of hepatic metabolism, in Petersdorf R.G., et al. (eds.): *Harrison's Principles of Internal Medicine,* ed. 10. New York, McGraw-Hill Book Co., 1983, pp. 1773–1779.
7. Stone H.H.: Pre and postoperative care of the hepatic surgical patient. *Surg. Clin. North Am.* 57:409–419, 1977.
8. Calibes B., Schenker S.: Laboratory tests, in Schiff L., Schiff E.R. (eds.): *Diseases of the Liver,* ed. 5. Philadelphia, J.B. Lippincott Co., 1982.
9. Wirthlin L.S., VanUrk H., Malt R.B., et al.: Predictors of surgical mortality in patients with cirrhosis and non-variceal gastro-duodenal bleeding. *Surg. Gynecol. Obstet.* 139:65–68, 1974.
10. Rosen M., Latto I.P., Ng W.S.: *Handbook of Percutaneous Central Venous Catheterization.* Philadelphia, W.B. Saunders Co., 1981.
11. Plummer M.L.: Bleeding problems in obstetric anesthesia, in James F.M. III, Wheeler A.S. (eds.): *Obstetrics and the Complicated Patient.* Philadelphia, F.A. Davis Co., 1982.
12. Shires T., Coln G., Carrico J., et al.: Fluid therapy in hemorrhagic shock. *Arch. Surg.* 88:688–693, 1964.
13. Messmer K.: Hemodilution. *Surg. Clin. North Am.* 55:659–678, 1975.
14. Takashi M., Safar P.: Treatment of massive hemorrhage with colloid and crystalloid solutions. *JAMA* 149:297–302,
15. Eurenius S., Smith R.M.: The effect of warming on the serum potassium content of stored blood. *Anesthesiology* 38:482–484, 1973.
16. Monafo W.W.: Volume replacement in hemorrhage, shock and burns, in Lefer A.M., Saba T.M., Mela L.M. (eds.): *Advances in Shock Research.* New York, Alan Liss, 1980, vol. 3, pp. 47–56.
17. Moffitt E.A.: Blood substitutes. *Can. Anaesth. Soc. J.* 22:12–19, 1975.
18. Gruber U.F., Sturm V., Messmer K.: Fluid replacement, in Ledingham IMcA (ed.): *Shock: Clinical and Experimental Aspects.* Amsterdam, Excerpta Medica, 1976, pp. 231–256.
19. Moyer C., Butcher H.: *Burns, Shock and Plasma Volume Regulation.* St. Louis, C.V. Mosby Co., 1967.
20. Virgilio R.W., Smith D.E., Zarins C.K.: Balanced electrolyte solutions: Experimental and clinical studies. *Crit. Care Med.* 7:98–106, 1979.

21. Lowe R.J., Moss G.S., Jilek J., et al.: Crystalloid versus colloid in the etiology of pulmonary failure after trauma: A randomized trial in man. *Crit. Care Med.* 7:107–112, 1979.
22. Shoemaker W.C., Hauser C.J.: Critique of crystalloid versus colloid therapy in shock and shock lung. *Crit. Care Med.* 7:117–124, 1979.
23. Simpson R.: Drug therapy in patients with liver disease, in Brown B.R. Jr. (ed.): *Anesthesia and the Patient with Liver Disease.* Philadelphia, F.A. Davis Co., 1981.
24. Cooper N., Brazier J.R., Hottenrott C., et al.: Myocardial depression following citrated blood transfusion. *Surgery* 107:756–763, 1973.
25. Olinger C.N., Hottenrott C., Mulder D.G., et al.: Acute clinical hypocalcemia myocardial depression during rapid blood transfusion and postoperative hemodialysis. *J. Thorac. Cardiovasc. Surg.* 72:503–511, 1978.
26. Loranto C., Howland W.S.: A reevaluation of massive blood replacement, in Howland W.S., Schweitzer O. (eds.): *Clinical Anesthesia: Management of Patients for Radical Cancer Surgery.* Philadelphia, F.A. Davis Co., 1972, pp. 34–42.
27. Litwin M.S., Hurley M.J.: Blood filtration. *Ann. Surg.* 10:105–122, 1978.
28. Howland W.S., Schweitzer O., Boyan C.P.: The effect of buffering on the mortality of massive blood replacement. *Surg. Gynecol. Obstet.* 121:777–782, 1965.
29. Collins J.: Problems associated with the massive transfusion of stored blood. *Surgery* 75:274–275, 1974.
30. Mollison P.L.: *Blood Transfusion in Clinical Medicine,* ed. 6. Oxford, Blackwell Scientific Publications, 1979, chaps. 13 and 15.
31. Strunin L.: *The Liver and Anaesthesia.* Philadelphia, W.B. Saunders Co., 1977.
32. Strunin L.: Anesthetic management of patients with liver disease, in Wright R., Alberti, K.G.M., Karran S., et al. (eds.): *Liver and Biliary Disease.* Philadelphia, W.B. Saunders Co., 1979, pp. 1097–1111.
33. Morgenstern L.: Postoperative jaundice, in Schiff L., Schiff E. (eds.): *Diseases of the Liver,* ed. 5. Philadelphia, J.B. Lippincott Co., 1982.
34. Sherlock S.: *The Liver and Biliary System,* ed. 5. Oxford, Blackwell Scientific Publications, 1975.

15 / Chronic Obstructive Pulmonary Disease

JEFFREY GLASSROTH, M.D.
BARRY A. SHAPIRO, M.D.

CHRONIC OBSTRUCTIVE PULMONARY DISEASE (COPD) is an imprecise term encompassing a wide variety of chronic respiratory conditions. In this chapter the acronym COPD is used to refer to *chronic bronchitis and emphysema*, although most of the information is applicable to other conditions such as asthma, cystic fibrosis, and bronchiolitis.

Regardless of type or degree of underlying pathology, all COPD patients demonstrate several common characteristics: (1) chronically increased airway resistance, resulting in increased work of breathing[1]; (2) decreased efficiency of inspiratory muscles secondary to chronic thoracic hyperinflation[2]; and (3) impaired pulmonary gas exchange due to ventilation-perfusion (V/Q) mismatching and, particularly in emphysema, alveolar-capillary destruction.[3] There is reason to believe that some of these patients have central ventilatory drive dysfunction resulting in diminished responsiveness to increasing arterial P_{CO_2} or decreasing arterial P_{O_2}.[4]

Patients with stable COPD often manifest arterial hypoxemia (arterial P_{O_2} <80 mm Hg on room air); however, CO_2 retention (compensated respiratory acidosis) is less common. Although CO_2 retention is most often seen in patients with severe COPD, some retain CO_2 with moderate disease while others remain normocarbic despite severe airway obstruction. Some event or series of events, when superimposed on these gas exchange deficiencies, may destabilize this precarious homeostasis, exacerbating the patient's symptoms and causing clinically significant deterioration. Acute respiratory failure superimposed on chronic respiratory failure is a common challenge in critical care medicine. This condition is compatible with arterial blood gas measurements revealing a P_{O_2} below 55 mm Hg, a P_{CO_2} above 50 mm Hg, and a pH below 7.35, particularly when concomitant metabolic acidosis has been excluded.

Although acute respiratory failure superimposed on COPD is a catastrophic event, appropriate therapy is often lifesaving.[5, 6] Indeed, a 2-year survival as high as 72% may be expected when mechanical ventilation is not required.[7] Furthermore, there is evidence that these patients have a life expectancy comparable to that of stable outpatients with the same severity of COPD who have not experienced acute respiratory failure.[7]

PATHOPHYSIOLOGY OF ACUTE RESPIRATORY FAILURE IN COPD

It is traditionally assumed that a specific event precipitates acute respiratory failure in the COPD patient. Most commonly these are bacterial or viral respiratory infections, myocardial failure, sedative drugs, dehydration, electrolyte imbalance, inappropriate oxygen therapy, air pollution, and, less commonly, an increased metabolic demand due to a nonrespiratory febrile illness. Although the precise pathophysiologic mechanisms responsible for acute respiratory failure in COPD are poorly understood, a hallmark is the acute increase in arterial Pa_{CO_2}.

Respiratory Drive

It is commonly thought that stable COPD patients with hypercarbia simply make less effort to ventilate than their counterparts who do not retain CO_2 because the "respiratory centers" of CO_2 retainers is somehow less responsive to increments in Pa_{CO_2}.[8, 9] There is controversy as to whether respiratory drive is reduced or increased in COPD patients with CO_2 retention, and recent data suggest that this concept of central CO_2 hyporesponsiveness may be an oversimplification.[10] In any event, it is clear that suppression of respiratory drive with sedative drugs is likely to have disastrous consequences. The potential role for respiratory stimulants is far less clear: if respiratory drive is decreased, the. stimulants may be useful; if respiratory drive is increased, the stimulants at best may be ineffective and at worst may further increase the work of breathing. More information is required before any recommendations can be made.

Respiratory Pattern

Comparison of severe but stable COPD patients with and without CO_2 retention reveals no significant difference in minute ventilation; i.e., CO_2 retainers "breathe" just as much as their normocapneic counterparts. However, CO_2 retainers display a more shallow and rapid breathing pattern, resulting in significant increases in the V_D/V_T.[11, 12] When these observations were extended to COPD patients with acute respiratory failure, it was found they also have relatively well-maintained levels of minute ventilation but breathe in a rapid, shallow fashion. In addition, the respiratory drive of these acutely CO_2-retaining patients may far exceed that of normal subjects. As the acute respiratory failure and CO_2 retention subside, the ventilatory pattern normalizes (becoming slower and deeper), which reduces the proportion of dead space ventilation.[13] Thus, regardless of responsiveness to CO_2 in the stable state, recent evidence suggests that many COPD patients in acute respiratory failure are expending great effort to breathe. The physiologically inefficient rapid, shallow breathing pattern may be the most significant factor responsible for the acute CO_2 retention and respiratory acidosis.

It is known that a rapid and shallow respiratory pattern can be produced experimentally by stimulating airway "irritant" receptors or the juxtacapillary (J) receptors of the interstitial space. Clinical counterparts of these experimental models would be acute bronchitis or air pollution triggering airway receptors and left heart failure producing interstitial edema to stimulate J receptors. Thus, we are starting to gain insights into the mechanisms by which precipitants of acute respiratory failure in COPD might act.

Ventilatory Muscle Fatigue

Rapid and shallow breathing patterns might also arise in an attempt to minimize ventilatory muscle work and thereby limit ventilatory muscle fatigue. Ventilatory muscles are subject to fatigue just as are other skeletal muscles,[2, 14] and there is reason to believe that the COPD patient is even more susceptible to fatigue than normal people. There is a maximum inspiratory pressure any individual can achieve. When normal subjects repetitively generate 50%–60% of this maximum pressure with each breath, they consistently develop ventilatory muscle fatigue within several minutes. Hyperinflation of normal subjects reduces the critical ratio of inspiratory pressure to maximum at which fatigue occurs.[14]

Chronic hyperinflation in COPD patients may well make them more prone to fatigue because the inspiratory muscles are at a disadvantageous position on their tension-length curve, decreasing the maximum inspiratory pressures attainable by these muscles.[2, 15] This may have an additive effect in reducing the absolute inspiratory pressure at which ventilatory muscle fatigue occurs. Although adequate inspiratory pressures might be achieved without fatigue in the stable COPD patient, the superimposition of factors such as increased airway resistance or increased ventilatory demand created by an acute febrile illness might produce ventilatory muscle fatigue. Clearly, much more information concerning these issues is required.

Nutritional Status

If ventilatory muscle fatigue is important to the development of respiratory failure, one ought to consider the availability of energy substrate to those muscles. Nutritional surveys demonstrate considerable malnutrition in advanced COPD.[16] Ventilatory muscles appear to be affected to the same extent as other muscle groups by nutritional depletion, resulting in impaired ventilatory muscle function and ventilatory mechanics.[17, 18] It is not known whether nutritional factors alone are sufficient to produce respiratory failure in the COPD patient or whether it is possible to reverse nutritional deficiencies in the ventilatory muscles of the COPD patient.

THERAPY OF ACUTE RESPIRATORY FAILURE IN COPD

Specific management related to reversing the precipitants of acute respiratory failure is essential. However, hours to days are sometimes required for such therapy to produce substantial results. Therefore, immediate therapy to decrease airway resistance and improve pulmonary gas exchange is essential in all of these patients, regardless of precipitating events. Airway resistance is diminished by bronchodilator therapy and removal of secretions (bronchial hygiene therapy); gas exchange is improved by oxygen therapy and ventilatory assistance if required.

Bronchodilator Therapy

Bronchodilators should be administered to all COPD patients in impending or acute respiratory failure. Although many COPD patients do not respond to bronchodilators during periods of relative stability, most of these patients develop some degree of bronchospasm when stressed. In addition, the various agents used to achieve bronchodilation have beneficial effects other than bronchodilation. For example, theophylline may improve diaphragmatic efficiency[19] and inhaled β-agonists may improve the ciliary clearance of mucus.[20]

Aminophylline

Theophylline accomplishes bronchodilation indirectly by inhibiting the enzyme (phosphodiesterase) that destroys bronchiolar smooth muscle cell cyclic adenosine monophosphate (AMP). The pharmacokinetics of theophylline are well known and regimens for its safe administration have been developed. Intravenous (IV) administration of aminophylline is preferred with a loading dose of 3–6 mg/kg over 20–30 minutes, followed by a constant infusion of 0.3–0.9 mg/kg/hour. A theophylline serum concentration between 10 and 20 μg/ml is recommended with maximal physiologic response at the higher range. The loading dose should be diminished or omitted and lower rates of infusion used in patients who have been taking theophylline up to the time of the acute exacerbation and in those with significant cardiac or liver dysfunction. Table 15–1 lists common drugs that interact with theophylline.

β₂ Agonists

β₂ agonists complement theophylline in bronchodilation by increasing synthesis of bronchial smooth muscle cyclic AMP by stimulating the synthetic enzyme adenyl cyclase. Therefore, they are recommended for coincident administration with theophylline in the COPD patient in acute respiratory failure. Of particular benefit are the inhaled β₂-specific agents, which offer the best potential for benefit with the least chance of side effects. Currently available β₂ agents are listed in Table 15–2. Inhalation bronchodilator treatments should be given every 2–4 hours during the acute phases of the patient's illness, depending on the anticipated half-life of the particular β agonist used.

There are a number of delivery systems available for aerosolizing drugs. Intermittent positive pressure breathing (IPPB) is seldom necessary since

TABLE 15–1.—INTERACTIONS BETWEEN THEOPHYLLINE
AND COMMONLY USED DRUGS

DRUG	EFFECT ON THEOPHYLLINE CONCENTRATION	PROBABLE THEOPHYLLINE INTERACTION
Barbiturates	Decreased	Microsomal enzyme induction
Cigarettes*	Decreased	Increased metabolism
Cimetidine	Increased	Microsomal enzyme inhibition
Erythromycin	Increased	Inhibition of metabolism
Phenytoin	Decreased	Enzyme induction (?)
Propranolol	Increased	Decreased clearance

*May be a factor despite recent cessation of smoking.

TABLE 15–2.—β₂ AGONISTS CURRENTLY AVAILABLE
FOR AEROSOL THERAPY

GENERIC NAME	BRAND NAMES	DURATION OF EFFECT
Albuterol	Ventolin, Proventil	2–6 hr
Isoetherine	Bronkosol	1–4 hr
Metaproterenol	Alupent, Metaprel	2–6 hr

these patients are capable of initiating a reasonable inspiratory tidal volume. In general, the simplest and cheapest means of delivering the drug aerosol is advised.

Corticosteroids

Adrenal corticosteroids have been claimed to be useful in reducing air flow resistance in COPD patients with acute exacerbations not caused by pneumonia. Intravenous Solumedrol (methylprednisolone sodium succinate), 0.5 mg/kg every 6 hours for the initial 72 hours of hospitalization, has been shown to produce significant improvements in air flow.[21] The mechanisms by which corticosteroids produce this acute improvement is unknown. In appropriate patients corticosteroids should be given early, since it is usually several hours before they begin to act. Early steroid use may obviate the need for mechanical ventilation in some patients. The use of steroids in this acute setting should not be confused with their use in stable COPD patients, in whom the potential benefit is less well documented.

BRONCHIAL HYGIENE THERAPY

The COPD patient with acute pulmonary inflammation usually produces significant amounts of mucus that increase air flow resistance unless mobilized from the airways. An intact cough mechanism is undoubtedly the most efficient means of raising these secretions, and adequate systemic hydration is the second most important factor. Thick tenacious secretions can be rendered less viscous with hydration. Aerosol therapy may be used to facilitate this process, but only when appropriately administered in conjunction with bronchodilators, assistance in coughing and deep breathing and adequate systemic hydration.

When a COPD patient in acute respiratory failure is unable to mobilize secretions adequately despite optimal therapy, tracheal intubation may be required. This is seldom necessary and should be considered only after other therapies have been attempted.

OXYGEN THERAPY

All COPD patients with acute respiratory failure require oxygen therapy. The goal is to restore the patient's arterial oxygenation status to a level which ensures adequate hemoglobin saturation while approximating the patient's stable baseline. Usually this requires an arterial PO_2 of 50–60 mm Hg.

The classic explanation for CO_2 retention with oxygen administration has been suppression of the hypoxic drive. In its simplest form, this situation is thought to result from a central CO_2 response that is blunted by chronic CO_2 retention, leaving only hypoxia-sensitive peripheral chemoreceptor mechanisms intact to drive ventilation.[4] When increased FI_{O_2} results in augmentation of the arterial P_{O_2}, a decrease in hypoxic stimulation occurs, causing hypoventilation. Experience in acute respiratory care resulted in abandonment of that "traditional wisdom" in favor of a more complex concept in which additional factors such as changes in the work of breathing, hypoxic vasoconstriction, denitrogenation, and hemoglobin-oxygen affinity relationships are potentially involved.[10, 22]

Suffice it to say that oxygen administration, though clinically necessary, has the risk of augmenting CO_2 retention, and the risk increases with increasing concentrations of inspired oxygen. Since great care must be taken to avoid significant CO_2 retention, precise and consistent inspired oxygen concentrations (FI_{O_2}) are essential. It is recommended that premixed, high flow gas delivery systems (e.g., air entrainment masks) be utilized until the patient's condition improves. It is generally prudent to initially administer an FI_{O_2} of about 0.24. If no significant increment in CO_2 retention results and the Pa_{O_2} is still inadequate, the FI_{O_2} can be safely increased to 0.28. This procedure should be continued in increments of 0.03 to 0.05 FI_{O_2}. The effects of each FI_{O_2} increment must be evaluated by clinical assessment as well as by arterial blood gas measurement.

CARDIOVASCULAR SUPPORT

Tissue oxygenation also depends on adequate cardiovascular function and blood flow. Thus, care must be taken to provide appropriate fluid therapy and inotropic support when necessary. These patients may be polycythemic despite adequate hydration. Hematocrits above 55%–60% can result in hyperviscosity of the blood and can threaten blood flow and tissue oxygen delivery. Phlebotomy is recommended to reduce the red blood cell (RBC) volume to a hematocrit below 55%. No more than a single unit of blood should be removed in one 24-hour period. Phlebotomy should not be substituted for adequate hydration. If the patient has a significant anemia (i.e., hematocrit <30%), RBCs should be administered to optimize oxygen-carrying capacity and the cause of the blood loss evaluated.

VENTILATORY ASSISTANCE

The ability to treat acute respiratory failure in the COPD patient without initiating positive pressure ventilation has contributed greatly to the long-term survival of this patient population. However, despite aggressive and appropriate therapy, a small but significant number of patients do require mechanical assistance of ventilation.

In the event that adequate levels of arterial oxygenation cannot be attained without an unacceptably high level of CO_2 retention and attendant respiratory acidosis, the institution of mechanical ventilation must be seriously entertained. Considerable attention has been given to identifying characteristics of those COPD patients who will ultimately fail conservative management and require mechanical ventilation. It appears that patients with either marked hypoxemia (Pa_{O_2} <45 mm Hg) or significant degrees of respiratory acidemia (pH <7.30), marked alterations of mental status, or obvious thoracoabdominal paradoxical breathing suggesting ventilatory muscle fatigue will frequently require mechanical ventilation.[23, 24] While it may still be reasonable to attempt management without mechanical ventilation, these patients will require very close observation, and if they do not begin to improve promptly, intubation and mechanical ventilation are probably indicated.

Once the physician is committed to positive pressure ventilation, it is essential to maintain the patient's baseline arterial P_{CO_2}. Such "eucapneic" support assures appropriate acid-base and electrolyte maintenance and also facilitates the weaning process. It is recommended that a P_{CO_2} level providing a pH between 7.40 and 7.45 be maintained.

Arterial P_{O_2} levels above 55 mm Hg are of no consequence if the patient is receiving full ventilatory support. However, if only partial support is being provided (i.e., significant effective work of breathing is being provided by the patient), an arterial P_{O_2} approximating the patient's baseline must be maintained. With the above exceptions, principles of ventilator management are similar to those for the general intensive care patient.

CASE STUDY

A retired 63-year-old male truck driver with an 80 pack-year smoking history was brought to the emergency room by ambulance. He had a 6-year history of a chronic productive cough and had had numerous pulmonary function tests demonstrating severe airway obstruction that was not reversible following inhalation of bronchodilators. One year prior to admission his FEV_1 was .78 L and FVC was 2.2 L (FEV_1/FVC = 33%). On the basis of his chronic cough and pulmonary function tests he was diagnosed as having chronic bronchitis. Arterial blood gases measured 1 year prior to admission showed an arterial P_{O_2} of 52 mm Hg, a P_{CO_2} of 54 mm Hg, and a pH of 7.42 on breathing room air. He had been managed with inhaled bronchodilators and oral theophylline, which together provided some improvement in symptoms. He was relatively active and able to walk several blocks and to bowl occasionally without distress. He had no other significant medical problems except for a peptic ulcer

20 years ago. He had no known allergies.

About 10 days prior to admission he noticed increased sputum production and dyspnea after walking less than one block, and his appetite decreased. His sputum became yellow and then somewhat gray, and he began to notice slight swelling in his legs. On the night of admission he began having difficulty raising sputum and complained of severe dyspnea. His wife noted he was audibly wheezing and called a local ambulance company to transport him to the hospital.

On arrival in the emergency room he was somnolent but arousable. His rectal temperature was 100° F, BP was 170/100 mm Hg, pulse was 110 beats per minute and regular, and respirations were 28/minute and shallow. He was diaphoretic with decreased skin turgor. Head and upper respiratory tract examination showed conjunctival injection bilaterally. Diffuse expiratory wheezes were heard bilaterally. He was sitting up and using accessory muscles to breathe. Heart sounds were distant; no gallop was noted. Mild pretibial edema was present. The neurologic examination showed no evidence of abnormality.

Initial laboratory tests disclosed the following values: hemoglobin, 17 gm/dl; hematocrit, 52%; and WBC, 12,200/mm^3 with 58% neutrophils, 5% band forms, 20% lymphocytes, 4% monocytes, and 3% eosinophils. An electrocardiogram (ECG) revealed a sinus tachycardia with right axis deviation and low voltage in the limb leads. Electrolyte, BUN, and glucose levels were normal; the bicarbonate concentration was 34 mEq/L. Arterial blood gas values obtained shortly after admission on room air showed a pH of 7.32, a P_{CO_2} of 72 mm Hg, and a P_{O_2} of 44 mm Hg. No acute infiltrate was evident on an anteroposterior portable chest radiograph.

Discussion

The patient's presentation and history suggest chronic CO_2 retention secondary to severe COPD. Since the pH is 7.32 despite a high P_{CO_2}, preexisting metabolic alkalosis exists. Intubation and ventilatory assistance may be avoidable if (1) the work of breathing can be decreased, (2) myocardial work can be diminished, and (3) the ventilatory status can be improved.

A major step toward relieving both the work of breathing and myocardial work would be to improve the arterial oxygenation. The severe arterial hypoxemia and presumptive alveolar hypoxia may significantly increase pulmonary vascular resistance, thereby increasing cardiac work load. Appropriate oxygen therapy may potentially decrease myocardial work and improve alveolar oxygen tensions without decreasing ventilation. To avoid variations in the $F_{I_{O_2}}$ as ventilatory patterns change, a Venturi-type device should be used to titrate the inspired oxygen concentration.

Decreasing the bronchospasm and facilitating the removal of airway secretions would greatly decrease airway resistance and the work of breathing. Evaluation and appropriate treatment of the presumed pulmonary infection are necessary. Despite dependent edema and cor pulmonale, there is evidence that the patient may be volume depleted. Adequate fluid management is essential.

A major point is that with proper therapy, cardiopulmonary collapse is not imminent. There is a good chance that intubation and ventilatory assistance may be avoided. However, the patient requires close cardiopulmonary monitoring and must be placed in an intensive care environment until his condition stabilizes.

Case Study Continued

A 24% air entrainment mask was applied and an IV line established. A blood specimen was obtained for serum theophylline determination and then a 3 mg/kg loading dose of aminophylline was administered over 20 minutes, followed by a constant infusion of 0.5 mg/kg/hour. An acetaminophen suppository was administered and the patient was transported to the intensive care unit. Although the patient was more alert, he was still audibly wheezing, preferred to sit up, and was using accessory muscles. A radial arterial line was inserted for BP monitoring and serial blood gas determinations. A coughed sputum specimen was obtained for wet preparation and Gram stain. Vital signs were as follows: BP, 150/90 mm Hg; pulse, 100 beats per minute and regular; respirations, 24/minute and less shallow. Arterial blood gas analysis with the patient breathing 24% oxygen disclosed a pH of 7.35, a P_{CO_2} of 66 mm Hg, and a P_{O_2} of 50 mm Hg.

Discussion

The patient remained alert and cooperative. Oxygen therapy improved arterial oxygenation without deterioration in the P_{CO_2}. Of course, some of this improvement may be attributed to the aggressive bronchodilator therapy. Many believe that steroid therapy is an important adjunct to bronchodilator therapy in this type of patient. Solumedrol, 0.5 mg/kg IV every 6 hours for 3 days, would be an acceptable regimen. Similarly, the administration of an aerosol bronchodilator every 2–4 hours may be helpful.

Two options are available at this point in terms of oxygen therapy: either 24% oxygen can be continued or the F_{IO_2} can be increased to 28%. This decision depends on the apparent rate of improvement and the clinical stability of the patient. As long as an arterial P_{O_2} above 55–60 mm Hg is not sought and careful evaluation of the ventilatory status is constantly accomplished, either option is appropriate.

Case Study Continued

The sputum wet preparation showed numerous polymorphonuclear cells, and the Gram stain showed mixed flora, including gram-negative diplococci consistent with *Hemophilus*. Ampicillin, 1 gm every 6 hours, was initiated.

The F_{IO_2} was increased to 28%, with arterial blood gas values determined after 30 minutes and then hourly (or immediately, if the clinical status were to deteriorate). Additionally, metaproterenol, 0.33 cc in 2.5 cc diluent, in conjunction with ultrasonic aerosol therapy, was initiated every 4 hours when the patient was awake, and Solumedrol was started.

Four hours after admission and 30 minutes following the ultrasonic treatment, the patient was perceptibly more comfortable. His use of accessory mus-cles had decreased, and he was able to cough up large amounts of yellow-green sputum. Diffuse expiratory wheezing was still present. Bedside spirometry showed an FVC of 1.3 L and an FEV_1 of 0.450 L. The serum theophylline level measured in the emergency room was reported as 7.8 μg/ml and the aminophylline infusion rate was left at 0.5 mg/kg/hour. The BP was 130/90 mm Hg, the pulse rate was 95 beats per minute and regular, respirations were 20/minute, and the temperature was 99° F. Arterial blood gas analysis on 28% oxygen disclosed a pH of 7.39, a P_{CO_2} of 55 mm Hg, and a P_{O_2} of 63 mm Hg.

Discussion

The patient's condition was obviously stabilizing. The primary concerns now are to optimize medical therapy and prepare for discharge from the intensive care unit to the general floor area. Specifically, the aminophylline infusion rate has to be adjusted, the aerosol therapy and inhaled bronchodilator therapy tapered, and the patient switched to oral fluid intake. Since the respiratory pattern was stable and the cardiopulmonary homeostasis improved, arterial blood gas monitoring should be decreased to an as-needed basis, with oxygen delivery attempted via a more comfortable mode (nasal cannula) as soon as appropriate. This should be accomplished prior to transfer from the intensive care unit.

Case Study Continued

Sixteen hours after admission the patient looked and felt much improved. He had slept several hours and was hungry. Although diffuse audible wheezes were present, the FVC had increased to 1.8 L and the FEV_1 to 0.6 L. A repeat serum theophylline level was 16.4 μg/ml and the infusion rate was decreased to 0.3 mg/kg/hour. Arterial blood gas values on 1 L per nasal cannula were pH, 7.41; P_{CO_2}, 58 mm Hg; and P_{O_2}, 57 mm Hg.

Thirty hours after admission the patient remained stable and was transferred to the general medical service.

He was switched to an oral theophylline preparation and oral antibiotics. Bronchodilator treatments were decreased to four times daily.

He continued to do well and by the fourth hospital day the oxygen was discontinued and arterial blood gas analysis on room air showed a pH of 7.41, a P_{CO_2} of 55 mm Hg, and a P_{O_2} of 52 mm Hg. However, on the sixth hospital day he complained of increased cough and shortness of breath, and felt feverish. Physical examination revealed a rectal temperature of 101.4° F, a BP of 150/90 mm Hg, a pulse rate of 110 beats per minute and regular, and respirations of 26/minute. Chest examination showed scattered expiratory wheezes and an area of increased breath sounds at the right base. A chest x-ray film confirmed the presence of a right lower lobe infiltrate. Arterial blood gas analysis on room air revealed a pH of 7.35, a Pco_2 of 60 mm Hg, and a Po_2 of 46 mm Hg. One liter of oxygen was given via a nasal cannula, following which arterial blood gas values were pH, 7.36; Pco_2, 58 mm Hg; and Po_2, 53 mm Hg.

Sputum Gram stain revealed many neutrophils and clusters of gram-positive cocci. Blood and sputum cultures were obtained and a tentative diagnosis of staphylococcal pneumonia was made. The ampicillin was discontinued, and oxacillin, 1 gm IV every 4 hours, was begun. Acetaminophen was given to reduce fever and ultrasonic nebulizer with bronchodilator treatments were increased from four times daily to every 4 hours while awake. A serum theophylline level obtained the previous day was 13.8 µg/ml.

Although the development of staphylococcal pneumonia represents a major setback for this patient, his ability to maintain near-baseline blood gas values and his general clinical condition led the physicians to decide to delay transfer to the intensive care unit. Over the next 16 hours the patient's rectal temperature remained below 101° F with antipyretic therapy. He began to raise less sputum with bronchial hygiene treatments. Arterial blood gas values remained stable while the tachypnea and tachycardia worsened. The patient began to appear fatigued and complained of increasing shortness of breath. The FVC had decreased to 1.1 L, while the FEV_1 was 0.55 L.

A decision was made to transfer the patient to the intensive care unit, where an arterial line was placed and nasal oxygen changed to a high-flow Venturi system delivering 28% oxygen. Arterial blood gas values deteriorated over the next 8 hours to a pH of 7.32, Pco_2 of 64 mm Hg, and Po_2 of 44 mm Hg on 28% oxygen. Vital signs were BP, 155/100 mm Hg; pulse, 130 beats per minute; and respirations, 30/minute. The patient had no appetite and was unable to sleep. A repeat chest x-ray film showed extension of the right lower lobe infiltrate.

Discussion

Although the patient's alveolar ventilation remained reasonable, it was being maintained at a significant cost in terms of work of breathing. Several factors were quite different now compared to the previous acute episode in the emergency room. First, the oxygenation deficit was significantly worse; second, airway resistance and vascular volume deficits (which can be reasonably rapidly reversed) were already optimally treated; third, the hospital-acquired pneumonitis was most likely more virulent and more difficult to treat than the presenting acute bronchitis; and fourth, ventilatory muscle fatigue appeared to be a greater factor at this time than when the patient was first admitted to the hospital. Note that the FVC was less than on admission, although the FEV_1 was better. This most likely represented a significant diminution of ventilatory reserve.

The primary factors indicating the need for mechanical ventilation are that respiratory muscle fatigue is apparently developing and the acute pathology is not rapidly reversible. A decision to mechanically ventilate would offer the following advantages: (1) assume the work of breathing, thereby allowing the patient to rest the fatiguing ventilatory muscles; (2) decrease myocardial demands by assuming the work of breathing; (3) allow the patient to sleep; (4) allow aggressive bronchial hygiene therapy via the endotracheal tube; and (5) provide time for the antibiotic therapy to be effective. Potential complications of such intervention are (1) difficulty with intubation, (2) embarrassment of venous return, requiring IV fluid loading, (3) contamination of the lower airways secondary to intubation, (4) barotrauma, and (5) difficulty weaning from the ventilator.

Case Study Continued

The procedure for a blind nasal intubation was explained to the patient and adequate topical anesthesia of the nasopharynx, oropharynx, and larynx was accomplished. An 8.5-mm internal diameter tube was placed without difficulty and positive pressure ventilation initiated with a self-inflating hand ventilator. Within 2 minutes the patient was fully apneic and asleep although easily arousable. BP was 110/70 mm Hg, pulse rate was 115 beats per minute, and 250 ml of crystalloid was infused over 10 minutes, which resulted in a BP of 120/80 mm Hg and a pulse rate of 105 beats per minute.

The patient was placed on a volume-cycled ventilator with an IMV circuit at a tidal volume of 15 ml/kg at a rate of 9/minute and an FI_{O_2} of 0.35. Arterial blood gas analysis then showed a pH of 7.48, a PCO_2 of 46 mm Hg, and a PO_2 of 110 mm Hg. The ventilator rate was decreased to 8/minute and repeated arterial blood gas analysis showed a pH of 7.45, a PCO_2 of 50 mm Hg, and a PO_2 of 105 mm Hg. Vital signs were stable and the patient was sleeping when not disturbed. A chest x-ray film confirmed placement of the endotracheal tube to the middle third of the trachea. The tidal volume was decreased to 13 ml/kg; repeated arterial blood gas analysis showed a pH of 7.41, a PCO_2 of 54 mm Hg, and a PO_2 of 101 mm Hg.

Discussion

Intubation was accomplished by the blind nasal technique with topical anesthesia and without sedation. The use of a fiberoptic bronchoscope to accomplish the intubation is appropriate, depending on the experience and preference of the intubating physician. The advantage of having the patient awake during the procedure is that the patient receives no sedation prior to intubation and continues to ventilate spontaneously. Thus, the chances of maintaining adequate gas exchange and cardiovascular function during the procedure are optimized, especially if difficulty is encountered in establishing the airway. A nasal tube is preferable because it is easier to stabilize and is better tolerated by the awake patient than an oral tube.

If an awake nasal technique is not desirable or possible, the next safest method is to preoxygenate and ventilate, administer IV sedation, and with or without muscle relaxation attempt oral intubation with direct laryngoscopy. When the patient's condition stabilizes, a nasal tube can be sited to replace the oral tube.

Since a primary reason for instituting positive pressure ventilation is to rest the respiratory muscles, full ventilatory support is preferable. This patient did what most patients with fatigue do—he became apneic shortly after the work of breathing was provided. With tidal volumes of 12–15 ml/kg, ventilator rates of 8/minute or more usually provide full ventilatory support. Since most patients will make some spontaneous breathing efforts from time to time, some flexibility in technology is desirable so that these efforts will not result in a need for heavy sedation and/or paralyzation. This flexibility in administering full ventilatory support is accomplished by use of either assist/control, IMV, or SIMV modes. The choices among these modes depend primarily on physician preference, since most patients can be adequately supported with any of them.

It must be appreciated that maintaining this patient at *his* acid-base baseline is essential (eucapneic ventilation). This was accomplished by first decreasing the ventilator rate to 8/minute and then decreasing the tidal volume. As a rule, tidal volumes of less than 12 ml/kg are not desirable.

As long as full ventilatory support is the goal, an arterial P_{O_2} above 60 mm Hg is not undesirable since it will tend to keep this patient's spontaneous efforts to a minimum. However, as soon as the patient is expected to do some of his work of breathing (partial ventilatory support), the $F_{I_{O_2}}$ should be decreased to bring the P_{O_2} to the 50–60 mm Hg range, which is normal for this individual.

Case Study Continued

During the next 48 hours the patient remained febrile and the arterial P_{O_2} fell to the 60s on an $F_{I_{O_2}}$ of 35%. Chest x-ray findings remained unchanged, and large amounts of sputum were suctioned from the endotracheal tube. Sputum cultures confirmed the presence of S. *aureus* sensitive to oxacillin. A small bore feeding tube was inserted to accomplish enteral alimentation with a goal of maintaining a slightly positive nitrogen balance.

By 72 hours following initiation of ventilatory support there was significant evidence that the pneumonia was resolving in that (1) an afebrile state for 24 hours ensued, (2) arterial P_{O_2} increased to 90 mm Hg with a consistent $F_{I_{O_2}}$ of 35%, (3) the copious secretions from the endotracheal tube diminished and contained fewer WBCs, and (4) the WBC count had significantly diminished. The patient was able to produce an FVC of 0.9 L with a negative inspiratory force of -15 cm H_2O in 20 seconds, and when removed from the ventilator, his spontaneous respiratory rate was 32/minute with a tidal volume of 150–225 ml (2–3 ml/kg).

Discussion

All evidence suggested that the acute pneumonitis was resolving and that the patient was increasing his ventilatory reserves. However, there was still significant acute pulmonary pathology that would take several more days to reverse. Alimentation had begun to maintain a reasonable nutritional status.

Since it was not yet reasonable to expect the patient to assume all his work of breathing without significant cardiopulmonary stress, removal from the ventilator at this point would have been premature. However, some clinicians prefer to allow the patients to assume some of their work of breathing (partial ventilatory support), while others prefer to keep the patient on full support. Assist modes of ventilation do not allow for partial support, only IMV and SIMV allow partial support.

Case Study Continued

The patient was placed on an IMV of 4/minute during the day and 6/minute at night. The F_{IO_2} was decreased to 28% and the representative arterial blood gas values were pH, 7.42; PCO_2, 54 mm Hg; and PO_2 of 55 mm Hg. BP was 125/90 mm Hg, and the pulse was 100 beats per minute. Spontaneous ventilation ranged from 10 to 20/minute with tidal volumes of 150 to 400 ml.

On the sixth day of ventilatory support the decision was made that the patient should be able to maintain spontaneous ventilation, as his FVC was 1.6 L with a negative inspiratory force of −30 cm H_2O. The chest x-ray film showed further resolution of the pneumonic infiltrate. The WBC count was normal, and the hemoglobin value was 14.6 gm/dl. The serum theophylline level was 13.0 μg/ml. He had been in a 50° head-up position during the day since partial ventilatory support had been instituted.

Following a bronchial hygiene treatment with bronchodilator and endotracheal suctioning, the patient was placed on a T piece circuit at an F_{IO_2} of 28%. Both BP and pulse rate increased less than 10% and the patient appeared comfortable without complaint. One hour after he was removed from the ventilator, arterial blood gas analysis showed a pH of 7.39, a PCO_2 of 57 mm Hg, and a PO_2 of 60 mm Hg. The patient was alert and did not desire to go back on the ventilator. The F_{IO_2} was decreased to 24% and 1 hour later there was no change in vital signs and arterial blood gas analysis showed a pH of 7.42, a PCO_2 of 52 mm Hg, and a PO_2 of 55 mm Hg. FVC was 1.6 L and FEV_1 0.76 L after a bronchodilator treatment.

The patient was extubated and placed on a 24% air entrainment mask. Vital signs were unchanged and he was very happy the tube was out and he could talk, even though it was in a hoarse whisper. He did well for the following 48 hours, including resuming eating, and was transferred from the intensive care unit 9 days after initiation of ventilatory support.

Discussion

There are several acceptable methods for "weaning" from the ventilator, However, none of these methods is successful until the patient's acute pathology has reversed and he possesses adequate ventilatory reserves. Once the decision to wean is made, the process should be accomplished as rapidly as is compatible with patient safety. The process seldom requires more than 4 hours unless (1) the baseline ventilatory reserve was borderline before the acute insult occurred, (2) the nutritional status is poor, or (3) emotional factors produce a "fear" or "desire" resulting in wanting to stay on the ventilator.

Although patients with severe COPD often require prolonged weaning times, this is by no means the rule. With proper medical care and appropriate respiratory therapy, most of these patients readily come off the ventilator when the acute insult has been adequately reversed.

REFERENCES

1. Rochester D.F., Braun N.M.T., Laine S.: Diaphragmatic energy expenditure in chronic respiratory failure: The effect of assisted ventilation with body respirators. Am. J. Med. 63:223–232, 1977.
2. Roussos C., Macklem P.T.: The respiratory muscles. N. Engl. J. Med. 307:786–797, 1982.
3. Wagner P.D., Dantzker D.R., Dueck R., et al.: Ventilation—perfusion inequality in chronic obstructive pulmonary disease. J. Clin. Invest. 59:203–216, 1977.
4. Tenney S.M.: Ventilatory response to carbon dioxide in pulmonary emphysema. J. Appl. Physiol. 6:477–484, 1954.
5. Roger R.M., Weiler C., Ruppenthal B.: Impact of the respiratory care unit on survival of patients with acute respiratory failure. Chest 62:94–97, 1972.
6. Petty T.L., Lakshminarayan S., Sahn S.A., et al.: Intensive respiratory care unit: Review of ten years' experience. JAMA 233:34–37, 1975.
7. Martin R.T., Lewis S.W., Albert R.K.: The prognosis of patients with chronic obstructive pulmonary disease after hospitalization for acute respiratory failure. Chest 82:310–314, 1982.
8. Altose M.D., McCauley W.C., Kelsen S.G., et al.: Effects of hypercapnia and inspiratory flow-resistive loading on respiratory activity in chronic airway obstruction. J. Clin. Invest. 59:500–506, 1977.
9. Mountain R., Zwillich C., Weil J.: Hypoventilation in obstructive lung disease: The role of familial factors. N. Engl. J. Med. 298:521–525, 1978.
10. Milic-Emili J., Aubier M.: Some recent advances in the study of the control of breathing in patients with chronic obstructive pulmonary disease. Anesth. Analg. 59:865–873, 1980.
11. Sorli J., Grassino A., Lovange G., et al.: Control of breathing in patients with chronic lung disease. Clin. Sci. 54:295–304, 1978.
12. Javaheri S., Blum J., Kazemi H.: Pattern of breathing and carbon dioxide retention in chronic obstructive lung disease. Am. J. Med. 71:228–234, 1981.
13. Aubier M., Murciano D., Fournier M., et al.: Central respiratory drive in acute respiratory failure of patients with chronic obstructive pulmonary disease. Am. Rev. Respir. Dis. 122:191–199, 1980.
14. Roussos C.S., Fixley M., Gross D., et al.: Fatigue of inspiratory muscles and their synergic behavior. J. Appl. Physiol. 46:897–904, 1979.
15. Macklem P.T., Roussos C.S.: Respiratory muscle fatigue: A cause of respiratory failure? Clin. Sci. Mol. Med. 53:419–422, 1977.

16. Hunter A.M., Carey M.A., Larsh H.W.: The nutritional status of patients with chronic obstructive pulmonary disease. *Am. Rev. Respir. Dis.* 124:376–381, 1981.
17. Rochester D.F., Braun N.M.T., Arora N.S.: Respiratory muscle strength in chronic obstructive pulmonary disease. *Am. Rev. Respir. Dis.* 119 (suppl. 2):151–154, 1979.
18. Askanazi J., Weissman C., Rosenbaum S.H., et al.: Nutrition and the respiratory system. *Crit. Care Med.* 10:163–172, 1982.
19. Aubier M., DeTroyer A., Sampson M., et al.: Aminophylline improves diaphragmatic contractility. *N. Engl. J. Med.* 305:249–252, 1981.
20. Wanner A.: Clinical aspects of mucociliary transport. *Am. Rev. Respir. Dis.* 116:73–125, 1977.
21. Albert R.K., Martin T.R., Lewis S.W.: Controlled clinical trial of methylprednisolone in patients with chronic bronchitis and acute respiratory insufficiency. *Ann. Intern. Med.* 92:753–758, 1980.
22. Aubier M., Murciano D., Milic-Emili V., et al.: Effects of the administration of O_2 on ventilation and blood gases in patients with chronic obstructive pulmonary disease during acute respiratory failure. *Am. Rev. Respir. Dis.* 122:747–754, 1980.
23. Bone R.C., Pierce A.K., Johnson R.L.: Controlled oxygen administration in acute respiratory failure in chronic obstructive pulmonary disease. *Am. J. Med.* 65:896–902, 1978.
24. Gilbert R., Ashutosh K., Auchincloss J.H., et al.: Prospective study of controlled oxygen therapy: Poor prognosis in patients with asynchronous breathing. *Chest* 71:456–462, 1977.

Subject Index